Nutrition Support for Infants and Children at Risk

Nestlé Nutrition Workshop Series
Pediatric Program, Vol. 59

Nutrition Support for Infants and Children at Risk

Editors

Richard J. Cooke, Memphis, TN, USA
Yvan Vandenplas, Brussels, Belgium
Ulrich Wahn, Berlin, Germany

KARGER

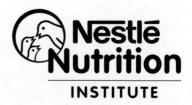

Nestec Ltd., 55 Avenue Nestlé, CH–1800 Vevey (Switzerland)
S. Karger AG, P.O. Box, CH–4009 Basel (Switzerland)   www.karger.com

Printed in Switzerland on acid-free paper by Reinhardt Druck, Basel
ISSN 1661–6677
ISBN-10: 3–8055–8194–7
ISBN-13: 978–3–8055–8194–3

Library of Congress Cataloging-in-Publication Data

Nestlé Nutrition Workshop (59th : 2006 : Berlin, Germany)
  Nutrition support for infants and children at risk / editors, Richard J. Cooke, Yvan Vandenplas, Ulrich Wahn.
        p. ; cm. – (Nestlé Nutrition Workshop series pediatric program, ISSN 1661-6677; v. 59)
  Includes bibliographical references and index.
  ISBN-13: 978-3-8055-8194-3 (hard cover : alk. paper)
  ISBN-10: 3-8055-8194-7 (hard cover : alk. paper)
 1. Nutrition disorders in infants–Congresses. 2.   Nutrition disorders in children–Congresses. 3.   Children–Nutrition–Congresses. I.   Cooke, Richard J. II.   Vandenplas, Yvan. III.   Wahn, U. (Ulrich). IV.   Nestlé Nutrition Institute. V.   Title. VI.   Series: Nestlé Nutrition workshop series. Paediatric programme; v. 59.
  [DNLM: 1.   Child Nutrition–Congresses. 2.   Infant Nutrition–Congresses. 3.   Child. 4.   Food Hypersensitivity–Congresses. 5.   Gastrointestinal Diseases–Congresses. 6.   Infant, Premature. 7.   Infant. W1 NE228D v.59 2007 / WS 120 N468n 2007]
  RJ399.N8N47 2006
  618.92′39–dc22   2006034919

KARGER   Basel · Freiburg · Paris · London · New York · Bangalore · Bangkok · Singapore · Tokyo · Sydney

Contents

Contents

Nutrition for Preterm Infants

Preface

The first manifestation of atopic diseases in many cases is atopic dermatitis, which may or may not be associated with IgE-mediated allergic reactions to food proteins, particularly hen's egg and cow's milk. Prospective birth cohort studies have provided clear evidence for the fact that infantile IgE responses to food protein may not just indicate infantile food allergy, but also have to be considered as the earliest markers for the atopic march resulting ultimately in persistent allergic inflammation of the upper or lower airways (bronchial asthma). For the pediatric allergist it is important to understand the mechanism regulating IgE responses as well as potential options for interventions aiming at primary or secondary prevention.

For decades breastfeeding was considered as the optimum measure for preventing food allergy in childhood. However, recent data indicate that the effects regarding the atopic march are limited. Different approaches include the use of hypoallergenic formulae, in which the allergenic activity has been reduced by enzymatic treatment. Prospective well-controlled trials have indeed suggested that this approach of preventative intervention has a role at least in the prevention of early atopic dermatitis. Other attempts in modulating infantile immune responses are represented by the addition of probiotics (lactobacilli) or prebiotics (oligosaccharides) to infant formulae. The long-term effects of these approaches are still under investigation.

I am particularly pleased that allergic diseases in childhood are acknowledged by a wide spectrum of pediatricians, nutritionists and public health authorities as a major health problem for children in the 21st century. Therefore, the challenge of prevention and early intervention needs to be met not only by pediatric allergists, but by all pediatricians, who share responsibility for a child's health from infancy to adolescence.

U. Wahn

Preface

There is universal consensus that quantity and quality of nutrition is relevant for general health, both in the short and the long-term. However, the gastrointestinal tract, whose most relevant function is the absorption of nutrients, is diseased in many situations. Acute gastroenteritis causes transient but sometimes severe alterations of gastrointestinal function. Other diseases, such as food allergy, celiac disease and Crohn's disease, cause further chronic alterations. Fundamental research has highlighted in recent years the molecular basis of some diseases causing chronic enteropathy such as microvillous atrophy. Extrapolation of this new knowledge in rare etiologies of severe chronic enteropathies to the enteropathy as it occurs in cow's milk protein allergy offers an interesting insight in the latter. After the molecular aspects, the main causes of chronic enteropathy were developed. Chronic enteropathy in developing countries is still a major cause of death of children (>1 million deaths/year). The etiologies of enteropathy differ in the developed and developing world. A direct interaction exists between intestinal mucosal injury, malnutrition and impaired immunity. Recovery from chronic enteropathy is dependent on proper nutritional management and rehabilitation. Parenteral nutrition is the final nutritional option in intestinal failure. In intestinal failure, parenteral nutrition can be live-saving but is at the same time potentially dangerous. The earlier (partial) enteral nutrition can be introduced, the better: 'If the gut works, use it'. Minimal enteral feeding decreases the need for total parenteral nutrition by optimizing intestinal adaptation. New semielemental diets directly influence inflammation and food intolerance. Nutrition has become more than an ingestion of calories and nutrients; the concept of 'functional food' opens a new area of research, of major interest in many different diseases such as gastrointestinal infection, celiac disease, or inflammatory bowel disease. Immunologic properties of lipids, nucleotides and probiotics have become a topic of research. It has become obvious that the strain specificity of probiotic organisms is of major importance. New semielemental diets are well tolerated and accepted. Many diseases affect gastrointestinal function by altering the barrier function. Also medications, such as antimycotic drugs, cause mucosal injury. Noninvasive techniques may provide a better way to assess the effects of stress and also a simple way to assess nutritional interventions. Finally, interest will be given to nutrition in the cholestatic patient. Children with chronic liver disease are not only prone to severe malnutrition, they also have special nutritional needs. The topics in the second part of the symposium (Gastrointestial Disorders) highlight that nutrition has become more than feeding. Nutrition has functional properties, which means that feeding actively intervenes with therapy.

Y. Vandenplas

Nutrition plays a critical role in the promotion of normal health and prevention of disease. Nowhere is this more important than during infancy and childhood, where even short periods of malnutrition may have long-lasting effects on growth, development and health in adult life. During infancy and childhood, there are several high-risk scenarios for the development of malnutrition and these are the focus of the current workshop.

Although the incidence of prematurity has not changed smaller and more immature infants are now surviving, presenting a series of unique challenges to the neonatologist. It takes time to establish adequate dietary intakes in the 'sick' immature infant. Once established, adequate intakes are rarely maintained throughout hospital stay. In effect, all infants accrue a nutritional deficit, the smaller the infant the greater the deficit.

Nutritional requirements are not well defined in preterm infants. It was assumed that needs were similar for all low-birth-weight infants. Yet, recent data suggest that needs change with advancing maturity and one formulation may not meet all requirements. Requirements are also based upon needs for maintenance and normal growth; no allowances are made for 'catch-up' growth.

Furthermore, sensitive, accurate and precise measures of nutritional outcome are not well defined in these infants. Weight gain is the primary reference for assessing adequacy of intake but this tells little about the composition of gain, a critical consideration when interpreting the relationship between early growth and later health.

The net effect of these uncertainties is that 100% of very-low-birth-weight infants are growth retarded at hospital discharge, the smaller and more immature the infant the greater the degree of growth retardation at initial hospital discharge. In the section on Nutrition for Preterm Infants, many of these issues will be reviewed, as will strategies for improving growth in these high-risk infants.

R.J. Cooke

Foreword

The 59th Nestlé Nutrition Pediatric Workshop on 'Nutrition Support for Infants and Children at Risk', held in Berlin in early April 2006, represents an important milestone in this workshop series since it is 25 years since the 1st Nestlé Nutrition Workshop entitled 'Maternal Nutrition in Pregnancy – Eating for Two' chaired by Prof. *John Dobbing* was published in 1981. Since then, two series of workshops have emerged giving rise to their respective books of proceedings, the so-called 'Blue Series' emanating from the pediatric workshops, with over 6,000 copies per workshop making it one of the largest medical publication in the world, and the 'Silver Series' resulting from our clinical and performance nutrition workshops. Moreover, we are proud to announce that the high quality of the 'Blue Series' has been recognized by the US National Libraries of Medicine, meaning that the scientific review articles they contain are now indexed on Medline.

The three topics covered within this workshop have already been addressed in previous Nestlé Nutrition Pediatric Workshops. The first of our workshops focusing on allergy took place in 1987, followed by two workshops in 1993 and 2003 dealing with aspects of intestinal immunology and the etiology, prevention and treatment of allergy. The 2nd Nestlé Nutrition Workshop on 'Acute Diarrhea: Its Nutritional Consequences in Children' was followed by 'Chronic Diarrhea' in 1983, 'Diarrheal Diseases' in 1993 and 'The Control of Food and Fluid Intake in Health and Disease' in 2002. As for nutrition for premature infants we held two workshops in 1992 and 1998 reviewing advances in this field. But nutrition of the premature infant has advanced considerably through modern intensive care medicine, and we now have to care for 500-gram premature infants needing proper nourishment after intensive care in order to grow and develop appropriately.

We are deeply indebted to the three chairpersons of this workshop, Prof. *Ulrich Wahn* from Berlin, Prof. *Yvan Vandenplas* from Brussels and *Richard Cooke* from Memphis, experts recognized worldwide in their respective fields of nutrition for allergy, gastrointestinal disorders and prematurity, for putting together this exciting workshop program. We also thank Dr. *Mike Possner* and his team from Nestlé Nutrition in Germany for the excellent logistical support and for enabling the workshop participants to enjoy the wonderful city of Berlin.

Prof. Ferdinand Haschke, MD, PhD   *Dr. Denis Barclay, PhD*
Chairman   Scientific Advisor
Nestlé Nutrition Institute   Nestlé Nutrition Institute
Vevey, Switzerland   Vevey, Switzerland

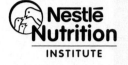

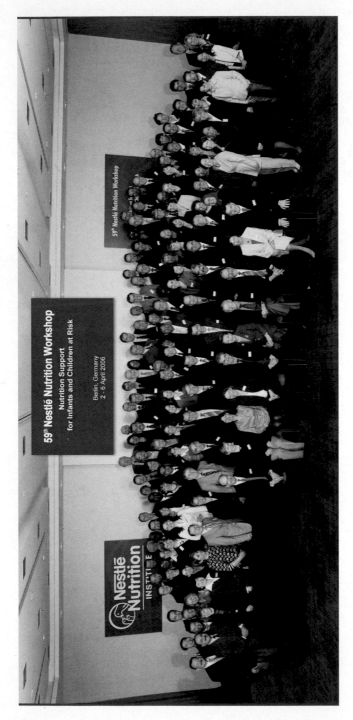

59th Nestlé Nutrition Workshop
Pediatric Program
Berlin, Germany, April 2–6, 2006

Contributors

Chairpersons & Speakers

Dr. Kirsten Beyer

Charité Universitätsmedizin
Department of Pediatric Pneumology
and Immunology
Augustenburger Platz 1
DE–13353 Berlin
Germany
E-Mail kirsten.beyer@charite.de

Prof. Richard J. Cooke

Division of Neonatology
University of Tennessee
Center for Health Sciences
853 Jefferson Ave
Memphis, TN 38163
USA
E-Mail rcooke@utmem.edu

Prof. Geoffrey Davidson

Centre for Paediatric and Adolescent
Gastroenterology
Women's and Children's Hospital
Children, Youth and Women's Health
Service
72 King William Rd.
North Adelaide, SA 5006
Australia
E-Mail geoff.davidson@
cywhs.sa.gov.au

Prof. J. George Fuchs

Pediatric Gastroenterology,
Hepatology and Nutrition
University of Arkansas
for Medical Sciences
4301 W. Markham Street, Slot #512-7
Little Rock, AR 72205
USA
E-Mail fuchsgeorgej@uams.edu

Prof. Ian J. Griffin

Research Center
Section of Neonatology
Department of Pediatrics
USDA/ARS Children's Nutrition
1100 Bates Street
Houston, TX 77030
USA
E-Mail igriffin@bcm.tmc.edu

Prof. Gideon Lack

King's College London
Paediatric Unit
Department of Medicine
4th Floor, North Wing
St. Thomas' Hospital
Lambeth Palace Road
London SE1 7EH
UK
E-Mail gideon.lack@kcl.ac.uk

Contributors

Prof. Peter J. Milla

Institute of Child Health
30 Guilford Street
London, WC1N 1EH
UK
E-Mail p.milla@ich.ucl.ac.uk

Prof. Anna Nowak-Wegrzyn

Division of Allergy and
Immunology
Department of Pediatrics
New York, NY 10029
USA
E-Mail anna.nowak-wegrzyn@
mssm.edu

Prof. Guy Putet

Néonatologie et reanimation
néonatales
Hôpital de la Croix Rousse
103 Grande Rue de la Croix Rousse
FR–69317 Lyon Cedex 04
France
E-Mail guy.putet@chu-lyon.fr

Dr. H.H.M. Edmond Rings

Division of Pediatric
Gastroenterology
Beatrix Kinderkliniek
University Medical Center Groningen
Postbus 30.001
NL–9700 RB Groningen
The Netherlands
E-Mail e.h.h.m.rings@bkk.umcg.nl

Dr. Frank Ruemmele

Pediatric Gastroenterology,
Hepatology and Nutrition
Hôpital Necker-Enfants Malades
149 Rue de Sèvres
FR–75743 Paris Cedex 15
France
E-Mail frank.ruemmele@
nck.ap-hop-paris.fr

Dr. Patti Thureen

Department of Pediatrics
University of Colorado
Health Sciences Center
Denver, CO 8022
USA
E-Mail patti.thureen@uchsc.edu

Prof. Yvan Vandenplas

AZ-VUB
Laarbeeklaan 101
BE–1090 Brussels
Belgium
E-Mail yvan.vandenplas@
az.vub.ac.be

Dr. Andrea von Berg

Research Institute for the Prevention
of Allergies and Respiratory Diseases
Wesel
Marien Hospital
Pastor-Janssen Strasse 8–38
DE–46483 Wesel
Germany
E-Mail Forschung1@
marien-hospital-wesel.de

Prof. Ulrich Wahn

Charité Universitätsmedizin
Department of Pneumology
Augustenburger Platz 1
DE–13353 Berlin
Germany
E-Mail ulrich.wahn@charite.de

Prof. Ekhard E. Ziegler

Department of Pediatrics
University of Iowa
200 Hawkins Drive
Iowa City, IA 52242-1082
USA
E-Mail ekhard-ziegler@uiowa.edu

Moderators

Prof. Christoph Fusch

Zentrum für Kinder-
und Jugendmedizin
Ernst-Moritz-Arndt-Universität
Greifswald
Soldmannstrasse 15
DE–17487 Greifswald
Germany
E-Mail fusch@uni-greifswald.de

Prof. Berthold Koletzko

Kinderklinik und Poliklinik
Abteilung Stoffwechselkrankheiten
und Ernährung
Dr. von Haunersches Kinderspital
Lindwurmstrasse 4
DE–80337 Munich
Germany
E-Mail Berthold.Koletzko@
med.uni-muenchen.de

Dr. Sibylle Koletzko

Abteilung für Pädiatrische
Gastroenterologie
Dr. von Haunersches Kinderspital,
Klinikum der Universität München
Lindwurmstrasse 4
DE–80337 Munich
Germany
E-Mail Sibylle.Koletzko@
med.uni-muenchen.de

Prof. Michael J. Lentze

Zentrum für Kinderheilkunde der
Universität Bonn, Allgemeine
Pädiatrie und Poliklinik
Adenauerallee 119
DE–53113 Bonn
Germany
E-Mail michael.lentze@
ukb.uni-bonn.de

Dr. Andrea von Berg

Research Institute for the Prevention
of Allergies and Respiratory
Diseases
Wesel
Marien Hospital
Pastor-Janssen-Strasse 8–38
DE–46483 Wesel
Germany
E-Mail vonberg@
marien-hospital-wesel.de

Invited attendees

Dr. Luis Bernardino/Angola
Dr. Ralf Heine/Australia
Prof. Wilhelm Kaulfersch/Austria
Dr. Patrick Degomme/Belgium
Dr. Marc Raes/Belgium
Dr. Cristina Jacob/Brazil
Dr. José Roberto de Moraes Ramos/
   Brazil
Dr. Marie-Josée Francoeur/Canada
Dr. Louis Beaumier/Canada
Dr. Kevan Jacobson/Canada
Dr. Sylvia Cruchet/Chile
Dr. Guofang Ding/China
Dr. Orjena Žaja Franulović/Croatia
Dr. Pavel Frühauf/Czech Republic
Prof. Luis Rivera/Dominican Republic

Dr. Rafael Aulestia/Ecuador
Prof. Gamal Aly/Egypt
Prof. Sanaa Shaaban/Egypt
Prof. Jean-Charles Picaud/France
Prof. Dietrich Berdel/Germany
Prof. Renate Bergmann/Germany
Dr. Stephan Buderus/Germany
Dr. Roland Hentschel/Germany
Dr. F. Jochum/Germany
Dr. Martina Kohl/Germany
Dr. Uta Lässker/Germany
Prof. Michael J. Lentze/Germany
Dr. Gesine Müller-Teicher/Germany
Prof. Michael Radke/Germany
Dr. Jutta Zimmermann/Germany
Prof. George Puplampu/Ghana

Contributors

Dr. Christos Costalos/Greece
Dr. Elisavet Diamanti/Greece
Prof. Eleftheria Roma/Greece
Dr. Eva Micskey/Hungary
Dr. Ekawaty Lutfia Haksari/Indonesia
Dr. Aryono Hendarto/Indonesia
Dr. Ruskandi Martaadmadja/Indonesia
Dr. Seyed Hossein Fakhraee/Iran
Dr. Farid Imanzadeh/Iran
Dr. Aliakbar Sayyari/Iran
Dr. Costantino de Giacomo/Italy
Dr. Silvia Salvatore/Italy
Dr. Leslie Gabay/Jamaica
Dr. Rose Kamenwa/Kenya
Dr. Leva Eglite/Latvia
Dr. Sonja Bojadzieva/Macedonia
Dr. Liang-Choo Hung/Malaysia
Dr. Ravi Chandran/Malaysia
Dr. Diego Benavides-
    Hernandez/Mexico
Dr. Francisco Javier Espinosa/Mexico
Dr. Thomas Mason/Mexico
Dr. Ignacio Ortiz/Mexico
Dr. Enrique Romero-Velarde/Mexico
Dr. Hans Hoekstra/The Netherlands
Dr. Frank Kneepkens/The
    Netherlands

Dr. Oscar Segreda/Panama
Dr. Efren Balanag/Philippines
Dr. William Bayhon Jr./Philippines
Prof. Maciej Kaczmarski/Poland
Prof. Jerzy Socha/Poland
Prof. Hania Szajewska/Poland
Dr. Jaime Marcal/Portugal
Dr. José Manuel Tojal
    Monteiro/Portugal
Prof. Silvia Stoicescu/Romania
Prof. Antonina I. Chubarova/Russia
Dr. Ali al Muhaideb/Saudi Arabia
Dr. Talal Iskandarani/Saudi Arabia
Dr. Peter Krcho/Slovakia
Dr. Anli Grobler/South Africa
Dr. Michele Zuckerman/South Africa
Prof. Félix Sánchez-Valverde/Spain
Prof. Maximo Vento/Spain
Dr. Alexander Rakow/Sweden
Prof. Christian Peter
    Braegger/Switzerland
Dr. Suwat Benjaponpitak/Thailand
Dr. Nihat Sapan/Turkey
Ms. Isabel Skypala/UK
Prof. Ramasubbareddy
    Dhanireddy/USA
Prof. Ricardo Sorensen/USA

Nestlé participants

Ms. Julie Muddiman/Australia
Ms. Lynn Weaver/Canada
Dr. Wilson Daza/Colombia
Dr. Louis-Dominique van Egroo/
    France
Dr. Regina Berwind/Germany
Ms. Mechthild Göbel/Germany
Ms. Beate Grum/Germany
Dr. Dagmar Kreft/Germany
Mr. Herwig Piepenbring/Germany
Mr. Mike Possner/Germany
Mr. Gustav Quast/Germany
Mr. Serge Dzeukou/Ghana
Mr. Panagiotis Bagkas/Greece
Mr. Fernando Infante/Mexico
Dr. Mihaela Cerbu/Romania
Dr. Olga Netrebenko/Russia

Dr. Bianca-Maria Exl-Preysch/
    Singapore
Dr. Anette Järvi/Sweden
Dr. Denis Barclay/Switzerland
Dr. Marie-Claire Fichot/ Switzerland
Dr. Clara Garcia/Switzerland
Prof. Ferdinand Haschke/Switzerland
Dr. Annick Mercenier/Switzerland
Mr. Urs Moser/Switzerland
Ms. Karin Rexeisen/Switzerland
Dr. Evelyn Spivey-
    Krobath/Switzerland
Dr. Peter van Dael/Switzerland
Dr. Thierry von der Weid/Switzerland
Ms. Zelda Wilson/UK
Mrs. Linda Hsieh/USA
Dr. José Saavedra/USA

Cooke RJ, Vandenplas Y, Wahn U (eds): Nutrition Support for Infants and Children at Risk.
Nestlé Nutr Workshop Ser Pediatr Program, vol 59, pp 1–15,
Nestec Ltd., Vevey/S. Karger AG, Basel, © 2007.

The Development of Atopic Phenotypes: Genetic and Environmental Determinants

Ulrich Wahn[a], *Erika von Mutius*[b], *Susanne Lau*[a], *Renate Nickel*[a]

[a]Department of Pediatric Pneumology and Immunology, Charité, Humboldt University, Berlin, and [b]v. Haunersches Kinderspital, Ludwig Maximilians University, Munich, Germany

Abstract

Atopic manifestations may be present from infancy to adolescence. Atopic dermatitis represents the first clinical manifestation followed by allergic symptoms of the upper or lower airways. IgE responses to alimentary or environmental allergens are hallmarks of atopy in childhood. Characteristically infantile IgE responses to cow's milk and hen's egg are the first immunological markers of atopy. In many cases they are followed by IgE responses to indoor or outdoor allergens, which suggests a high risk for the development of persistent asthma in childhood. During recent years a variety of genes for both asthma and atopic dermatitis have been described. Infantile diet, early exposure to environmental allergens and a variety of environmental and lifestyle factors may act as strong modulators of atopy during the first decade of life.

Copyright © 2007 Nestec Ltd., Vevey/S. Karger AG, Basel

Introduction

Atopic phenotypes such as hay fever, asthma and eczema are allergic conditions (table 1) that tend to cluster in families and are associated with the production of specific IgE antibodies to common environmental allergens. The process of sensitization may or may not be associated with the induction of clinical symptoms, which by themselves are characterized by inflammation, corresponding to hyperresponsiveness of skin or mucous membranes.

A prerequisite for allergic inflammation is a specific sensitization which requires antigen-presenting cells and their interaction with T lymphocytes. This interaction is provided by HLA class molecules and the T cell receptor together with co-stimulatory signals. T cells will then develop into either Th1 or Th2 cells. It is the Th2 cell which provides help for B lymphocytes to

1

Table 1. Atopic phenotypes in childhood

---

1 Atopic dermatitis
2 Seasonal allergic rhinoconjunctivitis
3 Bronchial hyperresponsiveness
4 Recurrent wheeze
5 Elevated concentrations of allergen-specific IgE in serum
6 Blood eosinophilia
7 Skin test reactivity to specific allergens
8 Food allergy
9 Elevated serum IgE

---

develop into IgE-secreting plasma cells. After secretion of IgE the molecule will bind with high affinity to the Fcε receptor on mast cells or basophils, expecting a new allergen contact. Subsequent allergen exposure with bivalent allergens may lead to cross-linking of cell-bound IgE and to an activation of the effector cells resulting in the release of preformed or newly generated mediators. These mast cell mediators either directly induce symptoms of anaphylaxis or contribute together with other cytokines to the adhesion or diapedesis of eosinophilic granulocytes, which themselves subsequently have the capacity to release proinflammatory mediators.

The Natural History of Atopic Diseases

Although wide individual variations may be observed, atopic phenotypes tend to be related to the first decades of life, and thereby to the maturation of the immune system. In general, no clinical symptoms are detectable at birth and although the production of IgE starts in the 11th week of gestation, no specific sensitization to food or inhalant allergens as measured by elevated serum IgE antibodies can be detected in cord blood with standard methods.

During the first months of life, the first IgE responses directed to food proteins may be observed, particularly to hen's egg and cow's milk [1]. Even in completely breastfed infants, high amounts of specific serum IgE antibodies to hen's egg can be detected. It has been proposed that exposure to hen's egg proteins occurs via mother's milk, but this needs further clarification.

Sensitization to environmental allergens from indoor and outdoor sources requires more time and is generally observed between the first and tenth year of life. The annual incidence of early sensitization depends on the amount of exposure. In a longitudinal birth cohort study in Germany (Multicenter Allergy Study, MAS) a dose-response relationship could be shown between early exposure to cat and mite allergens and the risk of sensitization during the first years of life.

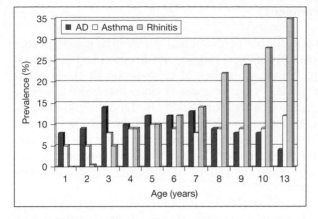

Fig. 1. Development of atopic dermatitis (AD), asthma and allergic rhinoconjunctivitis with age (MAS cohort, 1–13 years). Data from the German MAS study.

It has recently been demonstrated that strong infantile IgE antibody responses to food proteins have to be considered as markers for atopic reactivity in general and are predictors of subsequent sensitization to aeroallergens.

As far as clinical symptoms are concerned, atopic dermatitis in general is the first manifestation with the highest incidence during the first 3 months of life and the highest period prevalence during the first 3 years of life (fig. 1).

Seasonal allergic rhinoconjunctivitis is generally not observed during the first 2 years of life, although a minority of children will develop specific IgE antibodies during this early period. Obviously, at least two seasons of pollen allergen exposure are required before classical seasonal allergic rhinoconjunctivitis with typical symptoms in association with specific serum IgE antibodies becomes manifest.

Asthmatic wheezing may already be observed during early infancy. The majority of early wheezers turn out to be transiently symptomatic, whereas in a minority symptoms may persist throughout school age and adolescence. Still our understanding of the natural history of childhood asthma is limited and numerous data sets support the existence of various asthma subtypes in childhood [2, 3]. During the first 3 years of life, the manifestation of wheezing is not related to elevated serum IgE levels or specific sensitization and a positive parental history of atopy and asthma seems to be of minor importance during the first 2 years of life. Those who have persistent wheezing show an increasing association with sensitization to aeroallergens with age. In addition, the association with a positive family history for atopy and asthma in first degree relatives becomes more and more obvious.

3

The Domestic Environment

No other environmental factor has been studied as extensively as exposure to environmental allergens as a potential risk for sensitization and manifestation of atopy and asthma. From a number of cross-sectional studies performed in children and in adults, it has become obvious that there is a close association between allergen exposure, particularly in the domestic environment, and sensitization to that specific allergen. Longitudinal studies like the MAS study in Germany have clearly demonstrated that during the first years of life there is a dose-response relationship between indoor allergen exposure to dust mite and cat allergens and the risk of sensitization to cat and mites, respectively [4, 6].

However, as far as the manifestation of atopic dermatitis and asthma is concerned, the situation is much less clear. Earlier studies performed by Sporik et al. [7] suggested that in sensitized children exposure to dust mite allergens not only determines the risk of asthma, but also the time of onset of the disease. More recent investigations by the same group, however, suggest that other factors besides allergen exposure are important in determining which children develop asthma.

In recent years, however, the paradigm that exposure induces asthma with airway inflammation via sensitization has been challenged: in several countries the prevalence of asthma in children has been increasing independent of allergen exposure. In genetically manipulated mice, allergic sensitization, i.e. the production of specific IgE antibodies, is regulated differently from the manifestation of disease and airway inflammation: while IL-4 has been shown to be a crucial cytokine for the process of sensitization, other cytokines, particularly IL-5, obviously play a central role in the pathogenesis of murine eosinophilic inflammation.

Data sets obtained from the birth cohort study MAS 90 suggest that while domestic allergen exposure is a strong determinant for early sensitization in childhood it cannot be considered to be a cause of airway hyperresponsiveness or asthmatic symptoms during preschool age (fig. 2).

A number of intervention studies are currently being performed in cohorts followed prospectively from birth, examining the effect of indoor allergen elimination on the incidence of asthma. The results will have a strong impact on public health policies, since they will clarify whether it is meaningful to consider indoor allergen elimination an important element of primary prevention of various atopic manifestations. But even if it turns out that other factors play a major part in determining whether an atopic child will develop asthma, so that allergen elimination as a measure of primary prevention is inefficient, a reduction of allergen exposure will still remain a very important element in secondary prevention.

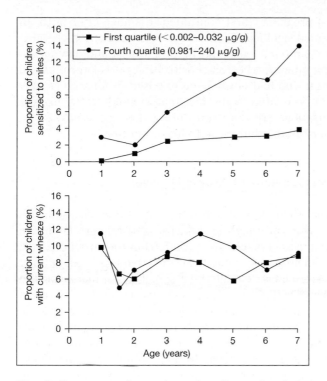

Fig. 2. Exposure to house dust mite allergen in relation to specific sensitization and prevalence of wheezing at age 1–7 years.

Pollutants and Tobacco Smoke as Adjuvant Factors

After guinea pig and mouse experiments suggested an increase of allergic sensitization to ovalbumin after experimental exposure to traffic- or industry-related pollutants, a strong association between allergic rhinitis caused by cedar pollen allergy and exposure to heavy traffic was reported from Japan. Other investigators were unable to describe any relationship between traffic exposure and the prevalence of hay fever or asthma.

The role of tobacco smoke, a complex mixture of various particles and organic compounds, has been extensively studied. The studies which have recently been reviewed consistently demonstrate that the risk of lower airway disease such as bronchitis, recurrent wheezing in infants as well as pneumonia is increased. Whether passive tobacco smoke exposure is causally related to the development of asthma is still disputed [8, 9].

Until recently there has been a lack of data about the risk of sensitization. In the prospective birth cohort study MAS in Germany it was reported that an increased risk of sensitization was found only in children whose mothers smoked up to the end of pregnancy and continued to smoke after birth. In this subgroup of the cohort, a significantly increased sensitization rate regarding IgE antibodies to food proteins, particularly to hen's egg and cow's milk, was only observed during infancy, whereas sensitization rates later on were not different from children who had never been exposed to tobacco smoke. These observations might be related to the fact that in children the highest urinary cotinine concentrations are detected during the first years of life, when the child spends most of the time close to his or her mother.

Lifestyle and the Development of Atopic Disease

Taking into account that the risk of atopic sensitization and disease manifestation early in life is particularly high in industrialized western countries and that within these countries concomitant variations in the socioeconomic status and the prevalence of atopy are evident, the question was brought up of what factor related to western lifestyle might be responsible for increasing the susceptibility to atopic sensitization [10]. Studies of Swiss as well as Bavarian and Austrian children have shown that the prevalence of symptoms of allergic rhinitis and of allergen-specific IgE antibodies is much lower among the offspring of farmers than among other children in these rural areas. In a recent Swedish study, the prevalence of atopy in children from anthroposophic families was found to be lower than in children from other families, which led the authors to conclude that lifestyle factors associated with anthroposophy may lessen the risk of atopy in childhood. Several studies focussing on differences between the former socialist countries and Western European societies reported lower prevalence rates for atopy in the former East, which was particularly striking in areas with little genetic difference like East and West Germany, where it was found that the critical period during which lifestyle mainly influences the development of atopy is probably the first years of life.

Recent observations from the MAS cohort study in Germany suggest that within the population of an industrialized country with a western lifestyle, high a socioeconomic status has to be considered as a risk factor for early sensitization and the manifestation of atopic dermatitis and allergic airway disease.

Can Early Exposure to Infections Be Protective?

One of the hypotheses which has attracted the most interest is that a decline in certain childhood infections or a lack of exposure to infectious agents during the first years of life, which is associated with smaller families in a middle-class environment of industrialized countries, could be causal for the recent epidemic in atopic disease and asthma. Although this area is obviously very complex, several pieces of information appear to support this hypothesis [11].

Studies from several countries provide indirect evidence for the hypothesis that early exposure to viral infections, although triggering lower airway symptoms during early life, may have long-lasting protective effects: children, who were born into families with several, particularly older, siblings, have been found to have a reduced risk of allergic sensitization and asthma at school age. Studies in children, who had attended day care centers during infancy, support this concept [12].

Recovery from natural measles infection reduces the incidence of atopy and allergic responses to house dust mite to half that seen in vaccinated children. Obviously, the fact that certain infections induce a systemic and nonspecific switch to Th1 activities could be responsible for an inhibition of the development of atopy during childhood [13].

Prenatal or perinatal bacterial infections should also be taken into account as potential modulators of the atopic march. Preterm birth in many cases is nowadays understood as the result of bacterial infections during pregnancy. The observation that infants with very low birth weight have a lower prevalence of atopic eczema and atopic sensitization could therefore fit this hypothesis.

The role of endotoxin exposure as a possible element of atopy prevention in early life has recently been discussed. Endotoxins consist of a family of molecules called lipopolysaccharides and are an intrinsic part of the outer membrane of Gram-negative bacteria. Lipopolysaccharides and other bacterial walls, which can also be found abundantly in stables, where pigs, cattle and poultry are kept, interact with antigen-presenting cells via CD14 ligation and elicit strong IL-12 responses. IL-12, in turn, is regarded as an obligatory signal for the maturation of naive T cells into Th2-type cells. Endotoxin concentrations were recently found to be highest in stables of farming families and also in dust samples from kitchen floors and mattresses in rural areas. These findings support the hypothesis that environmental exposure to endotoxin and other bacterial walls is an important protective determinant regarding the development of atopic diseases [14].

Another aspect is that the intestinal microflora might well be the major source of microbial stimulation of the immune system in early childhood. Also, the intestinal microflora could enhance Th1-type responses. The results of a comparative study of Estonian and Swedish children demonstrated that there are indeed differences in the intestinal microflora. In Estonia, the typical microflora includes more lactobacilli and fewer clostridia, which is associated with a lower prevalence of atopic disease [16].

Intervention studies are needed to demonstrate the relevance of these findings and to examine the effect of adding probiotics to infant formulas. In one recently published study from Finland, which unfortunately was not blinded, infants with milk allergy and atopic dermatitis had milder symptoms and fewer markers of intestinal inflammation if their milk formula was fortified with lactobacilli.

7

Observations from Japan suggesting that positive tuberculin responses in children predict a lower incidence of asthma, lower serum IgE levels and cytokine profiles bias toward Th1-type were supported by animal experiments which demonstrated that the IgE response to ovalbumin in mice could be downregulated by a previous infection with BCG. [17]

Although these observations on the relationship between immune responses to infectious agents and atopic sensitization and disease expression are most stimulating and challenging, conclusions regarding their relevance for the atopic march should be drawn with care. In different parts of the world, completely different infectious agents have been addressed in different study settings. It appears to be quite fashionable to join Rook and Stanford [15], who in a recent review article in *Immunology Today* pleaded 'give us this day our daily germs', but which germs at what time under which circumstances and what is the price we have to pay? Pediatricians should definitely resist questioning most successful immunization programs like the one for measles.

Genetic Factors

Multiple twin and family analyses strongly imply a genetic basis for asthma and atopy [5, 17]. A recent study of 11,688 Danish twin pairs suggested that 73% of asthma susceptibility is due to genetic factors [18]. However, atopy-associated phenotypes do not appear to follow any Mendelian inheritance pattern, which is characteristic of complex genetic (multifactorial) traits. The dissection of these traits is hampered by phenocopy, incomplete penetrance, and genetic heterogeneity. The complexity of the genetics of asthma and atopy is reflected by an increasingly large number of chromosomal regions showing (mostly weak to moderate) evidence for linkage, as well as various genetic variations in multiple candidate genes that are associated with asthma or associated phenotypes.

Multiple chromosomal regions showed evidence for linkage to asthma and atopy. Few regions show evidence for linkage in more than one population, which may be due to racial differences, a different definition of phenotypes or (most likely) insufficient numbers of affected sib pairs. Theoretically, at least 1,000 affected sib pairs seem to be required to avoid type 1 and type 2 errors in genetic analyses of complex traits.

A genome-wide linkage study in nuclear families of European origin with affected siblings with early age of onset atopic dermatitis revealed highly significant evidence for linkage on chromosome 3q21 (Z_{all} = 4.31, p = 8.42×10^{-6}). Moreover, this locus provided significant evidence for linkage of allergic sensitization under the assumption of paternal imprinting (hlod = 3.71; α = 44%), further supporting the presence of an atopy gene in this region [20].

Despite the high degree of inconsistent findings, it is intriguing that chromosomal regions linked to asthma have also shown evidence for linkage to other inflammatory and autoimmune diseases. Regions linked to atopic dermatitis have also been linked to psoriasis [21].

Candidate Gene Studies

This approach is chosen to test whether chromosomal regions containing distinct genes (of known biological function and location) are linked to disease, followed by mutational analysis of respective candidate genes. Commonly, genotyping of selected STRPs that map closely to candidate genes (e.g. IL-4) is performed in affected sib pairs (allele-sharing analysis) or trios [affected offspring and parents; transmission disequilibrium test (TDT) analysis] to establish linkage.

The most solid chromosomal regions showing evidence for linkage or associations with atopy-related traits are on chromosome 6p, 5q, 11q, 12q and 13q. These chromosomal regions contain many genes that are critically involved in the allergic inflammation. Screening for mutations/polymorphisms in the majority of the candidate genes has been performed. Multiple (mostly weak to moderate) associations with atopy-related traits have been reported [22–24].

Gene-Environment Interactions

The analysis of gene-environment interactions to date is hypothesis driven and stands at the very beginning [25]. The difficulties in quantifying and characterizing environmental risk factors for atopy (including onset and length of period of exposure) make these studies a challenge. Very high numbers of affected and unaffected subjects carefully characterized (longitudinally) for both the environmental setting and disease expression may be required to test for interactions between genetic variants and nongenetic influences.

However, recent genetic studies support the 'hygiene hypothesis', which postulates that atopy may be the result of a misdirected immune response in the absence of infection:

- Resistance to *Schistosoma mansoni* as well as *Plasmodium falciparum* blood levels was linked to chromosome 5q31–33, a region (containing the IL-4 cytokine gene cluster) that has shown strong evidence for linkage to atopy-associated traits. Furthermore, a major locus closely linked to the interferon-γ receptor gene appears to control the switch from a Th2 to a Th1 cytokine profile during *S. mansoni* infection.
- SNPs within the FcεRI-β gene have been related to IgE levels in heavily parasitized Australian aborigines indicating a protective role in parasitic infection. These SNPs have also been related to asthma, bronchial hyperresponsiveness, atopic dermatitis and atopy. FcεRI-β maps to 11q13, a region that showed evidence for linkage to asthma and associated traits in multiple studies.

9

- A polymorphism in the β_2AR encoding gene (Arg16) that has been related to asthma was also associated with higher levels of parasitic infection.

Conclusion

Asthma and atopy are complex multifactorial disorders. Major strides have been made in identifying chromosomal regions and candidate genes linked to asthma. However, the significant increase in the prevalence of atopy-related disorders over the last decades cannot be explained by changes in the genetic pool. It is rather likely that various preexisting genetic factors in a dramatically changing environment (decline of infectious diseases, change in diet, immunizations, and others) have rendered a large percentage of the population susceptible to asthma and atopy. Genetic variations that evolved to improve resistance to infections may very likely be misdirected to promote allergic inflammation in the absence of infection in western societies. Redundancies in host defense mechanisms may explain the large number of chromosomal regions as well as a steadily growing number of genetic variants related to atopy. Inconsistent findings summarized in this article may be explained by ethnic differences in host defense genes, but also by limitations to take gene-gene as well as gene-environment interactions into account. Large prospective multicenter studies in addition to retrospective collaborations may help to better understand genetic and environmental risk factors for atopy.

References

1 Kulig M, Bergmann R, Klettke U, et al: Natural course of sensitization to food and inhalant allergens during the first 6 years of life. J Allergy Clin Immunol 1999;103:1173–1179.
2 Worldwide variation in prevalence of symptoms of asthma, allergic rhinoconjunctivitis, and atopic eczema: ISAAC. The International Study of Asthma and Allergies in Childhood (ISAAC) Steering Committee. Lancet 1998;351:1225–1232.
3 Martinez FD, Wright AL, Taussig LM, et al: Asthma and wheezing in the first six years of life. N Engl J Med 1995;332:133–138.
4 Wahn U, Lau S, Bergmann R, et al: Indoor allergen exposure is a risk factor for sensitization during the first three years of life. J Allergy Clin Immunol 1997;99:763–769.
5 Schultz Larsen F: Atopic dermatitis: a genetic-epidemiologic study in a population-based twin sample. J Am Acad Dermatol 1993;28:719–723.
6 Lau S, Illi S, Sommerfeld C, et al: Early exposure to house-dust mite and cat allergens and development of childhood asthma: a cohort study. Multicentre Allergy Study Group. Lancet 2000;356:1392–1397.
7 Sporik R, Holgate ST, Platts-Mills TA, et al: Exposure to house-dust mite allergen (Der pI) and the development of asthma in childhood. A prospective study. N Engl J Med 1990; 323:502–507.
8 Strachan DP, Cook DG: Health effects of passive smoking. 5. Parental smoking and allergic sensitization in children. Thorax 1998;53:117–123.
9 Strachan DP, Cook DG: Health effects of passive smoking. 6. Parental smoking and childhood asthma: longitudinal and case-control studies. Thorax 1998;53:204–212.

10 Von Mutius E, Martinez FD, Fritsch C, et al: Prevalence of asthma and atopy in two areas of West and East Germany. Am J Respir Crit Care Med 1994;149:358–364.
11 Strachan DP: Allergy and family size: a riddle worth solving. Clin Exp Allergy 1997;27: 235–236.
12 Krämer U, Heinrich J, Wjst M, Wichmann HE: Age of entry to day nursery and allergy in later childhood. Lancet 1999;353:450–454.
13 Matricardi PM, Rosmini F, Ferrigno L, et al: Cross sectional retrospective study of prevalence of atopy among Italian military students with antibodies against hepatitis A virus. BMJ 1997;314:999–1003.
14 Cookson WOCM, Moffatt MF: Asthma: an epidemic in the absence of infection? Science 1997;275: 41–42.
15 Rook GAW, Stanford JL: Give us this day our daily germs. Immunol Today 1999;19:113–117.
16 Shida K, Makino K, Morishita A, et al: *Lactobacillus casei* inhibits antigen-induced IgE secretion through regulation of cytokine production in murine splenocyte cultures. Int Arch Allergy Immunol 1998;115:278–287.
17 Shirakawa T, Enomoto T, Shimazu S, Hopkin JM: The inverse association between tuberculin responses and atopic disorder. Science 1997;275:77–79.
18 Sandfort A, Weir T, Parae P: The genetic of asthma. Am J Respir Crit Care 1996;153:1749–1765.
19 Skadhauge LR, Christensen K, Kyvik KO, Sigsgaard T: Genetic and environmental influence on asthma: a population-based study of 11,688 Danish twin pairs. Eur Respir J 1999;13:8–14.
20 Lee YA, Wahn U, Kehrt R, et al: A major susceptibility locus for atopic dermatitis maps to chromosome 3q21. Nat Genet 2000;26:470–473.
21 Cookson WO, Ubhi B, Lawrence R, et al: Genetic linkage of childhood atopic dermatitis to psoriasis susceptibility loci. Nat Genet 2001;27:372–373.
22 Barnes KC: Atopy and asthma genes – where do we stand? Allergy 2000;55:803–817.
23 Cookson WO, Moffatt MF: Genetics of asthma and allergic disease. Hum Mol Genet 2000;9: 2359–2364.
24 Shirakawa I, Deichmann KA, Izuhara I, et al: Atopy and asthma: genetics variants of IL-4 and IL-13 signalling. Immunol Today 2000;21:60–64.
25 Sengler C, Lau S, Wahn U, Nickel R: Interactions between genes and environmental factors in asthma and atopy: new developments. Respir Res 2002;3:7.

Discussion

Dr. B. Koletzko: Thank you for a very stimulating and fascinating talk. I was particularly impressed by your observation that early specific sensitization to food allergens is a strong predictor of later respiratory disease. Is this related to your choice of putting IgE on top of your list of atopic phenotypes? From the clinical point of view, IgE is a rather frustrating molecule because we see a lot of patients with allergy who don't have elevated IgE, particularly if they have food allergy or GI manifestations. Moreover, we see a lot of patients with elevated IgE that don't have disease. In your MAS data you found that the frequency of IgE sensitization to food allergens was pretty stable between age 1 and 13 years, even though point prevalence of food allergy varies markedly during this age range. Thus I wonder whether you might be able to offer any better perspective for the future? Would there be an opportunity to develop a better algorithm where IgE may act as one factor, and the combination with other markers, such as genetic polymorphisms or environmental markers, might increase sensitivity and specificity of prediction?

Dr. Wahn: The reason why the prevalence of food allergies seems to decrease with age and not to increase was due to the fact that we always used the same panel of 4 food proteins, food allergens. This was the classical infant-type panel and Dr. Lack would immediately say why didn't you add peanut? We did not add peanut because 15 years ago nobody in this country was concerned about peanut. Now we would have added it. We actually took hen's egg, cow's milk, soy and wheat, which are the top 4 of the German list. Now I would say peanut has entered the top 4 even in this country where there is hazelnut exposure but not peanut exposure in babies. But one thing is quite clear, I don't think total IgE is a good predictor but the specific IgE responses indeed are. Whether this is a causal link between the early response and the subsequent sensitization to anything; whether phase A is a prerequisite for phase B or whether it is the other way round, and is just a co-expression of different atopic phenotypes that are not causally linked but just associated, I don't know. But for the group of cohort children we know that the concentration for food-specific IgE antibodies in the serum is important in two regards. If you have very high concentrations you are more likely to develop food allergy and not just sensitization, and if you have very high concentrations you are more likely to develop other IgE responses and even clinical phenotypes. Whether this has any preventional aspect, I don't know, I would even doubt it.

Dr. Szajewska: You only briefly mentioned parasites in the prevention and treatment. Could you please comment on whether or not you see any place for the use of parasite antigens in the treatment and/or prevention of all allergic disease?

Dr. Wahn: As I said many people are developing wild ideas. One candidate is *Trichuris suis* which is known to gastroenterologists and is involved in Crohn's disease and chronic inflammatory disease. We are about to start a placebo-controlled trial on both the prevention and intervention of atopic phenotypes in hay fever.

Dr. Szajewska: Also in children?

Dr. Wahn: We would never recommend this for treatment but we strongly recommend it for study.

Dr. Kaulfersch: You mentioned that there is no risk that allergic symptoms are enhanced in children due to vaccinations; but you listed vaccinations as a risk factor. So, I am still confused.

Dr. Wahn: Gruber [1] has studied this extensively and the answer is that the atopic child should have the same rights as any other child to get the whole panel of immunizations. There is no additional risk of developing any allergic phenotype even with injections such as those for measles and rubella, which in public opinion are always the bad guys. Some parent organizations still claim this without any evidence.

Dr. Saavedra: We typically establish respiratory phenotypes such as upper respiratory (rhinitis), lower respiratory (asthma) and skin (atopic dermatitis) as phenotypes. As gastroenterologists we feel a little left out because we think allergy of the GI system also has a phenotype. We don't quite understand these eosinophilia phenomena yet. But they clearly do respond to the protein management children get. So it seems to be one of those phenotypes, and from the nomenclatural point of view we also tend to confuse 'food allergy' as a phenotype, but we don't use 'aero-allergy' as a phenotype. Would you agree with that? It does look like there is a difference or an association between the first and latter manifestations, like atopic dermatitis which is associated with a higher incidence of other phenotypes later in life. With GI allergy some of it seems to be food related. Does the GI tract-associated lymphoid system handle things better than the respiratory tract lymphoid system, and therefore are there different associations? How can we ever decide if we begin with a food versus an air-borne allergen, or is it a GI manifestation versus lung manifestation? Those two organs are not only origins but also targets of the allergic march.

Dr. Wahn: I apologize for not pointing it out clearly enough, food allergy is a phenotype. I left it out because I know it will be covered elsewhere. If you compare it to the skin or the airway manifestation, we would also say it is an important phenotype. If you look at the first age window of let's say 0–5 years, food allergy is more important than hay fever for example. When it comes to all kinds of food-related allergic reactions according to our experience it is the second most important manifestation after the skin. Then all kinds of GI symptoms come before we see anything in the airways, but this might actually be due to the kind of patient who you see as a physician. What I am not so clear about and I would like to share my doubts with you, is what we see in the clinics. There apparently is a typical or characteristic sequential manifestation of certain phenotypes and a sequential manifestation of sensitization patterns. Food comes first, then comes inhalant; skin frequently comes before the GI tract, and then come the others. Is it just associated but independent? I would favor this now because many intervention studies aiming at secondary prevention have taken this window of opportunity between phenotype 1 and 2 and tried to intervene for example with the cetirizine, the H1 blocker, and they have failed to show anything. In my opinion it is not unlikely that we are facing independent, associated but not causally linked phenotypes and it will be very difficult to interfere at a later stage in order to block the atopic march.

Dr. S. Koletzko: I assume that language is only a marker for how many generations they have been in this country. But did you look for other environmental and also genetic markers?

Dr. Wahn: There are a couple of factors which account for this difference. We are in the process of starting a new Turkish cohort called the allergy prevention cohort. We want to understand more but this has to be done separately. A purely cross-sectional study with the school doctors generated hypotheses but did not prove anything, so now we want to understand whether it is related to nutrition or the domestic environment.

Dr. Fusch: One thing that considerably changed during the last 20 years in children is the oral exposure to antibiotics, especially aminopenicillin and erythromycin. What is the influence on allergy?

Dr. Wahn: There has also been a study by Niggemann et al. [2] in a variety of pediatric populations. My current conclusion is we don't have the answer to the question but there is something. Even if the exposure to a lot of antibiotics during the first year of life could be a slight modulatory factor, it still does not explain the whole epidemiologic trend. It could at least modulate this in terms of favoring manifestations. This has clearly been a candidate for anthroposophic research because this hypothesis was generated in a Swedish study. We don't have the final answer.

Dr. Sorensen: When you talk about atopic dermatitis being a risk factor for the atopic march, atopic dermatitis in the first year of life can be very different from one child to another. Very often it just persists for 1 or 2 months, in others it persists for an entire year. Did you see a relationship between the intensity and the persistence of atopic dermatitis and the risk for developing asthma?

Dr. Wahn: We have followed the natural history of all these children in the cohort with regard to their eczema persistence. Actually by the age of 7, 64% lost their eczema completely, 20% had persistent eczema from infancy to the 7th year of life, and 16% were intermediate, they had eczema which came and went away again. The prediction for persistence was actually the same as for the subsequent manifestation of asthma, which was severe in infancy, and food allergy. Once you had this you had a much lower chance of growing out of it. This was published last year in the *Journal of Clinical Investigation.*

Dr. Kamenwa: I would like to go back to the issue of infection being protective against developing allergy. I work in a developing country where we have a lot of infections, parasitic, bacterial and viral. In my work as a gastroenterologist, I see more and more gut allergy evolving, which we never saw before. It is possible that these infections are actually a risk factor for developing allergy. Now I hear that they could be protective. So I wonder if some specific infections could be protective while others put the children at risk. In my observation, children who have had previous GI infections, especially viral in etiology, appear to have a higher risk of developing allergy.

Dr. Wahn: This is what the data say so far. I also heard from other developing countries that allergies are really on the rise, particularly hay fever for example. I wouldn't tell anyone that infection might be good because it would be confusing. It is important for us to understand the right message. Certain infections might have long-term consequences on the infantile immune system. If this is true, we must understand the effect in order to mimic it and develop something which might be protective in the end; but so far this is not the final message.

Dr. Rivera: My question is related to the issue that we should learn something from infection and allergy. You mentioned the issue of hepatitis A and later on pertussis vaccine; as far as I know good work has been done with pertussis vaccine. I raise this question because we know the relationship of the worsening of wheezing and infection in children, and about hepatitis A and the so-called pertussis relationship. Do we have any scientific data about the difference in hepatitis A and pertussis in relation to infection?

Dr. Wahn: No, again we are just collecting data. It was Matricardi et al. [3] who did a study on Italian conscripts. All the data on these Italian conscripts are available, including their hepatitis A sero status. Two things are clear: the more older siblings they had in the family (if they were born in Italy when families still had many children), the more they were exposed to infections fairly early in their lives and the less likely they were to have developed airway allergies by the age of 18, and the same was true for hepatitis A. They concluded it was just oro-fecal infections which were protective. But then the tuberculosis investigators found that in countries where tuberculosis was still prevalent that allergies were relatively rare, not totally unknown, but relatively rare. Then animal experiments were made; we have several thousand allergic mice here at the Charité and we test for LPS or BCG for example. The mouse does not respond with IgE anymore; the mouse does not develop asthma anymore when exposed, and even if the mother is exposed before birth to LPS this helps her offspring. It is very difficult to come up with a final conclusion. It is an interesting field, research is ongoing, so let's keep an open mind and in the end we will understand.

Dr. Lack: I just want to push you a bit on your comments about the association between early egg allergy and the subsequent development of atopic disease, particularly asthma. You said you thought it was more likely to be an association between food allergies and development of asthma than causality. You also documented very nicely in your MAS study that there is very little inhalant allergen sensitization. If foods are relevant in the genesis of asthma and there is no inhalant sensitization around and the pathways for asthma being laid down very early in the first few years of life, then one could argue that allergy has nothing to do with it because aero allergens aren't there yet, food allergy is but it is irrelevant. I wonder whether there may be a causal link? It is very interesting that Heymann et al. [4] 20 years ago were already able to measure quantities of egg allergen and milk allergen in the dust of children's bed sheets. The same levels can actually be measured for house dust mites, and in fact in adults, in occupational asthma, egg and milk proteins can actually play a very significant role. Do you think there might be a link after all?

Dr. Wahn: I discussed it several times with those authors and they have some support for their idea that sensitization occurs via the skin and not via the route which we usually expect. We are having another meeting in which we will share our confusion on the atopic march. Spergel [5] has suggested that it starts in the skin and it ends up in the airways; this is true for the mouse but whether it is true for babies, we don't know. I would at the present time feel more comfortable with a rather conservative view. I also have to say that we were very enthusiastic about the ETAC and EPAAC trial which unfortunately turned out to be negative. So this confuses us even more. I am not so sure what we will end up with but we should at least leave the option open that the skin is more important than we think with regard to sensitization.

References

1   Gruber C: Childhood immunisations and the development of atopic disease. Arch Dis Child 2005;90:553–555.
2   Niggemann B, Illi S, Madloch C, et al: Histamine challenges discriminate between symptomatic and asymptomatic children. MAS-Study Group. Multicentre Allergy Study. Eur Respir J 2001;17:246–253.
3   Matricardi PM, Rosmini F, Ferrigno L, et al: Cross sectional retrospective study of prevalence of atopy among Italian military students with antibodies against hepatitis A virus. BMJ 1997;314:999–1003.
4   Heymann PW, Chapman MD, Aalberse RC, et al: Antigenic and structural analysis of group II allergens (Der f II and Der p II) from house dust mites (Dermatophagoides spp). J Allergy Clin Immunol 1989;83:1055–1067.
5   Spergel JM: Atopic march: link to upper airways. Curr Opin Allergy Clin Immunol 2005;5:17–21.

Cooke RJ, Vandenplas Y, Wahn U (eds): Nutrition Support for Infants and Children at Risk.
Nestlé Nutr Workshop Ser Pediatr Program, vol 59, pp 17–35,
Nestec Ltd., Vevey/S. Karger AG, Basel, © 2007.

Food Allergy to Proteins

Anna Nowak-Wegrzyn

Jaffe Food Allergy Institute, Department of Pediatrics, Mount Sinai School of Medicine,
New York, NY, USA

Abstract

Food allergy is defined as an immune system-mediated adverse reaction to food proteins. Class 1 food allergens are represented by peanut, egg white, and cow's milk; they are heat- and acid-stable glycoproteins that induce allergic sensitization via gastrointestinal tract and cause systemic reactions. Class 2 food allergens are homologous to proteins in birch tree pollen and class 2 food allergy develops as a consequence of respiratory sensitization to the cross-reactive pollen. Class 2 food allergens are very heat-labile and tend to induce reactions limited to oral allergy symptoms. In contrast, plant nonspecific lipid transfer proteins are resistant to heating and tend to induce systemic reactions. Analysis of IgE-binding epitopes with SPOT membranes revealed that cow's milk-, egg- and peanut-allergic subjects without IgE antibodies against certain sequential epitopes of the major allergens were more likely to achieve tolerance than subjects whose IgE antibodies were directed against those epitopes. Subsequently, peptide microarray showed a correlation between reaction severity and the intensity of IgE binding and the number of epitopes recognized of patients' immune responses against peanut allergens. Taken together, these data suggest that the epitope recognition pattern and intensity of IgE binding are important determinants of severity and duration of food allergy.

Copyright © 2007 Nestec Ltd., Vevey/S. Karger AG, Basel

Introduction

Food allergy is defined as an immune-mediated adverse reaction to food protein [1]. Nonimmune adverse food reactions (i.e. lactose intolerance) can mimic food allergy but their pathophysiology and treatment are distinctly different from those of food allergy (table 1). It is estimated that 6–8% of young children and 3.5% of adults in the USA have food allergy; a similar prevalence was reported from many Western European countries [2]. Almost any food can cause an allergic reaction, but more than 90% of food allergy in infants

Table 1. Adverse reactions to foods mimicking food allergy

Condition	Symptoms	Mechanism	Treatment
Lactose intolerance	Bloating, abdominal pain, diarrhea (dose dependent)	Lactase deficiency	Lactase replacement or lactose-free milk
Pancreatic insufficiency	Malabsorption	Deficiency of pancreatic enzymes	Enzyme replacement
Food poisoning	Pain, fever, nausea, emesis, diarrhea	Bacterial toxins in food	Supportive
Scombroid fish poisoning	Flushing, angioedema, hives, abdominal pain	In spoiled fish histidine is metabolized to histamine	Supportive
Auriculotemporal syndrome (Freye syndrome)	Facial flush in trigeminal nerve distribution associated with spicy foods	Neurogenic reflex, frequently associated with birth trauma to trigeminal nerve (forceps delivery)	None
Gustatory rhinitis	Profuse watery rhinorrhea associated with spicy foods	Neurogenic reflex	Avoidance of spicy food
Panic disorder	Subjective reactions, fainting upon smelling or seeing the food	Psychological	Pharmacologic treatment

and young children are caused by cow's milk, egg, peanut, soybean, wheat, tree nuts, fish and shellfish. In adults, shellfish, peanut, tree nuts and fish are most common, indicating that these food allergies are rarely outgrown by children. Allergies to cow's milk, egg, wheat and soy are typically outgrown by age 3–5 years; in contrast, peanut allergy may resolve by age 5 years in only about 20% of children [3, 4].

A recent US twin study estimated heritability of peanut allergy at 81%, but genetic factors alone cannot explain doubling of peanut allergy prevalence in the past two decades [5]. Peanut allergy increased up to 0.8% in the USA, UK and Canada, suggesting that environmental factors influence the expression of food allergy. The exact mechanisms by which the environment contributes to the development of food allergy are unclear; however, promoting peanut butter as healthy nutrition for pregnant and lactating women and for young children (increased exposure), presence of food ingredients in skin care preparations (cutaneous sensitization), and liberal use of antiacids (lowering gastric pH and decreased ability to digest food proteins) have been proposed as potential culprits.

Pathophysiology

Food allergy results from failed oral tolerance that is characterized by suppression of immune responses toward food proteins by the gut-associated lymphoid tissue [6].

In the past two decades many of the food allergens were identified and characterized, contributing to our understanding of how these proteins induce Th2-skewed immune responses. Traditional or class 1 food allergens induce allergic sensitization in the gastrointestinal tract and are responsible for systemic reactions. Recent data from experimental studies in mice as well as from epidemiological reports in humans suggest that cutaneous exposure to class 1 allergens (e.g. through inflamed skin of atopic dermatitis, AD) may also contribute to the development of allergy. Class 1 food allergens are typically heat- and acid-stable, water-soluble glycoproteins ranging in size from 10 to 70 kD, such as proteins in cow's milk, egg white, and peanut. In contrast, class 2 food allergens are heat-labile and susceptible to digestion. Class 2 food allergens are highly homologous with proteins in pollens (e.g. Mal d 1 in apple and Bet v 1 in birch tree pollen) and sensitization occurs in the respiratory tract as a consequence of sensitization to the cross-reactive pollen allergens (oral allergy syndrome) [7]. Class 2 food allergy affects approximately 50% of adults with birch tree pollen-allergic rhinitis. Cooking can reduce the allergenicity of fruits and vegetables by destroying conformational allergenic epitopes of pollen-homologous allergens. In contrast, high temperatures (e.g. roasting) can increase allergenicity of certain allergens such as peanut through the induction of glycosylated end-products and covalent binding that leads to new antigens or improved stability [8] (table 2).

In recent years, plant nonspecific lipid transfer proteins (nsLTPs) were identified as major allergens in fruits and vegetables [9]. In contrast to pollen-related food allergy, sensitization to plant food nsLTPs occurs independently of birch pollinosis and frequently results in systemic and severe reactions. Plant LTPs belong to the prolamin superfamily and possess eight conserved cysteines that are stabilized by four intra-chain disulfide bonds. The compact structure of nsLTPs renders them remarkably stable by virtue of resistance to high temperature and relative inaccessibility to proteases such as pepsin and trypsin. LTPs were shown to retain their allergenicity in processed foods such as pasteurized peach juice, beer, baked or boiled apple and fermented products such as wine. LTPs are also abundant in the skin and peel of fruits and vegetables whereas they are present in significantly lower concentrations in the pulp. In view of the high prevalence of sensitization to nsLTPs in the

Table 2. Factors determining Th2 immune responses to food proteins

Factor	Examples
Food protein-specific	
Stability to high temperatures	Roasting of peanuts results in formation of Ara h 1 trimers of increased allergenicity and increases in Ara h 2 trypsin inhibitory activity; retained allergenicity of nsLTPs in plant foods
Stability to low pH and proteases	Egg ovomucoid and peanut Ara h 2 have trypsinogen inhibitor activity; nsLTPs are resistant to pepsin and trypsin due to their compact structure
Adjuvant activity	Ara h 1 from peanut is a ligand for DC-SIGN and may skew dendritic cells toward promoting Th2 responses
Homology to other food allergens	50% cross-reactivity among tree nuts
Homology to environmental allergens	Rosaceae fruits (apple, peach, almond, plum) cross-reactive with birch tree pollen major allergen Bet v 1 Alpha-livetin in egg yolk cross-reactive with bird proteins (chicken serum albumin) in bird egg syndrome in people exposed to birds (parakeets, pigeons) Avocado, chestnut, banana, kiwi, papaya, fig, melon, passion fruit, pineapple, peach, and tomato cross-reactive with latex
Environmental exposure to high levels of food proteins	Occupational bakers' asthma to inhaled wheat flour or to egg proteins; egg-egg syndrome in which adults previously egg-tolerant develop symptoms upon egg ingestion following development of egg asthma in the occupational setting
Host specific	
Atopy	Tendency to generate IgE antibody responses to non-pathogenic environmental and food proteins
Increased intestinal permeability	Developmental (infants, young children) Viral gastrointestinal infections Drugs: tacrolimus, aspirin Alcohol Exercise (decreased splanchnic blood flow)
Exercise	Activation of tissue transglutaminase and formation of high-molecular-weight complexes of n-5 gliadin (an alcohol-soluble fraction of gluten) that have increased allergenicity
Antiacids	Development of IgE to hazelnut and clinical reactions to ingestion of hazelnut in adults receiving antiacid therapy

Mediterranean countries where no birch tree pollen is present, sensitization to nsLTPs likely occurs via the gastrointestinal route.

Considering that most food allergens are glycoproteins, attention has been turned to the role of food carbohydrate moieties in Th2 skewing. Complex carbohydrates are potent inducers of Th2 responses, and carbohydrate antigens can stimulate the production of different classes of glycan-specific antibodies, including Th2-associated IgG and IgE. Biological effects of carbohydrate antigens are dependent on the recognition of these antigens by carbohydrate-binding proteins (lectins). Cell-surface C-type lectin receptors, such as DC-SIGN, L-SIGN, the mannose receptor, macrophage galactose-binding lectin, and other lectins, such as the soluble collectins and galectin-3, recognize particular glycan antigens of schistosomes and allergens. Shreffler et al. [10] proposed that the major allergen from peanut, Ara h 1 may be a ligand for DC-SIGN on dendritic cells. DC-SIGN bound to a 65-kD protein from peanut extract in a calcium-dependent manner, whereas there was no precipitation of proteins from chemically deglycosylated peanut extract. Mass spectrometry confirmed that DC-SIGN ligand from peanut was Ara h 1. Ara h 1 activated human dendritic cells as measured by phenotype and T cell stimulation. These preliminary results suggest that Ara h 1 is a ligand for DC-SIGN and may play a role in differentiating dendritic cells to promote Th2 responses to peanut.

IgE antibodies produced by B cells may be directed at sequential epitopes comprised of sequential amino acids, or conformational epitopes comprised of amino acid residues from different regions of the allergen brought together by folding of the protein. Since food allergens are subjected to extensive chemical and proteolytic digestion prior to absorption and uptake by the cells of gut-associated lymphoid tissue, it has been assumed that in class 1 food allergy, immune responses are directed against sequential epitopes [1]. However, analysis of IgE-binding epitopes with the use of SPOTs membrane technology revealed that cow's milk-, egg- and peanut-allergic subjects who lacked IgE antibodies against certain sequential epitopes of the major allergens were more likely to achieve tolerance to these foods than subjects whose IgE antibodies were directed against those epitopes [11–14] (table 3).

In subsequent studies, Shreffler et al. [15] at the Jaffe Food Allergy Institute at Mount Sinai School of Medicine in New York utilized peptide microarray to characterize humoral responses to major peanut allergens. Reaction severity in patients correlated with the heterogeneity (intensity of IgE binding and number of epitopes recognized) of their immune responses against peanut allergens. In vitro sensitization of effector cells (basophils and rat basophil leukemia cell line SX38 transfected with human FcεRI) with more diverse IgE antibodies conferred greater reactivity to specific allergens. Taken together, these data suggest that the epitope recognition pattern (conformational vs. sequential, number of epitopes recognized) as well as intensity of IgE binding are important determinants of severity and duration of food allergy.

Classification of Food Allergy Disorders

Food allergy disorders may be classified based on the role of IgE antibody as IgE-mediated, non-IgE-mediated (cell-mediated) and mixed-IgE- and cell-mediated (table 4).

Table 3. IgE epitope recognition patterns in subjects with allergy to cow's milk, egg white and peanut

Study	Allergen	Patient population and methods	Results
Jarvinen et al. [11]	Cow's milk	10 patients with persistent CMA and 10 patients who subsequently outgrew their milk allergy; 25 decapeptides of α(s1)-casein, α(s2)-casein, κ-casein, α-lactalbumin, and β-lactoglobulin, comprising the core epitopes, synthesized on a SPOTs membrane; sera from individual patients were used for immunolabeling	Five IgE-binding epitopes (2 on α(s1)-casein, 1 on α(s2)-casein, and 2 on κ-casein) were not recognized by any of the patients with transient CMA but showed binding by the majority of the patients with persistent allergy. The presence of IgE antibodies against at least 1 of 3 epitopes (AA 123–132 on α(s1)-casein, AA 171–180 on α(s2)-casein, and AA 155–164 on κ-casein) identified all patients with persistent CMA
Jarvinen et al. [14]	Egg white	11 children with transient and 7 children with persistent egg allergy; the central decapeptides from each of the major IgE-binding epitopes of ovomucoid synthesized on a SPOTs membrane; immunolabeling was done with individual patients' sera	Both groups had a comparable range of egg-specific IgE levels, but none of the patients with transient egg allergy had IgE antibodies against these epitopes of ovomucoid: AA 1–10, 11–20, 47–56, and 113–122. In contrast, all 7 patients with persistent egg allergy recognized at least 4 of these immunodominant epitopes
Beyer et al. [12]	Peanut	15 patients with symptomatic peanut allergy and 16 patients who were sensitized but tolerant. Ten of these 16 patients had 'outgrown' their allergy. Eight peptides representing the immunodominant sequential epitopes on Ara h 1, 2 and 3 synthesized on SPOTs membranes and immunolabeled with individual patients' sera	Regardless of their peanut-specific IgE levels, at least 93% of symptomatic, but only 12.5% of tolerant patients, recognized 1 of the 'predictive' epitopes on Ara h 1 or 2. The cumulative IgE binding to the peanut peptides was significantly higher in patients with peanut allergy than in tolerant patients

| Shreffler et al. [15, 41] | Peanut | 77 patients with peanut allergy and 15 controls; overlapping 20-amino acid peptides covering the entire sequence of Ara h 1, 2 and 3 were used for microarray immunoassay | The majority of patients (97%) had specific IgE to at least one of the recombinant allergens, and 87% had detectable IgE to sequential epitopes. The analysis of individual patients revealed remarkable heterogeneity in the number and patterns of epitope recognition. High epitope diversity was found in patients with a history of more severe reactions |
| Lewis et al. [42] | Peanut | 40 peanut-allergic patients underwent DBPC low-dose OFC to peanut; serum peanut IgE (CAP-FEIA) and IgE-binding patterns (Western blot) to peanut proteins were analyzed | Seventeen IgE-binding bands were identified between 5 and 100 kD with 8 bound by >50% of patients. The total number of bands correlated significantly with OFC score and peanut IgE. Cluster analysis failed to reveal any association between particular protein or pattern of proteins |

AA = Amino acid; CMA = cow milk allergy; DBPC = double-blind placebo-controlled; OFC = oral food challenge.

Table 4. Classification of food-allergic disorders based on the role of IgE antibody in the pathophysiology

Disorder	IgE-mediated	Mixed mechanism, IgE- and cell-mediated	Non-IgE-mediated
Generalized	Anaphylactic shock, food-dependent exercise-induced anaphylaxis		
Cutaneous	Urticaria, angioedema, flushing, morbilliform rash, acute contact urticaria	AD Contact dermatitis	Dermatitis herpetiformis
Gastrointestinal	Oral allergy syndrome, immediate gastrointestinal food allergy	AEE AEG	Allergic proctocolitis Food protein-induced enterocolitis syndrome Celiac disease Infantile colic
Respiratory	Acute rhinoconjunctivits, bronchospasm	Asthma	Pulmonary hemosiderosis (Heiner's syndrome)

AD = Atopic dermatitis; AEE = allergic eosinophilic esophagitis; AEG = allergic eosinophilic gastroenteritis.

IgE-Mediated Food Allergy

Anaphylaxis represents the most severe form of IgE-mediated food allergy and is clinically defined as a food-allergic reaction involving two or more organ systems [16]. Symptoms start within seconds to 1–2 h following the ingestion and include feelings of 'impending doom', throat tightness, coughing or wheezing, abdominal pain, vomiting, diarrhea, and loss of consciousness. Cutaneous symptoms of flushing, urticaria, and angioedema are present in the majority of the anaphylactic reactions; however, the most rapidly progressive anaphylaxis may involve no cutaneous manifestations.

Peanut, tree nuts (i.e. almond, cashew, hazelnut, pecan, and walnut), fish, and shellfish are most often responsible for food-induced anaphylaxis in the USA.

Acute urticaria and angioedema are the most common manifestations of acute allergic reactions to ingested foods in children. Onset of symptoms may be rapid, within minutes of ingesting the responsible food. Skin involvement may be isolated or associated with other organ systems in food anaphylaxis. Acute IgE-mediated urticaria can be induced by skin contact with cow's milk allergy, raw egg white, raw meats, fish, vegetables and fruits. Skin contact reactions are typically local in nature but oral mucous membranes (e.g. kissing) or conjunctiva (e.g. eye rubbing) contact may lead to generalized reactions [17, 18].

Mixed-IgE-Mediated and Cell-Mediated Food Allergy Disorders

Food allergy is frequently seen in children with atopic dermatitis (AD). AD is a chronic inflammatory disease of the skin characterized by marked pruritus and a remitting and relapsing course. In a study of 64 patients with moderate to severe AD referred to a pediatric dermatologist in a tertiary medical center who underwent double-blind placebo-controlled food challenges, 35–40% of children were allergic to at least one food [19]. In adults with birch pollen sensitivity, ingestion of birch pollen-related foods (e.g. apple, carrot, celery) causes immediate and/or late eczematous reactions [20, 21]. Strict elimination of the causative food allergen results in significant improvement in dermatitis [19, 22].

Allergic eosinophilic esophagitis (AEE) and gastroenteritis (AEG) are characterized by infiltration of the gastrointestinal tract with eosinophils. Both, T lymphocytes and food-specific IgE antibodies are implicated in a subset of patients, especially infants and children; the role of food allergy in adults with AEE/AEG is controversial. Symptoms correlate with the extent of eosinophilic infiltration of the bowel wall [23]. AEE is seen most frequently in infants, children and adolescents and presents with symptoms of gastroesophageal reflux, such as nausea, dysphagia, emesis and epigastric pain, that fail to resolve with standard antireflux therapy. Patients typically have a negative pH probe; on esophageal biopsy more than 10–20 eosinophils per 40× high-power field are seen [24]. AEG can occur at any age, including young infants. Failure to thrive is common; in young infants AEG may cause gastric outlet obstruction with pyloric stenosis. Patients also present with abdominal pain, emesis, diarrhea, blood loss in the stool, anemia, and protein-losing gastroenteropathy.

Up to 50% of patients with these eosinophilic disorders are atopic and have detectable IgE sensitization to one or more foods; however, food-induced IgE-mediated immediate reactions are uncommon. Results of skin prick tests and serum allergen-specific IgE antibody tests correlate poorly with response to elimination of the food and thus must be interpreted with caution. Resolution of symptoms typically occurs within 3–8 weeks following the elimination of the responsible food allergen, frequently multiple foods, most commonly: cow's milk, soy, wheat, and egg. Because patients with AEE and AEG can react to single small peptides and trace amounts of the offending foods and testing may fail to identify all relevant allergens, a diet based on an amino acid formula may be necessary to achieve improvement [25–27].

Non-IgE-Mediated Gastrointestinal Food Allergy Disorders

Allergic proctocolitis typically starts in the first few months of life, with blood-streaked stools in otherwise healthy-looking infants and is considered a major cause of colitis under age 1 year [28]. Unlike other forms of gastrointestinal food hypersensitivity, proctocolitis is highly prevalent in breastfed infants, with more than 50% of infants in the published reports being exclusively breastfed. Food protein-induced proctocolitis is typically caused by cow's milk and soybean protein. Pathologic findings are limited to the colon and include focal acute inflammation with epithelial erosions and eosinophilic infiltration of the lamina propria, the epithelium and lamina muscularis. Most infants respond well to casein hydrolysate and only few require amino acid-based formulas. After 9–12 months of age, the infants typically tolerate an unrestricted diet.

Food protein-induced enterocolitis syndrome (FPIES) is most frequently seen in young infants who present with irritability, protracted vomiting, and diarrhea [29]. Vomiting generally occurs 1–3 h after feeding but continued exposure may result in bloody diarrhea, anemia, abdominal distention, and failure to thrive. FPIES is typically caused by cow's milk or soy-based formula but other foods such as grains (rice, oat), meats (turkey, chicken) and vegetables (pea) were reported [30, 31]. Patients rapidly recover with avoidance diets, but ingestion of the offending food proteins following a period of dietary elimination triggers subacute symptoms (median, 2 h) with an associated elevation of the peripheral blood polymorphonuclear leukocyte count.

Infantile colic is defined as unexplained paroxysms of irritability, fussing or crying that persist for more than 3 h per day, for more than 3 days per week and for at least 3 weeks. Prevalence of infantile colic has been recently estimated at 5–19%. Several studies demonstrated improvement of colic symptoms in a subset of babies fed with soy-based and extensively hydrolyzed hypoallergenic infant formulas, suggesting a possible role of an underlying transient hypersensitivity to one or several foods [32, 33].

It has been recently appreciated that up to 50% of gastroesophageal reflux symptoms in infants younger than 1 year is caused by hypersensitivity to dietary food proteins, mainly cow's milk and soybean [34].

Diagnosis

A careful medical history is crucial; however, it needs to be validated by laboratory tests and oral food challenges (OFCs), especially in chronic disorders such as AD or AEG. In such remitting and relapsing disorders, accurate identification of the offending food on the basis of history is particularly difficult and sometimes impossible [19].

Skin prick testing with commercial food allergen extract has a high negative predictive value >95%, whereas a positive skin test has only an average 50% positive predictive value. In infants and young children, a large skin prick test wheal (mean size 8–10 mm) is associated with a high >95%

likelihood of clinical reactivity to cow's milk, egg and peanut, confirmed by an OFC [35].

A number of laboratory immune assays (RAST, CAP system) have been developed for the detection of allergen-specific IgE antibody in the bloodstream. These assays have a similar performance to skin tests in that a negative test (specific IgE antibody <0.35 kIU/l measured by Pharmacia CAP system) has a high negative predictive value >95%. Clinical decision points indicating >95% likelihood of reaction were established for the most common food allergens, including milk, egg, peanut, tree nuts, and fish [36]. For example, a child older than 2 years with milk IgE antibody level ≥15 kIU/l is highly (>95%) likely to react during an oral milk challenge. Food-specific IgE antibody levels below the decision points indicate a decreasing likelihood of reaction that needs to be determined with OFC. Currently available diagnostic tests for IgE-mediated food allergy do not predict severity of reactions and chances of resolving food allergy with time. Considering data from studies in peanut, cow's milk and egg allergy on specific epitope recognition patterns correlating with severity of reactions and persistence of food allergy, these questions may be answered with novel approaches to diagnosis of food allergy that is based on a peptide microarray. This technique utilizes minute amounts of patient sera and can be highly automated; time and labor efficient. Hopefully peptide microarray will become incorporated into the clinical practice in the near future and allow for more precise and individualized diagnosis of food allergy.

Skin prick test and measurement of serum food IgE antibody concentration are not helpful in food allergy disorders with cell-mediated mechanism, such as FPIES, and have limited usefulness in disorders with mixed mechanism, such as AEE and AEG. Recently patch testing for the diagnosis of food allergy in children with AD and AEE has been investigated in a number of studies. Patch testing is typically used for the diagnosis of delayed contact hypersensitivity reactions in which T cells play a prominent role. In children with challenge-proven milk allergy, skin prick tests were positive in 67% of the cases with acute-onset reactions (under 2 h) to milk challenge, whereas patch tests tended to be negative [37]. Patch tests were positive in 89% of children with delayed-onset reactions (25–44 h), although skin prick tests were frequently negative. These results indicate that a combination of patch testing and detection of IgE could enhance the accuracy of the diagnosis of food allergy and eliminate the need for OFCs.

For gastrointestinal food allergy disorders such as AEE and AEG, the ultimate diagnosis is established by sampling of the mucosa and finding increased numbers of eosinophils. Noninvasive diagnostic tests are highly desirable but currently available laboratory techniques (e.g. peripheral eosinophil count, serum albumin and total protein level, fecal occult blood, fecal α_1-antitrypsin) offer limited insight into these conditions. Experimental tests for AEE/AEG include peripheral T lymphocyte proliferation assays, cytokine release upon food stimulation, inflammatory cytokines (interleukin-4, TNF-α) in serum and stool, as well as markers of eosinophil activation in stool (e.g. eosinophilic cationic protein). These tests require further evaluation and standardization before introduction into clinical practice.

Oral Food Challenges

OFCs remain the most accurate method for diagnosing food allergy, for both IgE-mediated as well as for non-IgE-mediated food allergy and for determining the threshold dose of food. Many protocols were developed; in one approach, during an OFC for an IgE-mediated food allergy, a premeasured amount of food (typically 8–10 g of dry food or 80–100 ml of liquid food) mixed with a masking food is administered in small increments every 10–15 min over 90 min. In a placebo-controlled challenge, two sessions (one with real food, one with placebo food) are separated by a 90-min break and completed on a single day or each session may be done on separate days. Double-blind, placebo-controlled food challenge is considered a gold standard for the diagnosis of food allergy and is preferred in the research setting. OFCs are stopped at the first sign of an objective reaction such as hives, rhinorrhea, sneezing, coughing, or vomiting. OFCs are always conducted under physician supervision in a controlled environment. Patients with AEE or AEG, whose food-induced symptoms are delayed and more insidious, may require prolonged challenges over several days.

Management of Food Allergy

Management of food allergy currently focuses on avoidance, prompt recognition and treatment of food-allergic reactions, and nutritional support.

Avoidance of food allergens focuses on dietary avoidance but attention must also be paid to exposure via skin (e.g. peanut oil in cosmetics), mucous membranes (e.g. kissing) or inhalation (e.g. peanut dust, steaming milk or fish). Accidental reactions are common; in children with peanut allergy, 50% reported reactions to peanuts despite avoidance over a 2-year period [38]. Individuals with a history of immediate allergic reactions, anaphylaxis, those with asthma, and those with allergy to foods typically associated with severe reactions (i.e., peanut, tree nuts, fish, shellfish) should be prescribed an epinephrine self-injector.

Children with food allergy, particularly those with multiple food allergies, are at risk of nutritional protein and calorie deficiency due to restricted diets and may require a hypoallergenic formula. Hypoallergenic formulas available in the US are either based on extensively hydrolyzed casein derived from cow's milk (Pregestimil, Nutramigen, Mead & Johnson; Alimentum, Ross) or on a mixture of single amino acids (Neocate, SHS; Elecare, Ross). Hypoallergenic formulas are well tolerated by children with IgE-mediated and with cell-mediated food allergy [25, 27]. Hypoallergenic formulas are also recommended for prophylaxis of food allergy in infants at risk of atopy.

Based on the observation that children with IgE-mediated immune responses directed predominantly at conformational epitopes are more likely to outgrow egg and cow's milk allergy, clinical trials of diets containing baked egg and baked milk (in which conformational epitopes are destroyed by high temperatures) are underway at the author's institution. Children undergo OFC to baked egg/milk to confirm tolerance and are followed prospectively for maximum 48 months or until they achieve tolerance to uncooked egg/milk. Clinical (weight, body fat, intestinal permeability, symptoms of AD, asthma, rhinitis, acute allergic reactions) and immunological parameters (allergen-specific IgE and IgG4 antibody levels, skin prick test) are monitored. The inclusion of baked egg/milk products results in substantial liberalization of the diet and improved nutrition. In addition, ingestion of baked egg/milk might promote tolerance and resolution of egg/milk allergy.

Oral immunotherapy for milk allergy and sublingual immunotherapy for hazelnut allergy have been reported but it is unclear whether such therapies result in a transient state of desensitization or permanent oral tolerance [39, 40].

The most promising future approaches to food allergy therapy include anti-IgE monoclonal antibody (TNX-901), Chinese herbs, vaccines containing heat-killed *Escherichia coli* expressing modified peanut proteins, and chimeric molecules with allergen and Fcγ. Considering a variety of approaches that are being investigated, effective prophylaxis as well as potentially curative therapy for food allergy seem to be within reach and bring hope to patients for whom no effective therapy is currently available.

References

1 Sampson HA: Update on food allergy. J Allergy Clin Immunol 2004;113:805–819.
2 Sicherer SH, Sampson HA: 9. Food allergy. J Allergy Clin Immunol 2006;117(2 Suppl Mini-Primer):S470–S475.
3 Wood RA: The natural history of food allergy. Pediatrics 2003;111:1631–1637.
4 Skolnick HS, Conover-Walker MK, Koerner CB, et al: The natural history of peanut allergy. J Allergy Clin Immunol 2001;107:367–374.
5 Sicherer SH, Munoz-Furlong A, Sampson HA: Prevalence of peanut and tree nut allergy in the United States determined by means of a random digit dial telephone survey: a 5-year follow-up study. J Allergy Clin Immunol 2003;112:1203–1207.
6 Chehade M, Mayer L: Oral tolerance and its relation to food hypersensitivities. J Allergy Clin Immunol 2005;115:3–12.
7 Vieths S, Scheurer S, Ballmer-Weber B: Current understanding of cross-reactivity of food allergens and pollen. Ann NY Acad Sci 2002;964:47–68.
8 Beyer K, Morrow E, Li XM, et al: Effects of cooking methods on peanut allergenicity. J Allergy Clin Immunol 2001;107:1077–1081.
9 Breiteneder H, Mills C: Nonspecific lipid-transfer proteins in plant foods and pollens: an important allergen class. Curr Opin Allergy Clin Immunol 2005;5:275–279.

10 Shreffler WG, Charlop-Powers Z, Castro RR, et al: The major allergen from peanut, Ara h 1, is a ligand of DC-SIGN. J Allergy Clin Immunol 2006;117:S87.

11 Jarvinen KM, Beyer K, Vila L, et al: B-cell epitopes as a screening instrument for persistent cow's milk allergy. J Allergy Clin Immunol 2002;110:293–297.

12 Beyer K, Ellman-Grunther L, Jarvinen KM, et al: Measurement of peptide-specific IgE as an additional tool in identifying patients with clinical reactivity to peanuts. J Allergy Clin Immunol 2003;112:202–207.

13 Chatchatee P, Jarvinen KM, Bardina L, et al: Identification of IgE- and IgG-binding epitopes on alpha(s1)-casein: differences in patients with persistent and transient cow's milk allergy. J Allergy Clin Immunol 2001;107:379–383.

14 Jarvinen KM, Beyer K, Bardina L, et al: Recognition of sequential and conformational structures of ovomucoid varies in patients with long-lasting and transient egg allergy. J Allergy Clin Immunol 2003;111:S351.

15 Shreffler WG, Beyer K, Chu TH, et al: Microarray immunoassay: association of clinical history, in vitro IgE function, and heterogeneity of allergenic peanut epitopes. J Allergy Clin Immunol 2004;113:776–782.

16 Sampson HA: Food anaphylaxis. Br Med Bull 2000;56:925–935.

17 Simonte SJ, Ma S, Mofidi S, Sicherer SH: Relevance of casual contact with peanut butter in children with peanut allergy. J Allergy Clin Immunol 2003;112:180–182.

18 Hallett R, Haapanen LA, Teuber SS: Food allergies and kissing. N Engl J Med 2002;346: 1833–1834.

19 Eigenmann PA, Sicherer SH, Borkowski TA, et al: Prevalence of IgE-mediated food allergy among children with atopic dermatitis. Pediatrics 1998;101:E8.

20 Reekers R, Busche M, Wittmann M, et al: Birch pollen-related foods trigger atopic dermatitis in patients with specific cutaneous T-cell responses to birch pollen antigens. J Allergy Clin Immunol 1999;104:466–472.

21 Breuer K, Wulf A, Constien A, et al: Birch pollen-related food as a provocation factor of allergic symptoms in children with atopic eczema/dermatitis syndrome. Allergy 2004;59:988–994.

22 Sampson HA, McCaskill CC: Food hypersensitivity and atopic dermatitis: evaluation of 113 patients. J Pediatr 1985;107:669–675.

23 Sampson HA, Anderson JA: Summary and recommendations: classification of gastrointestinal manifestations due to immunologic reactions to foods in infants and young children. J Pediatr Gastroenterol Nutr 2000;30:S87–S94.

24 Rothenberg ME, Mishra A, Collins MH, Putnam PE: Pathogenesis and clinical features of eosinophilic esophagitis. J Allergy Clin Immunol 2001;108:891–894.

25 Kelly KJ, Lazenby AJ, Rowe PC, et al: Eosinophilic esophagitis attributed to gastroesophageal reflux: improvement with an amino acid-based formula. Gastroenterology 1995;109:1503–1512.

26 Markowitz JE, Spergel JM, Ruchelli E, Liacouras CA: Elemental diet is an effective treatment for eosinophilic esophagitis in children and adolescents. Am J Gastroenterol 2003;98: 777–782.

27 Sicherer SH, Noone SA, Koerner CB, et al: Hypoallergenicity and efficacy of an amino acid-based formula in children with cow's milk and multiple food hypersensitivities. J Pediatr 2001;138:688–693.

28 Lake AM, Whitington PF, Hamilton SR: Dietary protein-induced colitis in breast-fed infants. J Pediatr 1982;101:906–910.

29 Powell GK: Milk- and soy-induced enterocolitis of infancy. J Pediatr 1978;93:553–560.

30 Sicherer SH, Eigenmann PA, Sampson HA: Clinical features of food-protein-induced entercolitis syndrome. J Pediatr 1998;133:214–219.

31 Nowak-Wegrzyn A, Sampson HA, Wood RA, Sicherer SH: Food protein-induced enterocolitis syndrome caused by solid food proteins. Pediatrics 2003;111:829–835.

32 Jenkins HR, Pincott JR, Soothill JF, et al: Food allergy: the major cause of infantile colitis. Arch Dis Child 1984;59:326–329.

33 Hill DJ, Hudson IL, Sheffield LJ, et al: A low allergen diet is a significant intervention in infantile colic: results of a community-based study. J Allergy Clin Immunol 1995;96:886–892.

34 Salvatore S, Vandenplas Y: Gastroesophageal reflux and cow milk allergy: is there a link? Pediatrics 2002;110:972–984.

35 Sporik R, Hill DJ, Hosking CS: Specificity of allergen skin testing in predicting positive open food challenges to milk, egg, and peanut in children. Clin Exp Allergy 2000;30:1540–1546.

36 Sampson HA: Utility of food-specific IgE concentrations in predicting symptomatic food allergy. J Allergy Clin Immunol 2001;107:891–896.
37 Isolauri E, Turnjanmaa K: Combined skin prick and patch testing enhances identification of food allergy in infants with atopic dermatitis. J Allergy Clin Immunol 1996;97:9–15.
38 Bock SA: Prospective appraisal of complaints of adverse reactions to foods in children during the first 3 years of life. Pediatrics 1987;79:683–688.
39 Patriarca G, Nucera E, Roncallo C, et al: Oral desensitizing treatment in food allergy: clinical and immunological results. Aliment Pharmacol Ther 2003;17:459–465.
40 Enrique E, Pineda F, Malek T, et al: Sublingual immunotherapy for hazelnut food allergy: a randomized, double-blind, placebo-controlled study with a standardized hazelnut extract. J allergy Clin Immunol 2005;116:1073–1079.
41 Shreffler WG, Lencer DA, Bardina L, Sampson HA: IgE and IgG4 epitope mapping by microarray immunoassay reveals the diversity of immune response to the peanut allergen, Ara h 2. J Allergy Clin Immunol 2005;116:893–899.
42 Lewis SA, Grimshaw KE, Warner JO, Hourihane JO: The promiscuity of immunoglobulin E binding to peanut allergens, as determined by Western blotting, correlates with the severity of clinical symptoms. Clin Exp Allergy 2005;35:767–773.

Discussion

Dr. Lentze: When you talk about the nonimmunological food allergens you mention a disease called fructase deficiency. I think you probably mean sucrase isomaltase deficiency because we don't have an enzyme called fructase.

Dr. Nowak-Wegrzyn: This is correct, thank you.

Dr. Wahn: You were explaining to us how important the IgE pattern is with regard to the epitopes of the allergen as far as the prognosis is concerned. We usually consider cow's milk allergy as an infantile allergic manifestation to food but occasionally it may become manifest only in adulthood. My personal prejudice is that the prognosis in adults is much worse than in children. They will never outgrow it apparently. Is there anything known about the epitopes relevant in adults? I always felt that casein plays more of a role.

Dr. Nowak-Wegrzyn: I am not aware of any studies that have been done on epitope recognition in adults with food allergy. All the data are from children and I agree with you that there could be different epitopes in adults. In adult food allergy mechanisms may be different. The primary failure to develop oral tolerance due to immaturity of the gastrointestinal tract, the inability to break down the proteins and increased intestinal permeability that is implied in childhood food allergy are unlikely to underlie food allergy in adults. So if somebody develops allergy at an older age there must be special circumstances. An example that comes to mind in adults is in the setting of heavy occupational exposure. For instance people who work in bakeries and are exposed by inhalation to aerosolized wheat may develop so-called baker's asthma, but some of them may go on to develop symptoms following ingestion of wheat. I don't think anybody is looking at the epitopes specific to adult food allergy and it definitely would be very interesting to see whether those are different.

Dr. Vandenplas: There are large differences in the prevalence of eosinophilic esophagitis between North America and Europe. You mentioned that 50% of the refluxing babies have eosinophilic esophagitis. If I exaggerate a little bit, I could say it does not exist in Western Europe. Certainly in our center, we are below 5%. Knowing that feeding is the same, reflux medication is the same, and that the condition is relatively easy to diagnose, does it not mean that 'environment' is by far the most important factor and that all the other factors we are studying are in fact only of minor importance? Can you speculate about that?

Dr. Nowak-Wegrzyn: Actually I did not include gastroesophageal reflux in the same category as allergic eosinophilic esophagitis (AEE). These are two separate disorders. AEE is an example of a mixed pathogenesis food allergy, and it is more common in older children, adolescents especially with pollen allergy [1]. The comment on gastroesophageal reflux was made in reference to non-IgE-mediated food allergy, specifically cow's milk allergy in infants younger than 1 year. We don't necessarily have biopsy data from those young infants to confirm that indeed it has anything to do with AEE. The studies that have focused on AEE emphasized that although the symptoms are similar, the patients with AEE fail to respond to standard antireflux therapy but improve with amino acid-based elemental formula [2, 3]. You made a very good point; there are animal models that show that inhalation of pollen produces AEE, and there are reports that show that patients with this disorder suffer exacerbation in the high pollen season, so there may be an environmental component involved [4, 5].

Dr. B. Koletzko: In your paper you referred to different methodologies or heat treatment and changes of antigen. In the table you presented you also refer to proton pump inhibitor treatment in relation to hazelnut allergy in adults. You are probably aware of the Vienna studies both on proton pump inhibitors and allergy. I wonder whether you have any comments to offer on the plausibility of the concept and the mechanisms behind it. Is it likely that this observation is simply related to an acid-induced denaturation of food allergens that reduce the allergenicity? If that would be so, is there also a potential for therapeutic or preventive use, for example considering fermentation of foods where acidity is somewhat enhanced even though to a lesser degree than in the fasting stomach? Are there any data that a fermented cow's milk product offers a lower allergy risk?

Dr. Nowak-Wegrzyn: There are data from animal models that if you use antacids the animals are more likely to develop hazelnut IgE antibody [6]. Adult patients with reflux have documented a new development of IgE antibody and the clinical reactivity to hazelnut [7]. I think that it is plausible; in the animal models when we encounter difficulties with sensitizing animals we actually add antacids to decrease the gastric pH. How close we are to using this as a principle for treatment I am not sure and many more studies are necessary to evaluate the utility of fermented foods.

Dr. B. Koletzko: Are there any studies looking at antigens in fermented vs. nonfermented foods, for example cow's milk products? Are you aware of any such investigations?

Dr. Nowak-Wegrzyn: No.

Dr. Fuchs: Can I follow up a little bit on the discussion that Dr. Vandenplas raised with regard to the role of allergy-related gastroesophageal reflux and esophagitis? If I may be so presumptuous as to speak for North America, we don't see 50% of children with reflux as having eosinophilic esophagitis. It is fairly rare, but I think most of us are convinced that it is a little bit more difficult to make a distinction between reflux esophagitis and eosinophilic esophagitis. There are certainly children that don't have reflux and still have eosinophilic inflammation of the esophagus. There are also children who have reflux esophagitis and eosinophilic inflammation which resolves completely with standard antireflux therapy. So clearly we have some phenotypic common expression, yet mechanisms that are really very different from one another. What I heard you say though, is not eosinophilic esophagitis but reflux, 50% of reflux, is related to the allergic response and that is clearly different from our current conceptual framework. I don't think we will find many North American gastroenterologists that would describe this sort of rate. I think there is evidence that about 10–20% of young infants with reflux seem to respond to an amino acid-based formula, but the precise mechanism has yet to be determined.

Dr. Nowak-Wegrzyn: A review article postulated that in up to 50% of infants younger than 1 year of age, gastroesophageal reflux may be associated with cow's milk allergy [8]. Maybe it is an exaggerated estimate, but it points out that there may be more reactions to the food than is being appreciated at this point. Considering a very aggressive use of antacids for treatment of gastroesophageal reflux in infants, this could be another potential mechanism why we see an increased prevalence of food allergy.

Dr. Fuchs: I think that is really a speculation at this point. Those of us who are more focused on reflux and esophagitis would be concerned if those were withheld for concern about precipitating allergy.

Dr. Wahn: Recently there was a study from Vienna confirming exactly what you said and they found a strong association between this kind of medication and the development of food allergy.

Dr. Vandenplas: Just to follow up on your comment; I think that the more the proteins are hydrolyzed, the more rapid their gastric emptying is. This has clearly been shown. So, if children have less reflux on extensive hydrolysates or amino acid formula, it may be because of the change in gastric emptying. In other words, the improvement obtained with extensive hydrolysates or with amino acid formula in reflux is not proof that a pathophysiologic mechanism is involved.

Dr. Heine: You dissected the IgE-mediated pathways very nicely. In gastroenterological food allergy often we don't find any increase in IgE, at least on serological testing, implying cell-mediated immune mechanisms. Is there any progress in identifying food protein epitopes that could explain why, for example, gastrointestinal food allergies are often transient?

Dr. Nowak-Wegrzyn: I am not aware of any studies in non-IgE-mediated food allergies looking at epitope recognition.

Dr. Heine: Do you feel that non-IgE food allergy is likely to align with the same recognition sites as IgE-mediated forms, or could this involve different parts of the protein?

Dr. Nowak-Wegrzyn: I think it could be different because the natural history seems to be so different.

Dr. Martaadmadja: I am a practician, not a researcher, so I would like to ask about the use of hypoallergenic formula given to allergic babies. Some of them have frequent defecation after having been given hypoallergenic formula which stops immediately after soy formula is used. Is there any other allergic factor in the hypoallergenic formula?

Dr. Nowak-Wegrzyn: Most of the children who are allergic to cow's milk tolerate soy-based formula. It is estimated that about only 12% will have problems when exposed to a soy formula [9].

Dr. Sorensen: It is commonly said that people in India and China have less peanut allergy because of different food preparation but there may also be a big difference in hygiene and the hygiene hypothesis may be the other explanation for it. What do you think is the most important part, the way the food is prepared or hygiene?

Dr. Nowak-Wegrzyn: This is a million dollar question. It is rather unlikely that a single factor can explain this discrepancy. Differences in food processing may account for part of it, but in addition the tendency of a population to develop an atopic type of reaction is crucial. So I agree with you that differences in hygiene are very important.

Dr. Rivera: At what point can we say that the so-called reflux in the newborn and low birth weight baby, which continues after the age of 6 months, is really a true reflux due to nonmaturity of the gastroesophagus or allergy?

Dr. Nowak-Wegrzyn: One practical way of approaching this issue is to focus on atopy risk factors such as atopic dermatitis and/or a family history of atopy in siblings or parents. When these risk factors are present, I would definitely consider evaluation for food allergy and/or an empirical trial of hypoallergenic infant formula. In contrast, in a child with symptoms of mild reflux and good weight gain, and no atopic predisposition, treatment with antacids is appropriate.

Dr. S. Koletzko: We are all puzzled by the results of the group from Vienna. They showed that increasing the intragastric pH with acid-suppressive drugs increases the risk of sensitization and allergic manifestation in adults. They could show this for cod fish and hazelnut. As pediatricians, we wonder if we increase the risk of cow's milk allergy when we treat bottle-fed infants with acid-suppressive drugs. From the physiological point of view, I have my doubts because after feeding the acid is buffered for at least 2 or sometimes 3 h, and by that time a lot of milk has already left the stomach. So the question is whether nature is prepared for that or not? Did you look in vitro if there is pH-dependent denaturation of these epitopes of cow's milk allergens.

Dr. Nowak-Wegrzyn: The short answer is no, and actually pH studies are not something we do and I am not aware of anyone looking at that recently.

Dr. Lack: I was intrigued to hear your comments about work on T cell responses to fruits even after denaturation, and I guess it is translated into a simple clinical question. What do you tell your patients with oral allergy syndrome and allergy to fruits to do? Do you tell them to continue eating cooked fruits that don't cause symptoms or do you recommend avoidance? On the one hand gastrointestinal inflammation or disactive T cell epitopes could potentially be caused, or pollen allergy could be maintained; on the other hand you might argue that by getting patients to eat a lot of raw and cooked fruit you might be inducing tolerance. Which way should we be going clinically?

Dr. Nowak-Wegrzyn: The data I presented came from a very recent study [10]. It is too early to make clinical recommendations but it is a very interesting insight into the pathophysiology. My current recommendation is based on clinical symptoms, so if a patient is asymptomatic with baked fruits I do not recommend their avoidance.

Dr. Saavedra: You mentioned that casein fractions in milk may be associated or be more predictive of long-term persistence of allergic symptoms. Why caseins? Should we be more concerned with bovine casein than with bovine whey from the point of view of atopic persistence? Does that have any potential preventive or therapeutic implication?

Dr. Nowak-Wegrzyn: It is not clear at this point why IgE antibodies against caseins would be a marker of more severe and/or more persistent milk allergy. I think they are more resistant to heating, and compared to whey proteins they have a better defined secondary structure. Maybe this makes casein an important allergen in terms of the differences in epitope recognition.

References

1 Rothenberg ME, Mishra A, Collins MH, Putnam PE: Pathogenesis and clinical features of eosinophilic esophagitis. J Allergy Clin Immunol 2001;108:891–894.
2 Orenstein SR, Shalaby TM, Di Lorenzo C, et al: The spectrum of pediatric eosinophilic esophagitis beyond infancy: a clinical series of 30 children. Am J Gastroenterol 2000;95: 1422–1430.
3 Kelly KJ, Lazenby AJ, Rowe PC, et al: Eosinophilic esophagitis attributed to gastroesophageal reflux: improvement with an amino acid-based formula. Gastroenterology 1995;109: 1503–1512.
4 Mishra A, Hogan SP, Brandt EB, Rothenberg ME: An etiological role for aeroallergens and eosinophils in experimental esophagitis. J Clin Invest 2001;107:83–90.
5 Fogg MI, Ruchelli E, Spergel JM: Pollen and eosinophilic esophagitis. J Allergy Clin Immunol 2003;112:796–797.
6 Scholl I, Untersmayr E, Bakos N, et al: Antiulcer drugs promote oral sensitization and hypersensitivity to hazelnut allergens in BALB/c mice and humans. Am J Clin Nutr 2005;81: 154–160.

7 Untersmayr E, Bakos N, Scholl I, et al: Anti-ulcer drugs promote IgE formation toward dietary antigens in adult patients. FASEB J 2005;19:656–658.
8 Salvatore S, Vandenplas Y: Gastroesophageal reflux and cow milk allergy: is there a link? Pediatrics 2002;110:972–984.
9 Zeiger RS, Sampson HA, Bock SA, et al: Soy allergy in infants and children with IgE-associated cow's milk allergy. J Pediatr 1999;134:614–622.
10 Bohle B, Zwolfer B, Heratizadeh A, et al: Cooking birch pollen-related food: divergent consequences for IgE- and T cell-mediated reactivity in vitro and in vivo. J Allergy Clin Immunol 2006;118:242–249.

Cooke RJ, Vandenplas Y, Wahn U (eds): Nutrition Support for Infants and Children at Risk.
Nestlé Nutr Workshop Ser Pediatr Program, vol 59, pp 37–47,
Nestec Ltd., Vevey/S. Karger AG, Basel, © 2007.

Hypoallergenicity: A Principle for the Treatment of Food Allergy

Kirsten Beyer

Charité, University Children's Hospital, Berlin, Germany

Abstract

Food allergy is a common disease with the treatment of choice being complete avoidance of the incriminated food. In cow's milk allergy a hypoallergenic milk substitute is necessary during infancy and childhood. Hypoallergenic formulas are produced through enzymatic hydrolysis of different sources such as bovine casein or whey followed by further processing such as heat treatment and/or ultrafiltration. According to the degree of protein hydrolysis the resulting products have been classified into 'extensively' or 'partially' hydrolyzed. Reduction of allergenicity should be assessed in vitro and in vivo. Hypoallergenic formulas might also be based on amino acid mixtures. These elementary diets can be considered as nonallergenic. Several novel therapies are currently being explored in food allergy. One of the most promising approaches is the immunotherapy with mutated proteins. For this approach, alteration of the IgE-binding sites through single amino acid substitution is performed resulting in reduced to complete loss of IgE binding. For the major peanut allergens such mutations were introduced into the cDNA sequences and successfully expressed as hypoallergenic recombinant proteins. In peanut-sensitized mice, the use of these modified proteins co-administered with adjuvant such as heat-killed *Escherichia coli* showed promising results for future therapeutic approaches.

Introduction

Food allergy is a major public health issue. About 6–8% of children and 1–2% of adults are affected. The prevalence rate is even higher in patients with atopic dermatitis with around one third of these children having a clinically relevant food allergy [1]. Despite the enormous diversity of the human diet, few foods are responsible for the vast majority of food-allergic reactions. Cow's milk, hen's egg, soy, wheat, peanut, tree nuts, fish and crustaceans are the most commonly offending foods. The characterization of these allergenic food proteins has increased dramatically within the last several years [2].

The majority of food-allergic reactions are IgE-mediated. Food proteins bind to the allergen-specific IgE molecules residing on mast cells and basophils and trigger the release of mediators, such as histamine, and an acute onset of symptoms occurs. Clinical reactions to these foods range from mild skin symptoms to life-threatening anaphylactic reactions.

The majority of children with food allergy will become tolerant later on in life. However, the natural course is different for each allergen. Most cow's milk-allergic patients will develop symptoms in the first year of life, but about 85% become clinically tolerant by their third year [3]. Hen's egg allergy appears to be more persistent with approximately half of the patients becoming tolerant in 3 years and up to two thirds of children in 5 years [4]. In contrast, peanut allergy tends to persist throughout adulthood; only about 20% of patients will lose their allergy [5, 6].

Today, the treatment of choice for food allergy is complete avoidance of the incriminated food. In the case of some food allergens there will be no nutritional problems; however, during infancy and childhood an alternative hypoallergenic milk substitute is necessary in children with cow's milk allergy. Moreover, a strict elimination diet is always difficult. Dietary failures occur frequently resulting sometimes in severe reactions. Therefore, new therapeutic approaches especially for the long-lasting peanut allergy are currently under development. One of these approaches is an immunotherapy with the mutated hypoallergenic proteins.

The following paragraphs will describe how hypoallergenicity can be used as a principle in the treatment of food allergy. First, current knowledge on the use of hypoallergenic formulas for the treatment of cow's milk allergy is described. Second, novel therapeutic approaches with mutated proteins are discussed.

Hypoallergenic Formulas for Cow's Milk Allergy

Cow's milk allergy is the most common cause of food allergy in the first years of life, affecting approximately 2–3% of children [7]. The majority of children outgrow their cow's milk allergy by 3–4 years of age [3]. Currently, the only treatment is strict avoidance; however, a hypoallergenic substitute is necessary at this young age.

Milk of another animal source such as goat or sheep cannot be recommended as a general substitute in cow's milk allergy. For example, many proteins in goat milk show a high similarity with cow's milk proteins resulting in a cross-reactivity of 92% [8]. Therefore, patients might react severely at first exposure. In contrast, cross-reactivity with mare's milk occurs only in about 4% [8]. Furthermore, soy formula may provide a safe and growth-promoting

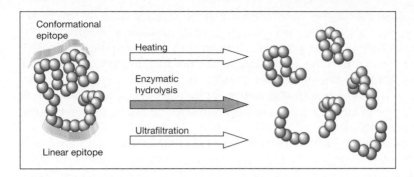

Fig. 1. Technologies to reduce the allergenicity of a protein. Hypoallergenic formulas are produced through enzymatic hydrolysis of different sources such as bovine casein, bovine whey or soy followed by further processing such as heat treatment and/or ultrafiltration.

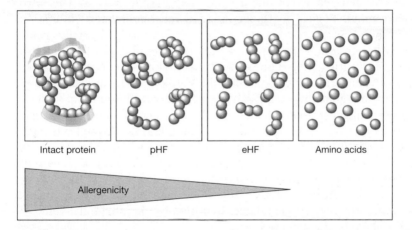

Fig. 2. Hypoallergenic formulas have been classified into 'extensively' (eHF) or 'partially' (pHF) hydrolyzed formulas according to the degree of protein hydrolysis. Hypoallergenic formulas might also be based on amino acid mixtures.

alternative for children with cow's milk allergy [9]. However, soy is a potent allergen itself and sensitization resulting in allergic reactions might occur.

For many years hypoallergenic formulas have been used in cow's milk allergy. As shown in figure 1 hypoallergenic formulas are produced through enzymatic hydrolysis of different sources such as bovine casein, bovine whey or soy followed by further processing such as heat treatment and/or ultrafiltration [10]. The resulting products have been classified into 'extensively' or 'partially' hydrolyzed formulas (fig. 2) according to the degree of protein hydrolysis [11]. The degree of hydrolysis may be characterized by biochemical techniques, such as the spectrum of peptide molecular weights or the ratio of alpha amino nitrogen to total nitrogen [10]. Assuming the theory that the shorter the peptides the less allergenic the product, much work has been done to determine the molecular weight of residual peptides in the hydrolysates [12]. As a practical guideline for industry the appropriate cutoff for the absence of larger peptides has been determined to be approximately 1,500 Daltons [12].

Anaphylactic reactions have been reported not only for partially hydrolyzed formula but also for extensively hydrolyzed ones; therefore, reduction of allergenicity should be assessed in vitro and in vivo [13]. Residual allergenicity can be explained by the degree of hydrolysis. Peptides representing IgE-binding sites might still be present. In addition, higher-molecular-weight particles that might be allergenic can occur in hydrolyzed formula through aggregation of smaller peptides [14]. Moreover, contamination with native proteins during production of the hypoallergenic formula is possible.

Reduction of allergenicity of dietary products may be assessed in vitro using various immunological methods, such as IgE-binding test, inhibition assays or immunoelectrophoresis methods [10]. Especially hypoallergenic formulas used for treatment in cow's milk allergy should undergo clinical in vivo testing. Skin testing should be the first step followed by challenge tests [15]. Suitable hypoallergenic formulas should be tolerated by at least 90% of infants with documented cow's milk allergy with 95% of confidence in double-blind placebo-controlled food challenges. It is recommended that trials should be performed in two independent centers, and be divided into IgE- and non-IgE-mediated cases before statistical treatment [15]. For each type of allergy ≥28 patients should be included in each trial [15]. If 1 patient reacts, 46 subjects must be included and the remaining 45 must be without reactions. In order to ensure long-term tolerance a normal daily intake during a period of 3 months is recommendable. In addition, the nutritional value of the products has to be documented.

Hypoallergenic formulas might also be based on amino acid mixtures (fig. 2). These elementary diets can be considered as nonallergenic. They do not need any clinical testing provided the production is sufficiently controlled assuring no contamination [15]. The hypoallergenicity and the nutritional value of such elementary diets have been documented [16].

Specific Immunotherapy for Food Allergy with Mutated Proteins

Currently the only treatment for food allergy is strict avoidance of the offending food. In the past years much effort has been made to develop new treatment methods. Specific immunotherapy using injections is commonly used for the treatment of inhalant allergies. However, for food allergy it is

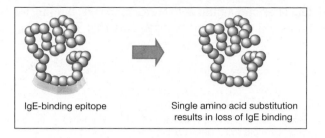

IgE-binding epitope

Single amino acid substitution
results in loss of IgE binding

Fig. 3. IgE-binding sites have been identified for many food allergens. Mutation through single amino acid substitution at these binding sites resulted in reduced to complete loss of IgE-binding.

currently not recommended because of the allergic side effects of the therapy. A study by Oppenheimer et al. [17] showed that patients with peanut allergy tolerated an increased amount of peanuts following a rush immunotherapy but an unacceptable rate of adverse systemic reactions occurred.

As traditional immunotherapy has been largely impractical for the treatment of food allergies, several novel therapies are currently being explored [18, 19]. One of the most promising approaches is the immunotherapy with mutated proteins. Within the last couple of years food allergens have been better characterized [2, 20]. IgE-binding sites have been identified for many of these food allergens [21–26]. With this knowledge attempts to alter IgE antibody binding through alteration of the amino acid sequences of the IgE-binding sites have started (fig. 3). Mutation through single amino acid substitution resulted in reduced to complete loss of IgE binding [26–29]. For the major peanut allergens Ara h 1, Ara h 2 and Ara h 3 such mutations were introduced into the cDNA sequences and successfully expressed as hypoallergenic recombinant proteins [18]. Most importantly, mutation of the IgE-binding sites appears to leave the T cell response unaffected [30].

In peanut-sensitized mice, the use of these modified proteins showed some protection; however, alone it did not appear to be adequate for the treatment of peanut allergy [19]. However, using co-administration of modified peanut proteins and heat-killed *Listeria monocytogenes* as an adjuvant resulted in much better protection [19]. However, although modified proteins reduce the concern regarding activation of mast cells during immunotherapy, the safety of subcutaneous injections of heat-killed *L. monocytogenes* remains to be determined. Another promising approach appears to be the rectal administration of mutated proteins with heat-killed *Escherichia coli* as an adjuvant. This novel immunotherapeutic approach has the benefit that expensive purification of the engineered proteins generated in *E. coli* is not necessary because it is administered into an environment replete with *E. coli* [19].

Although animal studies using mutated hypoallergenic proteins seem to be very promising, studies in humans will be necessary to prove the effect.

41

Heterogenicity in IgE-binding sites and amino acids critical for IgE binding as shown for cow's milk proteins [29] might lead to problems that need to be addressed in the future.

References

1 Eigenmann PA, Sicherer SH, Borkowski TA, et al: Prevalence of IgE-mediated food allergy among children with atopic dermatitis. Pediatrics 1998;101:E8.
2 Beyer K: Characterization of allergenic food proteins for improved diagnostic methods. Curr Opin Allergy Clin Immunol 2003;3:189–197.
3 Host A, Halken S, Jacobsen HP, et al: Clinical course of cow's milk protein allergy/intolerance and atopic diseases in childhood. Pediatr Allergy Immunol 2002;13(suppl 15):23–28.
4 Boyano-Martinez T, Garcia-Ara C, Diaz-Pena JM, Martin-Esteban M: Prediction of tolerance on the basis of quantification of egg white-specific IgE antibodies in children with egg allergy. J Allergy Clin Immunol 2002;110:304–309.
5 Hourihane JO: Recent advances in peanut allergy. Curr Opin Allergy Clin Immunol 2002;2: 227–231.
6 Skolnick HS, Conover-Walker MK, Koerner CB, et al: The natural history of peanut allergy. J Allergy Clin Immunol 2001;107:367–374.
7 Sampson HA: Food allergy. 1. Immunopathogenesis and clinical disorders. J Allergy Clin Immunol 1999;103:717–728.
8 Sicherer SH, Teuber S: Current approach to the diagnosis and management of adverse reactions to foods. J Allergy Clin Immunol 2004;114:1146–1150.
9 Zeiger RS, Sampson HA, Bock SA, et al: Soy allergy in infants and children with IgE-associated cow's milk allergy. J Pediatr 1999;134:614–622.
10 Host A, Halken S: Hypoallergenic formulas – when, to whom and how long: after more than 15 years we know the right indication! Allergy 2004;59:45–52.
11 Host A, Koletzko B, Dreborg S, et al: Dietary products used in infants for treatment and prevention of food allergy. Joint Statement of the European Society for Paediatric Allergology and Clinical Immunology (ESPACI) Committee on Hypoallergenic Formulas and the European Society for Paediatric Gastroenterology, Hepatology and Nutrition (ESPGHAN) Committee on Nutrition. Arch Dis Child 1999;81:80–84.
12 Walker-Smith J: Hypoallergenic formulas: are they really hypoallergenic? Ann Allergy Asthma Immunol 2003;90:112–114.
13 Niggemann B, Binder C, Klettke U, Wahn U: In vivo and in vitro studies on the residual allergenicity of partially hydrolysed infant formulae. Acta Paediatr 1999;88:394–398.
14 Rosendal A, Barkholt V: Detection of potentially allergenic material in 12 hydrolyzed milk formulas. J Dairy Sci 2000;83:2200–2210.
15 Muraro A, Dreborg S, Halken S, et al: Dietary prevention of allergic diseases in infants and small children. I. Immunologic background and criteria for hypoallergenicity. Pediatr Allergy Immunol 2004;15:103–111.
16 Sicherer SH, Noone SA, Koerner CB, et al: Hypoallergenicity and efficacy of an amino acid-based formula in children with cow's milk and multiple food hypersensitivities. J Pediatr 2001;138:688–693.
17 Oppenheimer JJ, Nelson HS, Bock SA, et al: Treatment of peanut allergy with rush immunotherapy. J Allergy Clin Immunol 1992;90:256–262.
18 Pons L, Palmer K, Burks W: Towards immunotherapy for peanut allergy. Curr Opin Allergy Clin Immunol 2005;5:558–562.
19 Li XM: Beyond allergen avoidance: update on developing therapies for peanut allergy. Curr Opin Allergy Clin Immunol 2005;5:287–292.
20 Teuber SS, Beyer K: Peanut, tree nut and seed allergies. Curr Opin Allergy Clin Immunol 2004;4:201–203.
21 Busse PJ, Jarvinen KM, Vila L, et al: Identification of sequential IgE-binding epitopes on bovine alpha(s2)-casein in cow's milk allergic patients. Int Arch Allergy Immunol 2002;129: 93–96.

22 Jarvinen KM, Chatchatee P, Bardina L, et al: IgE and IgG binding epitopes on alpha-lactalbumin and beta-lactoglobulin in cow's milk allergy. Int Arch Allergy Immunol 2001;126:111–118.
23 Chatchatee P, Jarvinen KM, Bardina L, et al: Identification of IgE and IgG binding epitopes on beta- and kappa-casein in cow's milk allergic patients. Clin Exp Allergy 2001;31:1256–1262.
24 Chatchatee P, Jarvinen KM, Bardina L, et al: Identification of IgE- and IgG-binding epitopes on alpha(s1)-casein: differences in patients with persistent and transient cow's milk allergy. J Allergy Clin Immunol 2001;107:379–383.
25 Rabjohn P, Helm EM, Stanley JS, et al: Molecular cloning and epitope analysis of the peanut allergen Ara h 3. J Clin Invest 1999;103:535–542.
26 Burks AW, Shin D, Cockrell G, et al: Mapping and mutational analysis of the IgE-binding epitopes on Ara h 1, a legume vicilin protein and a major allergen in peanut hypersensitivity. Eur J Biochem 1997;245:334–339.
27 Rabjohn P, West CM, Connaughton C, et al: Modification of peanut allergen Ara h 3: effects on IgE binding and T cell stimulation. Int Arch Allergy Immunol 2002;128:15–23.
28 Stanley JS, King N, Burks AW, et al: Identification and mutational analysis of the immunodominant IgE binding epitopes of the major peanut allergen Ara h 2. Arch Biochem Biophys 1997;342:244–253.
29 Cocco RR, Jarvinen KM, Sampson HA, Beyer K: Mutational analysis of major, sequential IgE-binding epitopes in alpha s1-casein, a major cow's milk allergen. J Allergy Clin Immunol 2003;112:433–437.
30 King N, Helm R, Stanley JS, et al: Allergenic characteristics of a modified peanut allergen. Mol Nutr Food Res 2005;49:963–971.

Discussion

Dr. Bojadzieva: I would like to ask if all these skin tests are valid for the first year of life, especially for the first 6 months of life? We know as pediatricians that sometimes cow's milk allergy can be only manifested with diarrhea, with other skin manifestations, and we also know that the immunologic reaction in the bowel is not the same as in the skin.

Dr. Beyer: In general it is possible to perform skin prick tests in children in the first year of life. However, age differences have to be taken into account [1]. In regard to gastrointestinal diseases, many of them are non-IgE-mediated. In these cases the skin prick test will not help you. Most important is the double-blind placebo-controlled food challenge test.

Dr. Sorensen: I was fascinated looking at the experiments with the mutated proteins that you discussed, but I am not sure really if you can say that you induce tolerance versus desensitization. Second, if you tolerize against the native protein, are you implying that you can use a mutated protein to then induce tolerance to the native protein?

Dr. Beyer: It is always a big discussion whether tolerance is induced. The aim is to use the modified proteins for specific immunotherapy to avoid immediate reactions. Whether tolerance can be induced has to be shown with future studies.

Dr. Sorensen: First of all I do not give allergy immunotherapy in general if I can avoid it. Second I think that the aim of immunotherapy is to induce tolerance, meaning that the time between the last deliberate allergen exposure of the individual and the challenge is long enough to exclude desensitization; that is then true tolerance.

Dr. Beyer: Common specific immunotherapy with aeroallergens is performed for about 3 years in which the individuals will gain tolerance that last for many years. This is what we aim for in food allergy with different approaches, e.g. therapy with mutated proteins or specific oral tolerance induction where children are fed with increasing amounts of food.

Beyer

Dr. Sorensen: I think that tolerance has to be differentiated. Is it clinical tolerance or T cell tolerance? That was discussed earlier but you may have intense T cell reactivity and clinical tolerance.

Dr. Lack: You spoke very nicely about the different amounts of protein fractions in hypoallergenic formulae. But of course the main hypoallergenic formula is breast milk which the WHO recommends until 6 months and we recommend as pediatricians. We know that it can contain cow's milk proteins and other food proteins and cause symptoms. How important do you think those are, what sort of levels do you think they can be detected at and how careful should we be about controlling maternal diet in our treatment?

Dr. Beyer: I would distinguish two things, treatment and prevention. We never would recommend a partially hydrolyzed formula for a therapeutic approach in a cow's milk-allergic child but it might be a completely different story for prevention. The same with breastfeeding, we recommend breastfeeding for a time period of 4-6 months. We know that what the mother eats is normally also found in the breast milk, however, we do not recommend dietary restrictions.

Dr. Lack: I am actually talking about treatment, not prevention.

Dr. Beyer: In case an infant is fully breast-fed but diagnosed for example with clinical relevant hen's egg allergy an elimination diet for the mother would be recommended because enough protein might get to the child with the breast milk to induce symptoms.

Dr. Heine: You mentioned the double-blind, placebo-controlled food challenge as the 'gold standard' of diagnosing food allergy, but in clinical practice it is often unreliable, and you may end up with dubious results or false-positives. How do you get around this issue, how can you actually confirm 100% whether, for example, someone is intolerant to extensively hydrolyzed formula?

Dr. Beyer: I think there is no 100% certainty. At the moment the double-blind placebo-controlled food challenges are the best way to go in most cases. There might be false positive reactions, this is why we perform it placebo controlled.

Dr. Mason: Have you any experience in the use of transfer factor in cow's milk allergy or in food allergy? Is it useful in this situation as a transfer factor in aeroallergens?

Dr. Wahn: This is an old immunological story. I think it addresses my age group a little bit. It was an attempt to provide immunomodulation and it is really interesting to hear that younger scientists don't know this anymore. Twenty years ago you would not have had to explain this.

Dr. Mason: Many pediatricians use it to treat aeroallergies and I don't know if they are using it in gastrointestinal allergies.

Dr. Haschke: This might be a slightly provocative remark. We are discussing formulas which can be used in treatment but we must be clear that less than 10% of children have access to these formulas. There are countries where even if people could buy the formulas, they are not available due to regulatory issues but most people have no access whatsoever. Now fortunately most children born in so-called Third World and emerging countries are breastfed for even longer than 6 months, which minimizes the problem to a certain extent. Industry is challenged to look for cheaper sources of so-called hypoallergenic proteins. So far we only have soy formulas which to a certain extent might help, but unfortunately we have never gone into detailed research looking for other sources like rice protein, which is probably an alternative and affordable choice and could be cheaply fortified with amino acids. What might be alternative protein sources for such formulas?

Dr. Beyer: It is a very difficult question because you have to consider a lot of things in relation to nutrition. Can nutrition for the child be provided by the different protein sources? It is really hard to do because the same clinical trials are needed to determine if the protein source is hypoallergenic.

Dr. S. Koletzko: You showed us this nice experiment changing only one amino acid in your proteins. Now does this happen in nature? In other words: if we talk about milk or egg, are they from the immunological point of view always the same or do we have spontaneous mutations between proteins from different cows and hens?

Dr. Beyer: Each of the proteins I just showed you has a lot of isoforms. Some of the isoforms are more allergenic than others. Comparing these different isoforms, it is interesting enough to see whether in nature there already are differences that account for less allergenicity. But it is very complex to do research this way because you would have to sequence all the different isoforms and this is very costly and time-consuming.

Dr. S. Koletzko: What does it mean from the clinical point of view? We perform a double-blind placebo-controlled egg challenge and no reaction occurs. We send the child home and it has a severe reaction to egg because there is a different protein in the egg?

Dr. Beyer: No, this is not the way. Normally the egg, as long it is from a hen, should behave the same whether it is eaten in Germany or in the United States. The same hen's egg protein has different isoforms that are more or less allergenic. Replacement of amino acid exists, but the content of the different isoforms are usually similar.

Dr. Kamenwa: You already answered my question because I was going to ask about alternatives in poor countries like mine because these formulas are actually very expensive for most of our population. My comment is on the prevalence of food allergies in the world. There are no data for Africa mainly due to little research if any in this area of food allergy in children. The prevalence is more or less the same. We have a lot of allergies to cow's milk protein, eggs and common weaning foods such as corn and bananas.

Dr. Beyer: I would be happy to include any data from other parts of the world because I think it is very important to know the main allergens. It is very interesting that cow's milk is a major allergen throughout the world.

Dr. Shaaban: Don't you think that there is a basis for genetics in food allergies? In Africa where I come from we consume a lot of peanuts and there is no prevalence of this allergy. You showed that there is some allergy to sesame seeds, and although we consume it we don't have this allergy. Have you ever thought about camel's milk? It is very expensive but very nutritious.

Dr. Beyer: Let's start with camel's milk first because this is a very interesting topic. In southern Germany, near Stuttgart, there is a camel farm. I talked to the farmers there because they see it as a source of hypoallergenic milk.

Dr. Shaaban: The cross-reactivity is not like goat's or sheep's milk?

Dr. Beyer: No, it is said that the cross-reactivity is more like mare's milk although I do not know studies about it so I have to be a bit cautious. However, we do not normally recommend such milk for children because we don't want to make them allergic to a new source. Regarding genetics and peanuts, you knowthat the genetic background is important. However, it is not everything. There must be other, e.g. environmental factors involved.

Dr. Balanag: As Dr. Haschke said earlier there are very limited alternatives if you don't have any other source of protein. You have given children less than 6 months of age soy-based milk. What is the importance of age as a risk factor?

Dr. Beyer: These of course are recommendations for Germany. We are a fortunate country that we have these products available on the market. This might be different of course in other countries. However, we know from a nutritional aspect that soy, especially in the first 6 months, might not be as good as cow's milk based formula. But before I would give anything to a child in a country where nothing else is available, I might switch to a soy formula to see if the child will tolerate it. What do you think, Dr. Koletzko?

Dr. B. Koletzko: Allow me to refer you to the recent comment of the ESPGHAN Committee on Nutrition on the use of soy protein-based formula [2]. The Committee appreciates that soy-based formulae are far cheaper than therapeutic hydrolysate formulae, and therefore for economical reasons it may be a choice for families that cannot afford hydrolysates under circumstances where the health care system does not offer reimbursement. However, in our comment we clearly emphasize soy formulae are a secondary choice for a number of reasons, including nutritional considerations. The high phytate content found in many soy formulae has been showed to reduce the bioavailability of zinc, iron and iodine. Soy formulae tend to have 10–100 times higher aluminum intake than cow's milk formulae, raising concerns about long-term effects. Moreover, soy formulae contain very high levels of phytoestrogens, supplying amounts in the order of 6–12 mg/kg/day to a 4-month-old infant fed such formulae. This results in about 100–300 times higher phytoestrogen levels in the serum of infants fed soy formulae than in breastfed infants, and 50–150 times higher levels than found in infants fed cow's milk-based formulae. In rodents such high serum levels of phytoestrogens significantly reduce antibody responses. Moreover, a follow-up study by Strom et al. [3] reported that the use of antiasthmatic drugs was twice as high in adult women who had been fed soy formula as infants than those fed cow's milk formula. A study by Ford et al. [4] reported that feeding soy formula is associated with later autoimmune disease of the thyroid. All these data do not provide hard and conclusive evidence, but they raise sufficient concern to let it appear prudent not to use soy formula preferentially in young infants during the first months of life.

Dr. Beyer: But would you also then recommend it if nothing else is available, even in children younger than 6 months of age?

Dr. B. Koletzko: I certainly agree that soy-based infant formula is far better than feeding unmodified animal milks, and that the level of concern is highest in younger infants.

Dr. Nowak-Wegrzyn: I have a comment pertaining to Dr. Lack's question regarding breastfeeding and allergy. It is very important to emphasize that breast milk is the gold standard for infant nutrition. It has been shown to be protective in several forms of food allergy. For instance we have never seen a severe form of food allergy such as food protein-induced enterocolitis in children who are breastfed. However it is also well documented that breast milk contains foods that mothers eat. Peanut, egg and milk proteins in the breast milk are predigested and different (less allergenic) from those proteins in the foods that are fed directly to the infants. So the recommendation regarding a restricted diet for the mother has to be based on whether the child developed food allergy while being exclusively breastfed. If this is the case, the child most likely is reacting to the sequential epitopes. These children tend to have more severe and long-lasting food allergy, and therefore extreme avoidance is necessary.

References

1   Verstege A, Mehl A, Rolinck-Werninghaus C, et al: The predictive value of the skin prick test weal size for the outcome of oral food challenges. Clin Exp Allergy 2005;35:1220–1226.
2   ESPGHAN Committee on Nutrition: Soy protein infant formulae and follow-on formulae. J Pediatr Gastroenterol Nutr 2006;42:352–361.

3   Strom BL, Schinnar R, Ziegler EE, et al: Exposure to soy-based formula in infancy and endocrinological and reproductive outcomes in young adulthood. JAMA 2001;286:807–814.
4   Ford P, Moses N, Fasano M, et al: Breast and soy-formula feedings in early infancy and the prevalence of autoimmune thyroid disease in children. J Am Coll Nutr 1990;9:164–167.

Cooke RJ, Vandenplas Y, Wahn U (eds): Nutrition Support for Infants and Children at Risk.
Nestlé Nutr Workshop Ser Pediatr Program, vol 59, pp 49–62,
Nestec Ltd., Vevey/S. Karger AG, Basel, © 2007.

The Concept of Hypoallergenicity for Atopy Prevention

Andrea von Berg

Research Institute at the Children's Department, Marien-Hospital Wesel,
Wesel, Germany

Abstract

Infancy represents the period in which an individual may be at the highest risk of sensitization. During the first year of life around 2.5% of neonates experience hypersensitivity reactions to cow's milk protein, which is highly associated with early exposure to cow's milk. Attempts to avoid sensitization in this very early period of life and to prevent allergic diseases focus on diets with reduced allergenicity and possibly on the induction of oral tolerance. Hydrolyzed infant formulas are characterized by a reduced allergenicity and thus recommended as substitute or supplementary to breastfeeding during the first 4–6 months of life for infants at high risk of developing atopic diseases. This concept of hypoallergenicity has been shown effective in clinical studies. Both partially and extensively hydrolyzed formulas have demonstrated a potential in protecting from allergic diseases, mainly atopic eczema and food allergy. The in vitro characterization of allergenicity by the degree of hydrolyzation and peptide size, however, does not necessarily predict the immunogenic effect in humans, as it could be shown that the preventive effect seems to be dependent on the process rather than on the degree of hydrolyzation, which could be best explained by a possible production of tolerogenic epitopes.

Introduction

The worldwide increase in the prevalence of allergy and atopic disorders especially in the pediatric population over the past several decades has become a cardinal target for the research of pediatric allergologists [1]. Results of large epidemiological studies have helped to better understand the natural course of allergic diseases and to identify at least some risk factors which play a role in the complex interaction between genetics and the environment [2].

Amongst others exposure to food allergens in early infancy often represents the most important risk factor in children with a genetically determined disposition for atopy.

Food proteins are per se immunogens, characterized by the capacity to either initiate the production of specific IgE antibodies and/or T cell immune responses, or to induce oral tolerance. Whether an immunogen is going to be allergenic or tolerogenic is influenced by the genetic disposition of an individual, by the dose and the time point of the first introduction of the immunogen and by environmental factors like passive smoke exposure, infections, the microbial gut composition and others, which can be either promoting or protecting against the development of allergy.

Infancy represents the period in which an individual may be at the highest risk of sensitization. In line with this is the development of food allergy and especially cow's milk allergy, which is highly associated with early exposure to cow's milk and quite common in early childhood; around 2.5% of neonates experience hypersensitivity reactions to cow's milk protein during the first year of life [3]. Thus, the counterregulatory processes of primary allergy prevention measures should exert their effects very early in life or even prenatally.

Consequently, the main approach in attempts to prevent allergic diseases focuses on elimination diets and on diets with reduced allergenicity in order to avoid sensitization in this very early period of life.

National and international guidelines for infant nutrition, therefore, concentrate on prolonged breastfeeding for 4–6 months and late introduction of solid foods for all children to prevent the development of allergic diseases. For high-risk children recommendations additionally include protein hydrolysates in case of insufficient breastfeeding during the first 4–6 months of life [4–8].

Breastfeeding always was and still is the gold standard for optimal infant nutrition and may – in addition – protect children from the development of atopic diseases, especially children at high risk of allergies as shown in a recent meta-analysis [8, 9]. However, it seems that the specific phenotype in the child's family history further modifies the effect of breastfeeding in those children at high risk. Results from the German Infant Nutritional Intervention study (GINI) clearly demonstrated that in children with a positive family history of atopic dermatitis the prevalence of atopic dermatitis in the exclusively breastfed offspring was significantly higher than in children with other atopic phenotypes such as asthma or allergic rhinitis in their immediate relatives [10].

Attempts to reduce the allergenicity of breast milk also included an allergen-reduced diet for the pregnant and the lactating mothers. The rational behind this is that specific IgE to food allergens [11] and T cell responses to milk and egg proteins as well as to inhaled allergens were detected in fetuses and in newborns [12]. The rational for an allergen avoidance diet for the lactating mother is based on several observations. Food allergens were detected in breast milk, and early sensitization to hen's egg and cow's milk protein as well as to other food allergens was observed in up to 6% of exclusively breastfed children [13]. In addition, in children with cow's milk allergy, the provocation with breast milk was positive in 16 out of 17 patients [14].

The reduction of milk, milk products and hen's egg in the maternal diet during the third trimester of pregnancy did not show any beneficial effect on early sensitization and prevention of early allergic manifestation [15]. This has recently been confirmed in a study, where rigorous dietary egg exclusion, starting already before 20 weeks of gestation (17–20 weeks), did neither eliminate the transplacental passage of egg allergen nor its passing into breast milk. It could be shown in this study that ovalbumin in blood and breast milk was not related to the maternal dietary intake or atopic predisposition [16].

The results of the studies with an allergen-reduced maternal diet during lactation are contradictory. The study by Hattevig et al. [17], where mothers avoided egg, cow's milk and fish during the first 3 months of lactation, showed a 50% reduction of eczema in the offspring at 3, 6 and 48 months of life, but not at 12 and 120 months of age. Sensitization to cow's milk and hen's egg was lower at 3 months only. This is in contrast to the study by Herrmann et al. [18], where mothers avoided eggs and cow's milk until their infants were 6 months of age, which did not result in any difference between the intervention and the control group regarding the cumulative incidence of eczema and sensitization to cow's milk and hen's egg.

According to the guidelines hypoallergenic formulas based on cow's milk protein are recommended for primary prevention in children at high risk of allergy who need a milk supplement to breastfeeding in the first 4–6 months of life [4–6, 8].

Hydrolyzed Infant Formulas

Hydrolyzed infant formulas as a milk substitute, primarily invented for infants with cow's milk allergy, have later been adapted for primary allergy prevention. The concept of introducing hydrolysates in an attempt to prevent allergic diseases focuses on the reduction of the antigenicity and allergenicity of milk proteins [19]. The residual allergenicity of an infant formula, defined as the capacity of the molecules (allergens) to initiate an allergic response, is affected by molecular weight, chemical complexity, 'foreignness', dose and other factors such as route of exposure and yet unknown species-specific genetic factors [20]. Different processing of foods can alter its antigenicity. Heat treatment of cow's milk protein does affect the conformational epitopes and facilitates their hydrolysis. To produce the least allergenic formulas, cow's milk protein can be modified by enzymatic hydrolysis with progressive destruction of sequential epitopes [21]. Dependent on the degree of enzymatic hydrolysis, ultraheating and ultrafiltration protein hydrolysates are differentiated in partially hydrolyzed (pHFs) or extensively hydrolyzed formulas (eHFs), and dependent on the protein source in whey and casein hydrolysates [partially hydrolyzed whey formula (pHF-W), extensively hydrolyzed whey formula (eHF-W), and extensively hydrolyzed casein formula (eHF-C)].

One way to classify the allergenicity of infant formulas is the molecular-weight profile. The molecular-weight profile of pHF ranges between 3,000 and 10,000 Da; peptides in the eHF have in >90% a molecular weight <3,000 Da. It could be shown that formulas containing considerable proportions of peptides >6,000 Da showed significantly more positive skin prick test results when compared to eHFs or an amino acid formula [22].

Allergenicity of a formula is also assessable by several in vitro and in vivo tests. Most suitable methods for determining the residual allergenicity of hydrolyzed infant formulas include tests for RAST or EAST inhibition and skin prick tests, while the protein content of the formula and the molecular weight alone have been shown not to be predictive for the clinical outcome [23].

According to data from the literature a declining ranking of infant formulas with regard to their allergenicity was found to be cow's milk formula, pHF-W, partially hydrolyzed casein formula, eHF-C and amino acid-based formula [23].

Hydrolyzed Infant Formulas for Therapy and Prevention

Hydrolyzed infant formulas, mainly based on cow's milk, have been intensively tested in numerous allergy prevention studies and in animal models. Both infant pHFs and eHFs could be demonstrated to be hypoallergenic, which means nothing but less allergenic.

However, by the definition of the American Academy of Pediatrics a hypoallergenic formula needs to fulfill three criteria: (1) the antigenicity of the protein must be reduced, (2) it should be successfully used in patients with documented cow's milk allergy and (3) the immunogenicity of the product must be reduced [5]. Following this definition, eHFs have a higher potential of being classified as hypoallergen than pHFs, because they can be successfully used in children with cow's milk allergy.

A further differentiation of hypoallergenic formulas in 'formula for therapy' and 'formula for prevention' was necessary, when a pHF, which was marketed as hypoallergenic, had caused anaphylactic reactions.

A formula suitable for being classified as a 'formula for therapy' of cow's milk allergy/intolerance has to fulfill several clinical and preclinical criteria. This includes a double-blind, placebo-controlled food challenge, followed by 7 days' feeding with the respective formula to prove that 90% (with 95% confidence) of children with documented cow's milk allergy/intolerance can tolerate the formula without developing allergic symptoms [5].

The definition of a hypoallergenic 'formula for prevention' of allergic diseases includes that the formula should be tested in a high-risk population defined by a positive family history, that children should be exclusively fed with the formula from birth to at least 6 months of age in a controlled randomized fashion and followed until 18 months of life with validated clinical scoring systems, where any allergic symptoms should be verified by double-blind placebo-controlled food challenge, and finally that a significantly lower prevalence of allergy should be documented in these children [5].

While several eHFs and amino-acid-based formulas fulfill the criteria of a 'formula for therapy', neither the eHFs nor the pHFs fulfill all criteria to be classified as 'preventive', because no clinical study exist which verifies all criteria according to the definition.

eHFs, primarily intended for the therapy of cow's milk allergy/intolerance some 60 years ago, have later been adapted for allergy prevention as well, while pHFs have always been reserved for the use in primary prevention due to their comparatively higher residual antigenicity.

Dietary primary allergy prevention aims at avoiding early sensitization to foods, mainly to milk proteins by induction of oral tolerance [24]. There is some scientific controversy as to whether a partial hydrolysate with its moderately reduced antigenicity or a hydrolysate with extensively reduced antigenicity is more beneficial for prevention. However, the optimal extent of hydrolysis and the amount of residual allergenicity needed to induce oral tolerance are not known.

In a mouse model it could be shown that prefeeding with a pHF-W had a suppressive effect on the IgE anti-β-lactoglobulin production at repeated feeding with cow's milk, while prefeeding with an eHF-W resulted in a similar antibody production to prefeeding with H_2O, which is interpreted by the authors as specific induction of oral tolerance due to the presence of tolerogenic peptides in the pHF-W [25, 26].

These and similar data are the reason for an ongoing discussion of whether the use of pHF should be recommended for allergy prevention in order to not only mimic as far as possible the amount of allergenic proteins like in breast milk, but also to induce oral tolerance, or whether the use of eHF is favorable to avoid an immunologic response. From the results of the GINI study, however, it must be suggested that factors – like the producing process itself – other than the degree of hydrolyzation alone are also associated with the expression of allergic reactions. Here the pHF-W and the eHF-C significantly reduced the incidence of atopic dermatitis, while the eHF-W had no preventive effect [10].

Some recent data from large intervention studies indicate less sensitization to cow's milk in children fed a partial hydrolyzed formula compared with children fed an eHF, which may be an indication for induction of specific oral tolerance [27]. Hence the guidelines on nutrition of infants at risk for allergy recommend both, eHF and pHF as a supplement for or a substitute to breast-feeding in the first 4–6 months.

Infant eHF and pHF in Clinical Studies

eHF fulfill the criteria to be classified as a formula for therapy, but they are also recommended by the American and the European Pediatric Societies for allergy prevention [4, 5].

The most intensively tested eHF is based on 100% casein (eHF-C). Its allergy-preventive effect has been investigated in several birth cohorts of high-risk infants and compared with breast milk, cow's milk formula and pHF [10, 27–34], and in two of these studies also with eHF-W [10, 27].

Most of the pHF's available today are based on 100% whey (pHF-W). The pHF's fulfill 2 of 3 criteria for the definition to be 'hypoallergenic' as recommended by the American Academy of Pediatrics [5]: they have a reduced antigenicity of the protein and induce limited immunological reactions. However, they are not suitable for the therapy of cow's milk allergy/intolerance. Nevertheless, in several clinical studies pHF has demonstrated a potential for prevention of allergic disease, and here mainly with regard to atopic dermatitis and food allergy [8, 28, 34–36].

Taking together the results of the intervention studies with hydrolysates, a preventive effect with regard to the prevalence and the cumulative incidence of allergic manifestations, mainly atopic dermatitis and food allergy could be demonstrated for both eHF and pHF [28].

In general it is not possible to compare these dietary intervention studies because of methodological differences in their design and their performance [28, 34, 36]. All of these studies were performed in children at risk of atopy; however, not always with the same level of risk (uniparental, biparental). All of the studies mentioned in the reviews tried to randomize the children to the study formula that would be fed as a supplement if breastfeeding was insufficient. However, some children were randomized before birth [29], some at birth [10], at weaning [30] or by the day of randomization (even, uneven) [27]. Not all of the studies were blinded, and only two of them were double-blinded [10, 30]. In case the formula is tested versus breast milk, blinding and randomization are not possible for ethical reasons. Additional differences between the studies are the result of the time of weaning and duration of feeding study formula, as well as of co-interventions such as recommendations for the diet of the lactating mother, solid food introduction, or avoidance of inhalant allergens. And not least important are the differences in the outcome definitions and the criteria for diagnosis in the various studies.

A direct comparison between eHF and pHF was performed only in two studies, showing that, with regard to the reduction of atopic dermatitis and food allergy, mainly cow's milk allergy, eHF was borderline significantly superior over pHF [27, 30, 34]. However, from results of the GINI study, where the allergy-preventive effect of three different hydrolysates (pHF-W, eHF-W and eHF-C) was compared with a regular cow's milk formula in children at high risk of atopic diseases, it became obvious that the effect of a formula was modified by the specific allergic phenotype in the child's immediate family. While the incidence of atopic dermatitis in children without atopic dermatitis in a first-degree family member was reduced with all 3 hydrolysates – and even significantly so with pHF-W, a significant reduction of atopic dermatitis in children with atopic dermatitis in the family could only be shown with eHF-C. This finding may have implications for the cost/benefit ratio, as pHF-W is much cheaper than eHF-C. The use of eHF-C should be reserved for infants at the highest risk of developing atopic dermatitis.

In conclusion, the concept of hypoallergenic infant formulas for atopy prevention in children at high risk of developing atopic diseases has been demonstrated efficacious in reducing the incidence of allergic manifestations, mainly atopic dermatitis and food allergy, in infancy and early childhood. So far there has been no evidence for a preventing effect of hypoallergenic infant formulas on respiratory allergic diseases.

References

1 Von Mutius E, Weiland SK, Fritzsch C, et al: Increasing prevalence of hay fever and atopy among children in Leipzig, East Germany. Lancet 1998;351:862–866.
2 Von Mutius E: The environmental predictors of allergic disease. J Allergy Clin Immunol 2000;105: 9–19.
3 Schrander JJ, van den Bogart JP, Forget PP, et al: Cow's milk protein intolerance in infants under 1 year of age: a prospective epidemiological study. Eur J Pediatr 1993;152:640–644.
4 Høst A, Koletzko B, Dreborg S, et al: Dietary products used in infants for treatment and prevention of food allergy. Joint statement of the European Society for Paediatric Allergology and Clinical Immunology (ESPACI) Committee on Hypoallergenic Formulas and the European Society for Paediatric Gastroenterology, Hepatology and Nutrition (ESPGHAN) Committee on Nutrition. Arch Dis Child 1999;81:80–84.
5 American Academy of Pediatrics. Committee on Nutrition. Hypoallergenic infant formulas. Pediatrics 2000;106:346–349.
6 Bauer CP, von Berg A, Niggemann B, Rebien W: Primäre alimentäre Atopieprävention. Allergologie 2004;13:120–125.
7 Fifty-Fourth World Health Assembly. WHA54.2. Agenda item 13.1. Infant and young child nutrition. Geneva, World Health Organization, 2004.
8 Muraro A, Dreborg S, Halken S, et al: Dietary prevention of allergic diseases in infants and small children. III. Critical review of published peer-reviewed observational and interventional studies and final recommendations. Pediatr Allergy Immunol 2004;15:291–307.
9 Gdalevich M, Mimouni D, Mimouni M: Breast-feeding and the risk of bronchial asthma in childhood: a systematic review with meta-analysis of prospective studies. J Pediatr 2001;139: 261–266.
10 Von Berg A, Koletzko S, Grübl A, et al: The effect of hydrolyzed cow's milk formula for allergy prevention in the first year of life: the German Infant Nutritional Intervention Study, a randomized double-blind trial. J Allergy Clin Immunol 2003;111:533–540.
11 Michel FB, Bousquet J, Greillier P, et al: Comparison of cord blood immunoglobulin E concentrations and maternal allergy for the prediction of atopic diseases in infancy. J Allergy Clin Immunol 1980;65:422–430.

12 Warner JA, Miles EA, Jones AC, et al: Is deficiency of interferon gamma production by allergen triggered cord blood cells a predictor of atopic eczema? Clin Exp Allergy 1994;24:399–400.
13 van Asperen PP, Kemp AS, Mellis CM: Immediate food hypersensitivity reactions on the first known exposure to the food. Arch Dis Child 1983;58:253–256.
14 Saarinen KM, Juntunen-Backman K, Jarvenpaa AL, et al: Breast-feeding and the development of cows' milk protein allergy. Adv Exp Med Biol 2000;478:121–130.
15 Fälth-Magnusson K, Kjellman NI: Allergy prevention by maternal elimination diet during late pregnancy – a 5-year follow-up of a randomized study. J Allergy Clin Immunol 1992;89: 709–713.
16 Vance GH, Lewis SA, Grimshaw KE, et al: Exposure of the fetus and infant to hens' egg ovalbumin via the placenta and breast milk in relation to maternal intake of dietary egg. Clin Exp Allergy 2005;35:1318–1326.
17 Hattevig G, Sigurs N, Kjellman B: Effects of maternal dietary avoidance during lactation on allergy in children at 10 years of age. Acta Paediatr 1999;88:7–12.
18 Herrmann ME, Dannemann A, Gruters A, et al: Prospective study of the atopy preventive effect of maternal avoidance of milk and eggs during pregnancy and lactation. Eur J Pediatr 1996;155:770–774.
19 Fritsche R: Animal models in food allergy: assessment of allergenicity and preventive activity of infant formulas. Toxicol Lett 2003;140–141:303–309.
20 Cordle CT: Control of food allergies using protein hydrolysates. Food Technol 1994;48:72–76.
21 Jost R, Fritsche R, Pahud JJ: Reduction of milk protein allergenicity through processing. Bibl Nutr Dieta 1991;48:127–137.
22 Bindels JG, Boerma JA: Hydrolysed cow's milk formulae. Pediatr Allergy Immunol 1994;5: 189–190.
23 Niggemann B, Binder C, Klettke U, Wahn U: In vivo and in vitro studies on the residual allergenicity of partially hydrolysed infant formulae. Acta Paediatr 1999;88:394–398.
24 Fritsche R: The role of immune tolerance in allergy prevention. Nestle Nutr Workshop Ser Pediatr Program 2005;56:1–14.
25 Fritsche R, Pahud JJ, Pecquet S, Pfeifer A: Induction of systemic immunologic tolerance to beta-lactoglobulin by oral administration of a whey protein hydrolysate. J Allergy Clin Immunol 1997;100:266–273.
26 Fritsche R: Animal models in food allergy: assessment of allergenicity and preventive activity of infant formulas. Toxicol Lett 2003;140–141:303–309.
27 Halken S, Hansen KS, Jacobsen HP, et al: Comparison of a partially hydrolyzed infant formula with two extensively hydrolyzed formulas for allergy prevention: a prospective, randomized study. Pediatr Allergy Immunol 2000;11:149–161.
28 Hays T, Wood RA: A systemic review of the role of hydrolyzed infant formulas in allergy prevention. Arch Pediatr Adolesc Med 2005;159:810–816.
29 Zeiger RS, Heller S: The development and prediction of atopy in high-risk children. J Allergy Clin Immunol 1995;95:1179–1190.
30 Oldaeus G, Anjou K, Bjorksten B, et al: Extensively and partially hydrolysed infant formulas for allergy prophylaxis. Arch Dis Child 1997;77:4–10.
31 Mallet E, Henocq A: Long-term prevention of allergic diseases by using protein hydrolysate formula in at-risk infants. J Pediatr 1992;121:S95–S100.
32 Halken S, Høst A, Hansen LG, Osterballe O: Preventive effect of feeding high-risk infants a casein hydrolysate formula or an ultrafiltrated whey hydrolysate formula: a prospective, randomized, comparative clinical study. Pediatr Allergy Immunol 1993;4:173–181.
33 Porch MC, Shahane AD, Leiva LE, et al: Influence of breast milk, soy, or two hydrolyzed formulas on the development of allergic manifestations in infants at risk. Nutr Res 1998;18: 1413–1424.
34 Osborne DA, Sinn J: Formulas containing hydrolyzed protein for prevention of allergy and food intolerance in infants. Cochrane Database Syst Rev 2003;4:CD003664.
35 Baumgartner M, Brown CA, Exl BM, et al: Controlled trials investigating the use of one partially hydrolyzed whey formula for dietary prevention of atopic manifestations until 60 months of age. Nutr Res 1998;18:1425–1442.
36 Schoetzau A, Gehring U, Wichmann HE: Prospective cohort studies using hydrolysed formulas for allergy prevention in atopy prone newborns: a systematic review. Eur J Pediatr 2001;160:323–332.

Discussion

Dr. Saavedra: When we look at strategies for prevention we probably should start thinking about breastfeeding. We continue to discuss breastfeeding as a way to prevent allergy, and in relative risk tables we use breastfeeding as the nonexclusive standard and then we look at the effect of breastfeeding in reducing allergy. Nobody would agree that the standard should be nonexclusive breastfeeding. The right question here is how does nonexclusive breastfeeding increase the risk of atopy. I think that this changes our mind set regarding where we need to go if we admit that there are risks associated with nonexclusive breastfeeding. It is not that breastfeeding reduces the risk of allergy, it is that nonexclusive breastfeeding increases it. For example these hydrolysates don't reduce or prevent allergy, they just cause less than what would be caused if we did not use these hydrolysates.

Dr. von Berg: You are absolutely right, it should be the other way round. We should have breastfeeding as gold standard and compare other foods in case breastfeeding is not sufficiently available. The aim of this study was not to compare hydrolysates versus breastfeeding, instead we wanted to find out in the case of insufficient breastfeeding, which kind of hydrolyzed formula is best for allergy prevention. This is one reason why the results in the breastfed group were not included in the analysis [1].

Dr. Wahn: I still like this GINI study, I think it is a wonderful study telling us a lot, and I recall the good old days of the study by Zeiger et al. [2]. It appears to me that the key messages are very similar. You followed 3 phenotypes, one was atopic dermatitis, one was asthma and one was specific sensitization. Please correct me if I am wrong, you saw a transient effect on the incidence of atopic dermatitis, the incidence afterwards was the same as the cumulated prevalence of atopy?

Dr. von Berg: Yes, the incidence was reduced in the first year with pHF-W and eHF-C, and in the second and third year the incidence was not different between the 4 study groups. This confirms the findings by Vandenplas et al. [3] and Zeiger et al. [2], who in their studies also saw the preventive effect developing early, in the first 6 and 12 months of life, respectively.

Dr. Wahn: You were unable to describe any effect on airway diseases, and this is also the case in Dr. Zeiger's study. You saw effects with regard to specific IgE responses as you found a reduced IgE response to cow's milk and also to hen's egg in one case.

Dr. von Berg: Yes, with pHF-W, we found a significant reduction of sensitization to cow's milk at 3 years.

Dr. Wahn: You saw no effect on inhalant allergens?

Dr. von Berg: We didn't see an effect on inhalant allergens, that is correct.

Dr. Wahn: If you saw something, an effect on hen's egg which was not related to the hydrolysates you gave, could you speculate on the effect? Is it really a nonspecific effect which has to do with some immunomodulation or regulatory processes or what is your interpretation with regard to the hen's egg and IgE response?

Dr. von Berg: At the age of 1 year about 30% of the cases of atopic eczema were associated with IgE, and most of them with specific sensitization to hen's egg. Interestingly, this hen's egg-associated atopic eczema was significantly reduced in the group of children fed eHF-C. If this finding is more than a statistical effect, then it has to be interpreted as a nonspecific effect likely to have something to do with immunoregulatory processes.

Dr. Fuchs: I find this fascinating. I am not an allergist or a dermatologist but in looking at the effect, as I understand it, the presence or absence of atopic dermatitis was the only clinical outcome variable. However, is all atopic dermatitis the same or does it vary in severity and, if you look at severity, are there more striking differences or do the differences become less significant?

Dr. von Berg: Atopic dermatitis is definitely not the same, one difference being whether it is associated with specific IgE responses or not. Regarding severity, we could not see marked differences between the study groups at 1 year; we have not yet looked at it after 3 years.

Dr. Wahn: In the EPAAC trial 2,500 children with atopic dermatitis were screened for specific IgE levels between their first and second birthday. It is quite clear that specific IgE responses are most likely related to severity.

Dr. von Berg: We have not yet related severity to IgE levels. We have just related severity to the 4 formulas.

Dr. Fuchs: I guess my patients would be more concerned not about the IgE levels but the degree of the atopic dermatitis.

Dr. Davidson: This is probably a naïve question from a pediatric gastroenterologist. The difference between hydrolyzed casein and hydrolyzed whey interests me because breast milk really is a combination of whey and casein and you would expect that that would be the ideal mix. So is there a good explanation as to why a whey hydrolysate or a casein hydrolysate may actually have some benefit?

Dr. von Berg: I give this question over to people who actually produce the formulas.

Dr. Saavedra: This an excellent question because it is probably one of the best demonstrations we have that not all hydrolysates are created equally or behave similarly. It is just a clear demonstration that the percentages of casein and whey from cow's milk are of course totally different from the percentages of casein and whey in breast milk. I use the analogy that casein in cow's milk is an excellent protein for making cheese, human casein isn't. So these proteins are not comparable chemically or physicochemically. Different amounts of certain types of casein are present in both cow's milk and human milk. The second major factor of course is hydrolysis. Not every method of hydrolysis is the same and currently each manufacturer has its own method, some use trypsin, some use a combination of enzymes, some use pancreatin, some use actual pancreatic glands, and some use no pancreatic enzymes at all. So of course these peptides are not going to look the same and I think this study does show that the 'degree of hydrolysis' may be less important than the 'method of hydrolysis' when it comes to allergy prevention.

Dr. von Berg: This is underlined by the fact that our extensively hydrolyzed whey showed no effect, while another extensively hydrolyzed whey formula in the study by Halken et al. [4] had an effect similar to that of extensively hydrolyzed casein.

Dr. Lack: I was interested to see your data on specific IgE to milk, which I don't think I've seen before. You showed the reduction in cow's milk which you say is the only significant reduction, is that right?

Dr. von Berg: Yes, at 3 years of age. We don't have the results at 6 years yet.

Dr. Lack: But what I don't understand is this 20- or 30-year-old belief that changing cow's milk composition is going to change asthma, eczema, other food allergies and inhalant allergens. I can understand how it would affect specific IgE to cow's milk, but by just taking out the protein how do you think it could affect egg or how could it affect inhalants if milk allergy was the main cause of asthma in older children?

Dr. von Berg: It neither affected the inhalant allergies nor did we expect this. However what one could perhaps expect is that if you prevent sensitization to food allergens then maybe you can avoid the allergic march from atopic dermatitis to inhalant allergies. We have now finished the 6-year follow-up in these children, where we performed lung function and looked at bronchial responsiveness in a subgroup. The results will show whether avoidance of sensitization to foods and/or atopic eczema will cause less asthma or airway inflammation.

Dr. Szajewska: I read your results which were published at 1 year of age [1]. I understand the results for atopic dermatitis at 3 years of age are very similar. If so the number needed to treat was 13, with quite a wide confidence interval (8–51) which means that one would need to treat 13 infants with extensively hydrolyzed casein formula to prevent one additional infant suffering from any allergic manifestation. I come from Poland, a country less rich than Germany, so my practical question is: do you really think with such a number needed to treat and such a wide confidence interval that this intervention is really the best way to prevent allergic diseases?

Dr. von Berg: At 3 years we calculated the cost-benefit relation on the basis of the number needed to treat. If you take all children with a family history for atopy together, there is no difference between the extensively hydrolyzed casein and the partially hydrolyzed whey, 12 versus 13 children, respectively. However if we look into the subgroup of children with the specific phenotype atopic eczema in the family then there was a big difference: 8 children had to be fed eHF-C compared to 47 fed pHF-W. Therefore, to prevent atopic eczema in children at risk in general I would recommend the partially hydrolyzed whey, which has a better taste and costs less. But for the subgroup of children with a very high risk of atopic eczema, that is atopic eczema in an immediate relative, eHF-C would most likely be more beneficial in preventing atopic eczema.

Dr. Szajewska: But my question was not whether to choose extensively hydrolyzed versus partially hydrolyzed formula but whether with this quite large number needed to treat and especially with a wide confidence interval, is it really worth doing this kind of intervention? It might be very expensive.

Dr. von Berg: If you look at prices the difference between the partially hydrolyzed whey and normal cow's milk formula is really not much. The difference comes up if you take the extensively hydrolyzed casein. Therefore I would suggest to carefully select whom you recommend the extensively hydrolyzed casein.

Dr. Wahn: Did you have a chance to look not only at the quality of the IgE response but also at the quantity? You obviously had a certain cutoff point above which you found an IgE response to egg or whatever. We know that there are decision points and if you have very high IgE responses then you might end up having just clinically relevant food allergy. Have you analyzed this?

Dr. von Berg: No, we have not yet related the level of IgE to disease.

Ms. Skypala: It interested me that you avoided the key food allergens also after a year. I wonder if you could speculate on how important this was in the results you had. What is your general view regarding the disparity between the American guidelines on the avoidance of key food allergens and the European guidelines that don't give such a recommendation?

Dr. von Berg: We recommended avoiding solid foods up to the 4th month and thereafter to introduce only one new solid food per week [1]. We have some data on solid food introduction for breastfed children and for children supplemented with regular cow's milk. It shows first that breastfeeding mothers hardly ever introduce solids in the first 4 months, while 30% of mothers in the cow's milk group did. The percentage of atopic eczema in both groups in our study is higher when solids are introduced later and lower when more diverse food groups are given [5]. This is totally different from the results in the older study by Fergusson et al. [8, 9]. Our interpretation of this finding is reverse causality [5, 7]. Because the decision of diversity and when to introduce solids first is driven not only by the family history of atopy, mainly atopic eczema or food allergy, but also by the presence of early skin symptoms of the baby. This has been nicely shown by Zutavern et al. [6] who analyzed data from our observational LISA study. There she showed that in those children who had no early skin symptoms egg and milk were equally often introduced before or after the 6th month, but if a child had early skin symptoms, then egg and milk were significantly more often introduced after the 6th month. So there is an association between early skin symptoms and the time of introduction of solid foods.

Dr. Wahn: Can I just add two sentences before everybody gets confused about this. You remember that Bergmann et al. [10] wrote a paper on the risk factors of prolonged breastfeeding. They showed that it is clearly reversed causation. Everyone knows that eczema becomes manifest between 2 and 6 months, and this is when mothers decide to prolong breastfeeding.

Dr. B. Koletzko: That is exactly why the paper of Zutavern et al. [6] is so important. Their data give strong dogmatic support to the recommendation that complementary feeding should not start before the first day of the 7th month with the aim of preventing allergy. I don't think we have any solid basis for that recommendation.

Dr. Micskey: How long do you recommend the use of different hydrolysates?

Dr. von Berg: Until 6 months. There is no evidence in any study that there is an effect of hydrolyzed formulas on allergy prevention beyond 6 months of life.

Dr. Beyer: I like the GINI study a lot but I was always puzzled that the extensively hydrolyzed whey formula did not give the result. It is not only the rate of hydrolysates or the proteins, it might also be the way the formulas are hydrolyzed. But let's turn it around. If you now recommend a partially hydrolyzed formula for prevention of atopic diseases and use a brand produced differently, you might see completely opposite results. So should we not require a standardization in producing formulas used for treatment or prevention in order to be able to compare the results between different companies?

Dr. Haschke: In part the methods are protected by patents so it would be very difficult to proceed according to one standard.

Dr. Beyer: Patents are a real problem in the whole research field. Many things we come across in patient care are due to this patent problem.

Dr. von Berg: What we recommend for allergy prevention is to use only those formulas that have shown a preventive effect in controlled studies, and there are very few [1]. It was very surprising that the extensively hydrolyzed whey did not have an effect. We actually gave the formulas to Hugh Sampson to find the reason for this, and even he has no explanation.

Dr. Saavedra: The important question from a practical point of view is how do we apply what we know. A very appropriate question is how many children need to receive an effective hydrolysate to see the effect in a population? If we use family history as a risk factor today, given the incidence of allergy, about 30% of the general newborn population would fall under the category of risk by family history. This means that 30% of the population would theoretically benefit from risk reduction. Obviously it is very hard to argue that family history should be the one criteria for obvious reasons. One reason is the large number of children needed to screen for only 30%. The second is that we cannot get the kind of history this research needs in real life, and in the US 30% of the time the father is neither available nor would he remember.

Dr. von Berg: Your question is why should only children at risk get a hydrolyzed formula or should not all children get it. Of course this is a question all of us have. There is only one study by Exl et al. [11] looking at health and skin problems in the general population, not specifically at allergy, in two areas of Switzerland. In one area where a partially hydrolyzed whey formula was recommended, the children had less health problems than in the other area where no feeding recommendations were given at all.

Dr. Wahn: The family history, usually you have the mother available, she knows certain things about the father whether he ever wheezed and so on. So this is quite reliable information and the family history isn't too complicated.

Dr. B. Koletzko: You have omitted the data by Chandra. At this time this is probably quite appropriate with all the questions we have as to the reliability of his data. I wonder whether the president of ESPGAN has any comment to offer as to whether this has already been looked into. Particularly as it is my understanding that the Cochrane review on this issue was very much based on Chandra's data which you now seriously question.

Dr. von Berg: This is the reason why I did not show them.

Dr. B. Koletzko: What would the Cochrane meta-analysis conclude if we were to take out Chandra's data?

Dr. von Berg: As far as I know the results are still showing a preventive effect of the partially hydrolyzed whey and of the extensively hydrolyzed casein formula.

Dr. Lentze: I have been asked whether ESPGAN has decided to withdraw the papers by Chandra from the *Journal of Pediatric Gastroenterology and Nutrition.* The journal has two societies, a European one and an American one. From the European side we recommended withdrawing the papers immediately and writing an article as to what was going on. The American side wanted to wait until there was an answer from Chandra but in my opinion we will never get an answer and I reckon that these papers will be withdrawn from the journal soon.

Dr. Haschke: I refer to a meta-analysis we have published, which included a total of 13 clinical trials with one partially hydrolyzed formula. As you indicated, after removing the Chandra data, the results remain the same.

Dr. von Berg: But I think until the situation is solved one should not take them into consideration in the meta-analysis.

Dr. Bayhon: I would like to know if there are any studies correlating the cord blood IgE level with the development of atopic dermatitis? Could these children with high cord blood IgE levels benefit from this milk formula?

Dr. von Berg: Dr. Wahn, I think you have looked at the level of total IgE.

Dr. Wahn: Yes we did. It must be certain that the cord blood IgE is not contaminated by maternal blood because then it can be an insufficient predictor of subsequent atopic manifestation. There was a time when we were hoping that we could screen cord blood IgE and use it for prediction and also for preventive measures, but it does not seem to be the case.

References

1 von Berg A, Koletzko S, Grübl A, et al: The effect of hydrolyzed cow's milk formula for allergy prevention in the first year of life: the German Infant Nutritional Intervention Study, a randomized double-blind trial. J Allergy Clin Immunol 2003;111:533–540.
2 Zeiger R, Heller S, Mellon M, et al: Genetic and environmental factors affecting the development of atopy through age 4 in children of atopic parents: a prospective randomized study of food allergen avoidance. Pediatr Allergy Immunol 1992;3:110–127.
3 Vandenplas Y, Hauser B, Van den Borre C, et al: The long-term effect of a partial whey hydrolysate formula on the prophylaxis of atopic disease. Eur J Pediatr 1995;154:488–494.
4 Halken S, Hansen KS, Jacobsen HP, et al: Comparison of a partially hydrolyzed infant formula with two extensively hydrolyzed formulas for allergy prevention: a prospective, randomized study. Pediatr Allergy Immunol 2000;11:149–161.
5 Schoetzau A, Filipiak-Pittroff B, Franke K, et al: Effect of exclusive breast-feeding and early solid food avoidance on the incidence of atopic dermatitis in high-risk infants at 1 year of age. Pediatr Allergy Immunol 2002;13:234–242.
6 Zutavern A, Brockow I, Schaaf B, et al; LISA Group: The timing of solid food introduction in relation to atopic dermatitis and sensitisation considering reverse causality: results from a prospective birth cohort study. Pediatrics 2006;117:401–411.

7 Zutavern A, von Mutius E, Harris J, et al: The introduction of solids in relation to asthma and eczema. Arch Dis Child 2004;89:303–308.
8 Fergusson DM, Horwood LJ, Beautrais AL, et al: Eczema and infant diet. Clin Allergy 1981;11:325–331.
9 Fergusson DM, Horwood LJ, Shannon FT: Risk factors in childhood eczema. J Epidemiol Community Health 1982;36:118–122.
10 Bergmann RL, Diepgen TL, Kuss O, et al: Breastfeeding duration is a risk factor for atopic eczema. Clin Exp Allergy 2002;32:205–209.
11 Exl BM, Deland U, Secretin MC, et al: Improved general health status in an unselected infant population following an allergen-reduced dietary intervention programme: ZUFF-STUDY-PROGRAMME. Part II. Infant growth and health status to age 6 months. Zug-Frauenfeld. Eur J Nutr 2000;39:145–156.

Cooke RJ, Vandenplas Y, Wahn U (eds): Nutrition Support for Infants and Children at Risk.
Nestlé Nutr Workshop Ser Pediatr Program, vol 59, pp 63–72,
Nestec Ltd., Vevey/S. Karger AG, Basel, © 2007.

The Concept of Oral Tolerance Induction to Foods

Gideon Lack

King's College London, Guys and St. Thomas' NHS Foundation Trust, London, UK

Abstract

The conventional wisdom is that early exposure to allergenic food proteins during pregnancy, lactation, or infancy leads to food allergies, and that prevention strategies should therefore aim to eliminate allergenic food proteins during pregnancy, breastfeeding, and early childhood. Prolonged exclusive breastfeeding and delayed weaning onto solid foods is therefore seen as an effective public health policy to prevent allergies. However, there is little epidemiological data to support this belief. Interventional studies on dietary elimination have failed to reduce IgE-mediated food allergies. Conversely, there is preclinical data and some clinical data to suggest that early cutaneous exposure to food protein through inflamed skin leads to allergic sensitization and that early oral exposure results in the induction of tolerance. New strategies to prevent food allergy in infants need to be put to test in randomized controlled interventional studies.

Despite increasing efforts to prevent food allergies in children, IgE-mediated food allergies are rising and now affect 4–7% of infants. At a global level, the World Health Organization's (WHO) strategy to prevent food allergies is to promote exclusive breastfeeding during the first 6 months of the infant's life and thus delay weaning onto solid foods [1]. In order to prevent specific food allergies, some countries recommend the avoidance of specific foods such as egg and peanut in atopic infants, and some national guidelines promote the avoidance of peanuts during pregnancy and lactation and in the first 3 years of childhood.

The evidence to support these guidelines is not entirely clear, and evidence for their efficacy is lacking. Studies of egg-allergic and peanut-allergic infants show that most affected cases react on first oral consumption of these foods, and therefore early oral exposure cannot explain the genesis of these allergies. Two birth cohort studies have failed to find an association between the development of peanut allergy and consumption of peanuts during pregnancy, lactation and infancy [2, 3]. Prospective randomized controlled interventional studies that remove food allergens from the maternal diet during the 3rd trimester and during lactation, and from the infant's diet in the first 3 years of life have consistently failed to show a significant long-term reduction in IgE-mediated food allergies, although they do show a transient improvement in eczema [4]. Similarly, prolonged exclusive breastfeeding has not been shown to prevent IgE-mediated food allergies [3].

Peanut allergy has become increasingly prevalent: recent studies demonstrate that the prevalence of peanut allergy has doubled in 10 years and approximates 1.3–1.5% [5]. Peanuts are a frequent cause of anaphylaxis for which there is no established treatment except allergen avoidance. Children with peanut allergy additionally have to avoid tree nuts since up to 50% have allergies to individual tree nuts. It is perhaps surprising that studies eliminating food allergens during pregnancy, lactation and infancy have consistently failed to reduce IgE-mediated food allergy in children. Three explanations for this failure with respect to peanut allergy include the following. (a) Allergen reduction measures have been insufficient in previous studies and elimination from the diet was not sufficiently rigorous. (b) Sensitization to food allergens does not occur through oral exposure but may occur via other routes. Indeed, the application of topical preparations containing peanut oil on infants with eczema during the first 6 months of life was associated with a high risk of developing peanut allergy [3]. A recent study has shown that even after washing hands and tabletops after eating peanuts, peanut protein was detectable in significant amounts (10 to several 100 μg) on hands and table surfaces [6]. (c) The paradigm of allergen avoidance is flawed and early oral exposure may be required to prevent the development of allergy. Oral tolerance induction is well recognized in murine models and even in the human literature [7, 8].

Murine studies exist showing that allergic sensitization to antigen can occur on cutaneous exposure. One study showed that exposure of mice to milligram quantities of ovalbumen on abraded skin led to significant anti-OVA IgE responses and positive intradermal tests [9]. More recently, it has been shown that cutaneous sensitization on the abraded skin of mice led to significant IgE responses to peanut and T cell responses to peanut [10]. This occurred even with the application of arachis oil to the skin of mice (less than 6 μg/ml of peanut protein).

Animal models demonstrate that a high early dose of oral protein antigen is highly effective in inducing tolerance to the respective antigen, even in the case of subsequent administrations of antigen in the presence of potent immune adjuvants. A literature search on oral tolerance induction in animal models has revealed 33 publications over the last 35 years in which a single oral dose of antigen was sufficient to induce tolerance. The phenomenon has been demonstrated for different antigens in different experimental models.

The data is consistent, uniformly showing that a single dose of oral protein administration effectively causes immunological tolerance and prevents the expression of related clinical disease. Oral tolerance induction in animal models is most potent in its effects on delayed type I hypersensitivity responses; prevention of antibody responses through induction of oral tolerance is less consistent. However, numerous publications point to the fact that a single dose of food allergen in mice (β-lactoglobulin, ovalbumen, peanut) is particularly effective in preventing the development of subsequent IgE-mediated responses. A most recent study [11] showed that naive mice orally tolerized to β-lactoglobulin were unable to mount significant IgE responses after subsequent sensitization with β-lactoglobulin injected with alum (intraperitoneally). Similarly, there were no significant T cell responses to β-lactoglobulin in the pretolerized animals.

Later in 2004, Strid et al. [12] fed mice a single intragastric feed of defatted peanut flour at doses varying from 0.2 to 100 mg per mouse. Seven days after the feed, animals were immunized with 100 μg of peanut antigen emulsified with complete Freund's adjuvant. Three weeks later, animals were given a recall immunization with 100 μg antigen. Mice were assayed for T cell proliferation to peanut, cytokine production, delayed-type hypersensitivity responses and antibody responses. Tolerizing doses of 100 mg of peanut protein resulted in significant reduction in delayed-type hypersensitivity responses and inhibition of proliferative responses to peanut. Animals tolerized to 100 mg of peanut protein showed significantly reduced interferon-γ and IL-4 production. Specific IgE responses to peanut following sensitization were almost completely prevented by the single tolerizing dose. However, very low 'tolerizing' doses of peanut below 2 mg per animal resulted in enhanced delayed-type hypersensitivity responses, T cell proliferative responses, cytokine production and IgE production. Doses between 2 and 20 mg of peanut protein induced no difference in T and B cell responses compared to sham-tolerized animals. Tolerance to peanut was only achieved at doses of 100 mg per animal. Oral tolerance to peanut was shown to be antigen specific. Tolerizing doses of peanut did not promote tolerance to ovalbumen and vice versa.

In the atopic march during infancy, atopic dermatitis (AD) usually precedes the development of IgE-mediated food allergy. Indeed, more severe AD is associated with a higher risk of food allergies, and in some studies, food allergen-specific T cells have been isolated from the lesional skin in patients with AD [13]. More recently, it has been shown in a prospective birth cohort study that low-dose exposure to peanut in the form of arachis oil applied to inflamed skin is associated with an increased risk of developing peanut allergy. While the use of such oils is not widespread in all countries, it is worth noting that food allergens can be measured in the environment and cutaneous sensitization to a variety of foods could occur through environmental exposure [6].

Table 1. Food allergies among allergy clinic patients

Country	Peanut allergy %	Dietary practice recommendations (infant peanut consumption)
UK (n = 191; Lack et al., 2004)	25	Avoidance
USA (n = 300) [18]	69	Avoidance
Israel (n = 992) [19]	2.1	High infant exposure
Philippines (n = 184) [20]	0	High infant exposure

There is evidence that cutaneous exposure to nickel causes allergic sensitization while oral exposure to nickel results in tolerance. Numerous studies, both prospective and retrospective, show that early cutaneous exposure to jewelry, particularly through ear piercing, is a risk factor for the development of contact dermatitis to nickel. Three independent studies [14–16], including one prospective birth cohort study, show that the early application of orthodontic braces made of nickel strongly protects against the development of contact dermatitis to nickel (in one study there was an odds ratio of 0.07). Indeed, the level of nickel in both saliva and serum of individuals increases significantly after the insertion of fixed orthodontic appliances and this is thought to result in oral tolerance. Similarly, parents exposed to pancreatic extract by inhalation or contact develop IgE-mediated allergic reactions but not the patients who were exposed to the extract by oral route [17].

It has been observed however that in African and Asian countries where peanuts are consumed throughout pregnancy and early childhood, peanut allergy is rarely seen compared to western industrialized societies such as the UK and USA where peanut allergy is high despite peanut avoidance during pregnancy and infancy (table 1) [18–20]. Differential predisposition to atopy due to both genetic and environmental factors could explain these differences.

There are no studies that examine the potential of oral tolerance induction to foods in the human infant. There is one adult study showing that feeding keyhole limpet hemocyanin (KLH) results in immunological tolerance to KLH antigen [8]. One study that attempted to induce tolerance to a food allergen [21] was conducted in patients who already had established milk allergy. The result of this study was promising: 71% of highly allergic children were able to tolerate a daily intake of 200 ml of milk after treatment. However, this was an uncontrolled study and therefore the possibility that these children would have shown spontaneous resolutions cannot be discounted. A more recent controlled study [22] showed that sublingual exposure to hazelnut in allergic individuals raised their allergic reactivity threshold to hazelnut.

In summary, the long-held view that allergic sensitization to food occurs through oral exposure and prevention of food allergy is best accomplished through elimination diets is being challenged. It is proposed that allergic sensitization to food may occur through low-dose cutaneous sensitization and that early food protein exposure may induce oral tolerance and prevent the development of food allergies. The validity of these hypotheses will need to be tested in randomized controlled, interventional studies.

References

1 Fifty-Fourth World Health Assembly. Provisional agenda item 13.1.1. Global strategy for infant and young child feeding: the optimal duration of exclusive breastfeeding. Geneva, World Health Organization, 2001.
2 Tariq SM, Stevens M, Matthew S, et al: Cohort study of peanut and tree nut sensitisation by age of 4 years. BMJ 1996;313:514–517.
3 Lack G, Fox D, Northstone K, Golding J: Factors associated with the development of peanut allergy in childhood. N Engl J Med 2003;348:977–985.
4 Zeiger RS, Heller S: The development and prediction of atopy in high-risk children: follow-up at age seven years in a prospective randomized study of combined maternal and infant food allergen avoidance. J Allergy Clin Immunol 1995;95:1179–1190.
5 Grundy J, Matthews S, Bateman B, et al: Rising prevalence of allergy to peanut in children: data from 2 sequential cohorts. J Allergy Clin Immunol 2002;110:784–789.
6 Perry TT, Conover-Walker MK, Pomes A, et al: Distribution of peanut allergen in the environment. J Allergy Clin Immunol 2004;113:973–976.
7 Ngan J, Kind LS: Suppressor T cells for IgE and IgG in Peyer's patches of mice made tolerant by the oral administration of ovalbumin. J Immunol 1978;120:861–865.
8 Husby S, Mestecky J, Moldoveanu Z, et al: Oral tolerance in humans. T cell but not B cell tolerance after antigen feeding. J Immunol 1994;152:4663–4670.
9 Saloga J, Renz H, Larsen GL, Gelfand EW: Increased airways responsiveness in mice depends on local challenge with antigen. Am J Respir Crit Care Med 1994;149:65–70.
10 Strid J, Hourihane J, Kimber I, et al: Disruption of the stratum corneum allows potent epicutaneous immunization with protein antigens resulting in a dominant systemic Th2 response. Eur J Immunol 2004;34:2100–2109.
11 Frossard CP, Tropia L, Hauser C, Eigenmann PA: Lymphocytes in Peyer patches regulate clinical tolerance in a murine model of food allergy. J Allergy Clin Immunol 2004;113:958–964.
12 Strid J, Thomson M, Hourihane J, et al: A novel model of sensitisation and oral tolerance to peanut protein. Immunology 2004;113:293–303.
13 van Reijsen FC, Felius A, Wauters EA, et al: T-cell reactivity for a peanut-derived epitope in the skin of a young infant with atopic dermatitis. J Allergy Clin Immunol 1998;101:207–209.
14 Kerosuo H, Kullaa A, Kerosuo E, et al: Nickel allergy in adolescents in relation to orthodontic treatment and piercing of ears. Am J Orthod Dentofacial Orthop 1996;109:148–154.
15 Mortz CG, Lauritsen JM, Bindslev-Jensen C, Andersen KE: Nickel sensitisation in adolescents and association with ear piercing, use of dental braces and hand eczema. The Odense Adolescence Cohort Study on Atopic Diseases and Dermatitis (TOACS). Acta Derm Venereol 2002;82:359–364.
16 Van Hoogstraten IM, Andersen KE, Von Blomberg BM, et al: Reduced frequency of nickel allergy upon oral nickel contact at an early age. Clin Exp Immunol 1991;85:441–445.
17 Twarog FJ, Weinstein SF, Khaw KT, et al: Hypersensitivity to pancreatic extracts in parents of patients with cystic fibrosis. J Allergy Clin Immunol 1977;59:35–40.
18 Sampson H, Ho D: Relationship between food-specific IgE concentration and the risk of positive food challenges in children and adolescents. J Allergy Clin Immunol 1997;100:444–451.
19 Levy Y, Broides A, Segal N, Danon YL: Peanut and tree nut allergy in children: role of peanut snacks in Israel? Allergy 2003;58:1206–1207.
20 Hill DJ, Hosking CS, Zhie CY, et al: The frequency of food allergy in Australia and Asia. Environ Toxicol Pharmacol 1997;4:101–110.

21 Meglio P, Bartone E, Plantamura M, et al: A protocol for oral desensitisation in children with IgE-mediated cow's milk allergy. Allergy 2004;59:980–987.
22 Enrique E, Pineda F, Malek T, et al: Sublingual immunotherapy for hazelnut food allergy: a randomized, double-blind, placebo-controlled study with a standardized hazelnut extract. J Allergy Clin Immunol 2005;116:1073–1079.

Discussion

Dr. Bergmann: In Germany, midwives visit mothers after delivery at home and help them with breastfeeding and the care of the newborn. Some recommend adding mother's milk to the baby's bath, even if the infant develops eczema. In my opinion, there is no study on the benefit of a breast milk bath for the prevention and treatment of eczema.

Dr. Lack: That is interesting. Certainly this is done with egg and in fact egg is used in shampoo. We have seen a few babies who presented with anaphylaxis to egg after the parents were advised to put egg white on their babies' skin.

Dr. Nowak-Wegrzyn: Your observations have been well documented, but how early is early and would you comment on milk allergy? It is hard to imagine more high-dose exposure to a food allergen than with cow's milk-based formula introduced on the first day of life but these children still develop allergy to cow's milk. So at what age would you consider to start feeding peanut? I hope that your studies will be able to answer this question.

Dr. Lack: Babies 4–11 months of age and generally the majority of children in the UK have not developed peanut allergy at this stage. Our study will be stratified because there will be some who already have low levels of IgE to peanut but a negative skin prick test. One of the questions is how far can you modulate in the very primary sense, and in a secondary sense once the IgE is detectable. Is it too late to intervene once the biologic ball has started rolling and IgE is present? We should be able to answer that hopefully. Milk is puzzling and as you pointed out, very often babies can have milk many times before they develop symptoms of milk allergy, which is very different to egg and peanut allergy. I think there are problems in milk allergy, one of which is that historically most studies have not separated the different phenotypes of milk allergy; so there is a quick onset of IgE mediated milk allergy, then eczema, and gastrointestinal symptoms and many of the studies lump them all together. It may be that milk is only started in a very partial form in combination with breastfeeding and a higher dose is needed. Milk is a bit of a puzzle, as is fish because a lot of people with fish allergy have of course eaten fish many times before they develop fish allergy. It is interesting that the fish allergen Gad c 1 is present in very low concentrations as a constituent of fish protein compared to other foods. So it may be that tolerance requires exposure to high concentration of allergens.

Dr. Beyer: How do the data from the United States fit in because almost 90% of the children are given peanut butter very early on? Although the recommendation is to avoid it in high-risk children, it is given and eaten there, and there is a high prevalence of peanut allergy in the USA. So how do you fit all these confusing data together?

Dr. Lack: I am actually not sure that this is the case in the United States. People don't always follow recommendations. In the United States 80–90% of children who react to peanuts do so on the first known exposure as in the rest of the world. Also it seems socially related. For example there is the WIC program in the United States where children from low socioeconomic groups are given nutritional supplementation and peanut butter earlier on. I have been told anecdotally that this group of children had the least peanut allergy. So there might be other confounding factors related to the socioeconomic status. I don't think the evidence is strong that American babies in general are eating huge amounts of peanut protein in the first 4–10 months of life.

Dr. Ruemmele: You succeeded in focusing on one single pathology. I think that is important when speaking about allergy and atopy, otherwise there is a mixture of different pathophysiological mechanisms, which is always quite difficult to compare. Do you consider that the route of antigen administration, cutaneous versus GI, decides whether a child develops an allergic disease or not, or is this too simplistic? Comparing allergy to celiac disease, as an example of an immune-mediated disorder, in both diseases there are clearly identified antigens, a T cell-mediated immune response on the level of the intestinal mucosal barrier. However, the immune responses are completely different with varying Th profiles. So how is it that proteins of cow's milk or whey provoke a Th2 or Th2-oriented immune response whereas in celiacs an Th1 immune-mediated response to gliadin is observed?

Dr. Lack: Yes, hypothetically I do believe that it is likely that sensitization occurs to the skin rather than the GI tract. Yes it is a simplistic hypothesis but I prefer to deal with something that I can understand at least in terms of translating it into human behaviour. What I think is going on is that there are two routes of antigen presentation, one is the oral route and the other is environmental, be it cutaneous or respiratory. In southern or western Africa or Asia, where there is higher environmental exposure, the babies will have eczema which induces sensitization, but at the same time there are oral tolerance signals through the GI tact. If environmental exposure is allowed to continue and cause sensitization but the tolerogenic signals to the GI tract are removed, then there is a potential for disaster. Removing peanuts and other foods from developing countries could result in malnutrition because they are a major source of proteins in these countries. The disjunction in routes of presentation leads to an allergic or a tolerant outcome. Peanut allergy is a Th2-mediated disease, which is not the case with celiac disease. There are epidemiological studies suggesting that early introduction of wheat may work both ways. One line of evidence suggests that wheat predisposes to celiac and other data suggests that it may be protective. Interpreting these studies is difficult. Even if it is shown that a food which is introduced early in life causes symptoms, this does not mean that the introduction of the food is causing the primary disease; it may simply mean that the disease is already there and the earlier the food is introduced the earlier symptoms are seen. If you have any thoughts on how celiac disease arises I will be grateful to hear them.

Dr. Ruemmele: It is amazing to see two different responses to major antigens of whey characterizing celiac disease or whey allergy; perhaps the antigens are not the same. One is Th1 and the other is Th2 disease; one is autoimmune and the other systemic allergic atopic disease. So what makes the switch? I don't have the answer but it is quite an interesting comparison.

Dr. Wahn: There was a time when I thought things were so easy and now they are so complicated; we are all getting confused. For clarification, when you showed this bell-shaped curve of environmental exposure you were implying that a lot of environmental exposure could be beneficial. Then you mentioned peanuts and said that the environmental exposure to peanuts is bad whereas oral exposure is potentially good. Is it just that things are totally different or are you still at the ascending part of the dose-response curve? Are you assuming that you will never reach the right side of the bell, or would you hypothesize that there is no bell with regard to peanut exposure?

Dr. Lack: Yes I think high-dose exposure or moderate- to high-dose exposure to peanut in the environment is problematic. I didn't show the data but it is interesting that children with egg allergy as a group had much lower exposure and they were all clustered down at the bottom in terms of environmental exposure, except for a very small subgroup who was way out and who had even more environmental exposure than the peanut group. What is high and what is low of course becomes a relative concept. I think that very high-dose exposure in its own right may tolerize but again is it tolerizing through the skin or is it tolerizing because there is a very high amount of the allergen in the environment and it gets into the saliva?

Dr. Wahn: But what doses are you using in your ITN prospective trial?

Dr. Lack: We are mirroring the natural pattern of introduction in terms of frequency, amount of snacks, and total protein amount because there is also a safety issue here. So we are not introducing something that has never been done before. We are mirroring this on the basis of other population-feeding studies.

Dr. Nowak-Wegrzyn: Regarding what you said about the introduction of peanut butter in America, I think it mostly occurs after 8 months of age, which is pretty early but it is not that early. We actually see a high percentage of young children sensitized and allergic to peanut in the inner city population. The question is about Bamba snack that you will use in your study. Is the peanut in Bamba processed differently from peanut butter?

Dr. Lack: We are not just feeding this Israeli snack, we are feeding other snacks including peanut butter and in fact peanut soup. We looked carefully at the amounts of major peanut allergens in peanut butter and in peanut-containing snacks, and a variety of peanut butters in different countries. We found no important differences. There are minor differences in protein content but IgE binding on these peanut snacks is the same, and in fact they are all made of roasted peanut butter. I don't think there really is an issue unless we get down to the variations in processing that Dr. Beyer was talking about that may affect hypoallergenic milk formulae. Sensitisation is not the same as allergy. It is very interesting that infants who are eating peanuts in high amounts may have moderate to high levels of specific IgE to peanut. This is another problem with studies; when we look for causality in large epidemiological studies, the production of IgE in a lot of these children is a normal tolerant phenomenon. We have to be very careful about distinguishing sensitization versus allergy.

Dr. Chubarova: How is it that children with eczema are recommended to apply an antigenic product on skin because there is a regular recommendation to avoid this? The theoretical question that I am especially interested in regards applying an antigen to a compromised skin barrier in children with eczema which can cause general sensitization and be realized at any locus. You are telling us that gastrointestinal allergy is not the main cause of the allergy. What about the risk?

Dr. Lack: There is no direct proof that these creams are causing peanut allergy. It would be unethical to randomize babies to receive these creams or not and I think very few parents would permit this. My advice is to avoid any topical preparation that contains a food protein that is known to be an allergen on eczematous skin. But another problem that we realize now is that these proteins are not just from these creams; they may be from the environment. Egg and milk and peanut are measurable in the environment; they are measurable in the air, on surfaces, hands and bed clothes, and we can't do much about this. If the environment were totally hypoallergenic with no milk protein at all, and no peanut and no egg, these food allergies might not exist. Kiwi allergy only developed in the UK after we started importing kiwi. If total environmental exposure and all forms of exposure could be brought down to zero then everything might be alright, but this is not practically possible.

Dr. Chubarova: Why have you taken eczema as independent risk factor because in that case you apply antigen to a compromised barrier?

Dr. Lack: It is a risk factor that we found in our studies and others have found it as well. Hill and Hosking [1] in Melbourne have shown very nicely that the severity of eczema directly correlates with the number of foods to which the infant is allergic and the number of days topical steroids are required. This increases the risk of food allergy; it is a risk factor. It is part of the atopic phenotype but the eczema is not being driven by these food allergies because these children aren't eating those foods.

Dr. Chubarova: That is exactly what I am saying, that the child has an allergic phenotype, maybe sensitization to some other antigen and then he gets another one. It is not surprising that he became sensitized to peanut. Everybody knows that when a child has an allergy to one antigen, the risk of allergy to other antigens increases.

Dr. Lack: That is true to a certain extent but not invariably so. Yes, there is an association between egg and peanut allergy; there is a much higher association between peanut, tree nut and sesame seed allergy; there is very little association between milk allergy and peanut allergy. Whether these differences can be explained by epitope spreading or common T cell epitopes, is not known. There are homologous sequences for some of the major allergens in peanuts and tree nuts and perhaps in sesame seeds. The acquisition of other food allergies may be related to structural similarities in a whole group of food proteins. It may also be that by tolerizing to one food there could be cross-tolerance to a group of structurally related foods. Just the way there is cross-sensitization between birch pollen and fruits, there may be cross-tolerance.

Dr. B. Koletzko: You deserve to be applauded for your intervention study. Are you taking into account whether some of these infants are still breastfed when peanut allergen is introduced? Swedish pediatricians claim that the risk for celiac disease is much lower when limited amounts of wheat protein are introduced while infants are still being breastfed, rather than introducing wheat protein after weaning. What is the practice in Israel? Is it possible that the introduction of peanut allergen during or after breastfeeding might affect the risk of developing an allergy to peanuts?

Dr. Lack: All geographical differences in PA might be explained on the basis of different breast-feeding patterns. Actually if that was the case, then it would be expected to have an influence in a nonallergen-specific way and a reduction in egg and milk allergy would be expected, but the levels of egg and milk allergy are very similar. There does not appear to be a difference in duration of breast-feeding in countries with very different prevalence of PA. It is interesting that the use of hypoallergenic formulae and soy formulae is also very similar in terms of the types introduced and the age at which they were introduced. Therefore we don't think that that is going to have an important effect. Adam Fox looked at maternal consumption during breastfeeding and his data didn't suggest that this was relevant.

Dr. Nowak-Wegrzyn: I want to go back to your comment on IgE sensitization to peanut in children with atopic dermatitis. Many children that we see with atopic eczema don't have obvious acute reactions when they eat milk or egg on a regular basis. However, if milk or eggs are removed from the diet for 2 weeks and are then reintroduced under supervision (oral food challenge), then acute reactions can be seen. If there is complete tolerance to food, it doesn't matter if it is eaten every day or once a year. I am curious whether these children with atopic dermatitis are truly permanently tolerant to peanut regardless of the frequency of peanut ingestion?

Dr. Lack: These infants are eating it very regularly and that is what is fascinating. At the moment the question is whether this is really allergy to peanut or is it low-affinity cross-reactive IgE to some other food? We are planning a study with Hugh Sampson as a collaborator, in which we will be able to look at IgE epitopes to peanut in sensitised and allergic children. We are also looking to see whether this is functional or nonfunctional IgE by purifying the IgE from the serum, adding the IgE to basophils and adding peanut antigen. One of the central questions in allergy is why sensitisation occurs in some children who remain asymptomatic despite exposure to allergen.

Reference

1   Hill DJ, Hosking CS: Food allergy and atopic dermatitis in infancy: an epidemiologic study. Pediatr Allergy Immunol 2004;15:421–427.

Cooke RJ, Vandenplas Y, Wahn U (eds): Nutrition Support for Infants and Children at Risk.
Nestlé Nutr Workshop Ser Pediatr Program, vol 59, pp 73–88,
Nestec Ltd., Vevey/S. Karger AG, Basel, © 2007.

Chronic Enteropathy: Molecular Basis

Frank M. Ruemmele

Pediatric Gastroenterology, INSERM U793, Hôpital Necker – Enfants Malades, Paris, France

Abstract

Major advances in the understanding of the pathophysiology of chronic and intractable diarrhea of infancy allow a new conceptual view of this heterogeneous group of disorders. Two major types of chronic 'intractable' enteropathies can be distinguished. (1) Congenital-constitutive forms are characterized by intrinsic enterocyte defects. To date three different types have been identified on a morphological-histological basis: microvillous inclusion disease, intestinal epithelial dysplasia and the so-called syndromatic diarrhea. These disorders are characterized by a high degree of consanguinity in the affected families. An autosomal recessive transmission was suggested, but the genes involved have not yet been identified. (2) Immunoinflammatory enteropathies starting within the first months of life, such as autoimmune enteropathies, can share the clinical picture of constitutive enteropathies; however, most often there are associated extraintestinal symptoms. A loss of function mutation in the *FOXP3* gene located on Xp11.23-q13.3 causes a distinct X-linked form of severe autoimmune enteropathy. The functional consequences of *FOXP3* mutations which point to a defect of regulatory T cells are currently under investigation. With the increasing understanding of the molecular basis of these distinct diarrheal disorders, new treatment strategies will emerge within the next years, giving new hope to these critically ill children and their families.

Copyright © 2007 Nestec Ltd., Vevey/S. Karger AG, Basel

Introduction

Over the past years, major advances in the understanding of the pathophysiology of chronic and intractable diarrhea of infancy have been made allowing a new conceptual view of this heterogeneous group of gastrointestinal (GI) diseases. Today, according to the mode of onset, the clinical presentation, the presence of systemic symptoms or of immunoinflammatory reactions different classifications of chronic enteropathies can be proposed (fig. 1). In 1968, the descriptive term 'intractable diarrhea of infancy' was

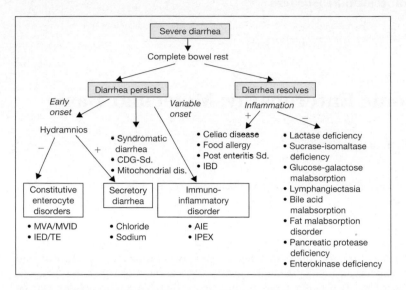

Fig. 1. Differential diagnostic approach for a child presenting with severe diarrhea with onset within the first days or weeks of life. CDG = Congenital disorders of glycosylation; dis. = disorder; IBD = inflammatory bowel disorder; Sd. = syndrome.

introduced by Avery et al. [1] for children who within the first 3 months of life presented with severe and abundant noninfectious diarrhea, which persisted despite bowel rest. Diarrhea becomes most often life threatening, and patients are only stabilized by the use of total parenteral nutrition. With the rapid improvement of techniques of artificial nutrition in the late 1970s these critically ill babies and infants, formerly condemned to die within the first days or weeks after the onset of symptoms, survived for the first time. Subsequently, distinct clinical pictures emerged and new pathologies were discovered, such as microvillous atrophy (MVA)/microvillous inclusion disease (MVID) or epithelial dysplasia/tufting enteropathy (TE).

In the present review, we suggest a classification of this heterogeneous group of chronic enteropathies according to the age of onset (congenital or within the first weeks/months of life) as well as according to the presence or absence of inflammatory or immune reaction. An important differential diagnostic criterion will be the persistence of diarrhea on complete bowel rest. Besides the clinical picture and presentation, we will discuss in the following the molecular basis, as far as known, for the different constitutive and immunoallergic GI pathologies. Pathologies causing electrolyte secretory diarrhea, malabsorption or malassimilation will not be discussed in this review. Infectious and postinfectious syndrome and other self-limiting pathologies causing protracted but not persistent diarrhea are also not part of this review, which is limited to chronic intestinal disorders defined by persistent or recurrent episodes of diarrhea over at least 3 weeks.

Congenital-Constitutive Diarrheal Disorders

Clinical Considerations

The typical clinical picture is abundant watery, sometimes mucous diarrhea starting within the first hours or days of life [2, 3]. Diarrhea can be so important that within a few hours a rapidly life-threatening situation develops due to massive dehydration and metabolic acidosis. The neonatal course (presence or absence of polyhydramnios) presents essential information contributing towards the differential diagnosis of a secretory (chloride or sodium) diarrheal disorder if polyhydramnios is present or a constitutive enterocyte disorder (absence of polyhydramnios). A major step in the differential diagnosis of congenital or early onset watery diarrhea is the response to complete bowel rest, as well as the determination of fecal and serum electrolytes. If diarrhea stops on total bowel rest it is most likely secondary to malabsorption or malassimilation (fig. 1), whereas, once defects in electrolyte transports are eliminated, massive and persistent diarrhea indicates a constitutive enterocyte disorder, such as MVA/MVID or intestinal epithelial dysplasia (IED)/TE or rarely syndromatic or phenotypic diarrhea.

In MVA/MVID, severe watery diarrhea typically starts within the first days of life [2–4]. This diarrhea becomes so abundant that within 24 h children can lose up to 30% of their body weight, resulting in profound metabolic acidosis and severe dehydration. MVID is most often severe and life-threatening. Accurate quantification of stool volumes reveals 150 to over 300 ml/kg/day with a high sodium content (over 100 mmol/l). Complete and prolonged bowel rest makes it possible to reduce stool volume moderately, but it nearly always remains above 150 ml/kg/day [4]. Typically, no additional clinical signs are associated with MVID; in particular, there are no malformations or involvement of other organs such as liver or kidney. However, a small number of children have massive pruritus secondary to elevated concentrations of biliary acids in the blood. Also, proximal renal tubular dysfunction was observed in some children with MVID/MVA. At clinical examination, no specific findings can be detected except enormous abdominal distension with fluid-filled intestinal and colonic loops. All children with congenital MVID urgently require total parental nutrition, which often causes rapidly evolving cholestasis and liver disease. A detailed multicenter analysis of 23 patients with MVID [4] distinguished two different forms and presentations of MVID on a clinical and morphological basis: the most frequent form, that is congenital early-onset MVID (starting within the first days of life), and some rare cases, that is late-onset MVID (with first symptoms appearing after 2 or 3 months of life). Intestinal failure is definitive in all children with early-onset

MVID and most with late-onset MVID. Some rare children with late-onset MVID were described who had a somewhat less severe course. In general, children with MVID are potential candidates for small bowel transplantation [5].

In IED/TE, massive watery diarrhea develops within the first days after birth in a way similar to MVA/MVID. Stool volumes are highly variable (100–200 ml/kg body weight/day) with stool electrolyte concentrations of sodium of 100–140 mmol/l [6, 7]. All children are highly dependent on parenteral nutrition. There is no past history of hydramnios or other antenatal or neonatal particularities. It is striking that in our experience most children with IED/TE have consanguineous parents and/or affected siblings and some of them died during the first months of life with severe diarrhea of unknown origin. Upon clinical examination, no malformations are observed; however, some children have somewhat rigid hair and a subgroup of patient shows clinical signs of photophobia. Distinct ophthalmologic examination reveals the presence of superficial keratitis in these children. The degree of severity of IED/TE is more variable compared to MVA/MVID with most children developing a severe course indicating lifelong and definitive intestinal failure. However, some patients have less severe disease and may acquire a certain degree of intestinal autonomy making it possible to reduce parenteral nutrition to three to four perfusions a week.

A distinct clinical group is the so-called phenotypic or syndromatic diarrhea. This disorder, first described by the group of Goulet [8] in Paris, is characterized by small for gestational age babies with severe persistent watery diarrhea associated with an abnormal phenotype, including facial dysmorphism, hypertelorism, and woolly, easily removable hair with trichorrhexis nodosa. In addition, immunological abnormalities were observed in all patients in the form of defective antibody responses despite normal serum immunoglobulin levels, and defective antigen-specific skin tests despite positive proliferative responses in vitro. The majority of patients followed in our center were the progeny of consanguineous marriages. The clinical course of these children is variable. Most of the children died in the past, but some of the survivors acquired a certain degree of intestinal autonomy.

Molecular Considerations

There is strong evidence that all these congenital/early-onset structural enterocyte disorders have a distinct genetic basis [2]. The clinical features suggest an autosomal recessive transmission. Since the gene(s) involved are not yet identified for these congenital inherited autosomal recessive diseases, no genetic or prenatal diagnosis is possible. The majority of children with MVA/MVID are of Turkish origin; however, we follow up a couple of children with MVA/MVID (most with several affected siblings) of Caucasian origin. Patients with IED/TE are most often of Arab origin, that is Middle East including Turkey or North Africa. The prevalence in Malta Island, in the Mediterranean Sea, seems high but the phenotype might be milder. Once again, a small number of IED patients

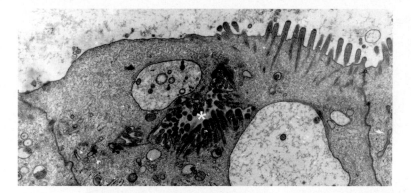

Fig. 2. MVA/MVID: electron-microscopic picture showing typical atrophic microvilli on a mature IEC of the duodenum as well as microvillous inclusions (asterisk).

followed up in our center are also of Caucasian origin without any evidence of consanguinity, indicating sporadic de novo mutations.

The precise molecular basis of MVA/MVID is still unknown. There is evidence of a major defect in membrane trafficking in intestinal epithelial cells (IEC), probably secondary to an altered structure of the cytoskeleton [9]. This disorder is morphologically characterized by the occurrence of so-called microvillous inclusions at the apical pole of enterocytes along with absent or atrophic microvilli on mature enterocytes easily visible on electron-microscopic analyses (fig. 2). The observation of morphologically normal microvilli on immature crypt cells in children with MVID indicates that the microvillous changes seen in differentiating and mature cells are of secondary nature or they are a consequence of yet unidentified events within the cell, such as membrane recycling or mechanisms controlling endo- or exocytosis [10, 11]. However, analysis of the membrane targeting of the disaccharidase sucrase-isomaltase revealed no abnormalities of the direct or indirect constitutive pathway. Another hypothesis suggesting a defect in the autophagocytosis pathway was proposed to explain the morphological and functional abnormalities in MVID. Very recent observations indicate a selective defect in glycoprotein exocytosis in patients with MVID [12]. These glycoproteins accumulate within the apical pole of enterocytes and form the characteristic secretory granules, easily observed on PAS staining on duodenal sections of patients with MVA/MVID (fig. 3).

In contrast to MVA/MVID which is most likely the consequence of an IEC membrane trafficking defect, IED/TE results from a regulatory defect of epithelial mesenchymal cell interactions, which are instrumental in intestinal development and differentiation. Alterations suggestive of abnormal cell-cell and cell-matrix interactions were seen in patients with IED without any evidence of abnormalities in epithelial cell polarization and proliferation [13].

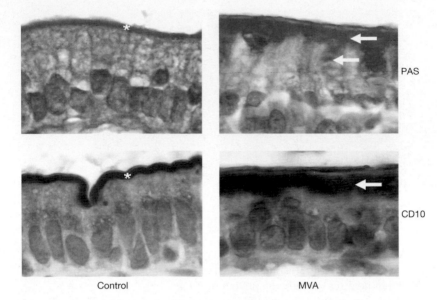

Fig. 3. MVA/MVID: high-power magnification of a duodenal section after periodic acid-Schiff (PAS) staining or anti-CD10 immunohistochemistry. As shown on both panels compared to normal controls, in MVA an enlarged intracytoplasmic band (arrow) at the apical pole of enterocytes can be seen along with an atrophic band instead of the normally well-defined small line representing the brush border (asterisk).

These alterations included abnormal distribution of the adhesion molecule α2β1 integrin along the crypt-villous axis. The α2β1 integrin is involved in the interaction of epithelial cells to various basement membrane components, such as laminin and collagen. To date, the pathophysiological mechanisms resulting in an increased immunohistochemical expression of desmoglein and the ultrastructural changes of desmosomes are unclear [13]. A major morphological feature of IED is the occurrence of epithelial tufts at the villi, along with crypt branching (fig. 4). Tufts correspond to rounded epithelial cells at the villous tips that are no longer in contact with the basement membrane. It can be speculated that a defect of normal enterocyte apoptosis at the end of their lifespan or an altered cell-cell contact is responsible for this effect. The primary or secondary nature of the formation of tufts remains to be determined. Mice with a disrupted gene encoding the transcription factor Elf3 display morphologic features resembling IED [14]. In this model, an abnormal morphogenesis of the villi was observed while progenitor crypt cells appear normal. IEC are characterized by a low transforming growth factor-β type 2 receptor expression, which is implicated in the differentiation of immature IEC.

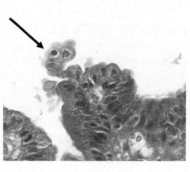
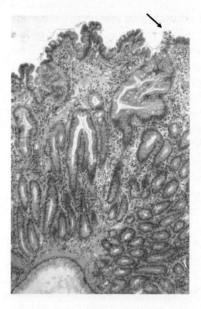

Fig. 4. IED or TE: partial villous atrophy with crypt hyperplasia and/or pseudocystic crypt appearance, branching pictures and disorganization of surface epithelium with typical tufts (arrow).

The molecular basis of phenotypic syndromatic diarrhea is completely unknown. The diagnosis of this syndrome is made by the association of different clinical symptoms. Characteristic or pathognomic histological alterations of the intestinal mucosa were not observed. Marked (subtotal to total) villous atrophy on duodenal biopsies along with a variable inflammatory infiltrate of the lamina propriety is seen in the majority of patients. In a recent study, we did not observe an increased expression of HLA molecules on IEC. To date, the genetic basis of this disorder remains unclear.

Immunological Inflammatory Diarrheal Disorders

Clinical Considerations

The neonatal course is completely normal. Onset of intestinal symptoms is within the first months of life and it is rarely isolated, in contrast to congenital early onset enterocyte disorders. Diarrhea is often bloody and most often systemic inflammatory symptoms exist, i.e. fever, elevated inflammatory markers in blood and stools. Changes in the mode of alimentation, such as withdrawal of breastfeeding, the introduction of cow's milk proteins, but sometimes even a simple viral infection or a vaccination, may precede the onset of GI symptoms. A main characteristic of inflammatory or autoimmune enteropathy (AIE) is a protein-losing enteropathy, seen in low serum albumin levels and a markedly enhanced α_1-antitrypsin clearance [15]. Complete bowel rest may improve diarrhea; however, in severe courses diarrhea often persists. This situation represents a diagnostic challenge, since the clinical pictures of children suffering from an early-onset enterocyte intrinsic defect and children with an immunological disorder overlap considerably. We recently evaluated the diagnostic value of measuring inflammatory markers in the stools to distinguish immunoinflammatory diarrheal GI disorders from constitutive enterocyte disorders in infants presenting with severe diarrhea within the first year of life [16]. The simple fecal test allowed with a specificity close to 100% to eliminate an inflammatory affection if fecal calprotectin levels were within the normal range. Contrary to autoimmune inflammatory enteropathies, allergic reactions always respond to and theoretically are healed on complete bowel rest. However, on re-alimentation, the symptoms reappear immediately if the causative antigen is re-introduced.

If a child presents with an AIE, the onset is often within the first 3 or 4 months in the form of severe diarrhea which can be bloody [15]. The majority of boys with AIE present in addition with severe atopic skin disease, hematological abnormalities along with endocrinopathy, such as insulin-dependent diabetes mellitus or thyroiditis. This association was described as IPEX (immune dysregulation, polyendocrinopathy, autoimmune enteropathy, X-linked) syndrome [15, 17, 18]. It is interesting to note that boys with IPEX also show severe immunoallergic symptoms with a strong Th2 response and hyper-IgE syndrome having some similarities with extremely severe food allergy. Isolated or oligosymptomatic forms of severe AIE exist in both, boys and girls. Prior to the onset of AIE/IPEX, these children develop completely normal, and no antenatal or neonatal particularities exist [19]. It is important to stress that the family history is most often positive for various autoimmune diseases. This indicates a particular genetic background, pointing to disease susceptibility genes. Another particularity is the exclusive occurrence of a subtype of AIE in boys, which indicates an X-linked mode of transmission. Inflammatory bowel disease (Crohn's disease or ulcerative colitis) is extremely rare in this age group; however, it has to be considered as a differential diagnosis.

The onset of food allergy-induced enteropathy/colitis is less severe compared to AIE/IPEX. However, severe forms exist as – in extreme cases – food protein-induced enterocolitis syndrome. Besides the presentation as upper GI disease, the onset is in the form of diarrhea and rectal bleeding combined with failure to thrive [20]. Often atopic skin and pulmonary symptoms are associated with the GI symptoms. The family history for atopy is often positive, and several affected children within one family are not exceptional. Once more this points to a particular genetic background and potential susceptibility genes. Systemic inflammatory symptoms are rare; however, inflammatory signs at the intestinal mucosal level are typical for this disease entity, as is the occurrence of protein-losing enteropathy. Biological exams help to make the diagnosis if IgE levels are enhanced with specific RASTs. However, food allergies are frequently related to delayed type 4 hypersensitivity reactions and show no biological or immunological abnormalities. Skin patch tests most often are not helpful in the diagnosis. Food allergy can share the clinical picture of celiac disease, which has to be ruled out combining serological and if necessary histological evaluations.

Molecular Considerations

Genetic mapping studies of several families with boys suffering from AIE made it possible to identify a disease causing mutation in a gene located on the X chromosome Xp11.23-q13.3 [21, 22]. This gene was named *FOXP3* and encodes a 48-kD protein of the forkhead (FKH)/winged helix transcription factor family, named scurfin. Scurfin is predominantly expressed in CD4+/CD25+ T cells with regulatory functions. Experimental data suggest that scurfin is implicated in the regulation and suppression of T cell activation [23]. In a recent review of boys with IPEX [17], a loss of function mutations was reported within the coding region of *FOXP3*, whereas in one family, a mutation in the 3'-untranslated region of *FOXP3* was observed. Two additional patients with typical clinical symptoms of IPEX did not show any mutations within the coding regions of *FOXP3*, suggesting that regulatory or conditional mutations may occur outside *FOXP3*, such as described by Bennett et al. [24] in the polyadenylation signal following the final coding exon of *FOXP3*. This may result in a decreased *FOXP3* messenger ribonucleic acid (RNA) expression, probably owing to nonspecific degradation of aberrant RNA. Similar to loss of function mutations in *FOXP3*, this results in a decreased or completely suppressed scurfin expression causing an altered biological function. In addition, it is possible that other forms of IPEX or AIE exist that are not related to mutations in the *FOXP3* gene and that are transmitted either with an X-chromosomal or an autosomic trait. Owen et al. [25] reported on two families with several members presenting with clinical IPEX. In one family a novel *FOXP3* mutation was identified with a single base deletion at codon 76 of exon 2, resulting in a frameshift mutation, whereas in the second family the FOXP3 locus was excluded by recombination and mutational analysis was negative. Since one girl was affected in this family, one can speculate about an autosomal locus.

The structure of the *FOXP3* protein, scurfin, suggests that it has deoxyribonucleic acid (DNA) binding activity and may serve as nuclear transcription factor. Schubert et al. [23] demonstrated that scurfin acts as a repressor of transcription and regulator of T cell activation. Intact scurfin represses transcription of a reporter containing a multimeric FKH-binding site. Such FKH-binding sites are located adjacent to nuclear factor of activated T cells (NFAT), regulatory sites in various cytokine promoters such as IL-2, or granulocyte-macrophage colony-stimulating factor enhancer. Therefore, intact

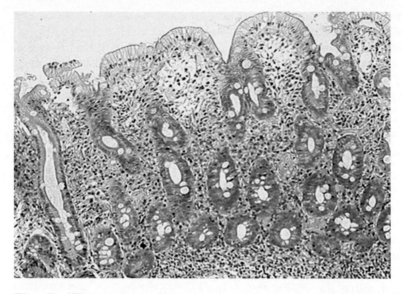

Fig. 5. AIE: complete villous atrophy and a major inflammatory infiltrate of mononuclear and some polynuclear cells within the lamina propria of the duodenum.

scurfy seems to be capable of directly repressing NFAT-mediated transcription of the IL-2 gene in CD4+ T cells upon activation [23]. In addition, scurfin seems to play an important role in thymic maturation of regulatory T cells. Nonfunctional (due to maturation or structural defects) or absent regulatory T cells cause highly overactivated T cell reactions, since the natural inhibitor fails. A tremendous T cell-mediated inflammatory reaction within the GI tract causes severe epithelial cell and mucosal destruction without villous atrophy and erosions or ulcerations (fig. 5).

In general, allergic reactions can occur as acute type 1 IgE-mediated or as delayed type 4 IgE-independent and Th2-cell-mediated reactions. Food allergy is often IgE independent and we are only beginning to understand some of the molecular events of food allergy-induced enteropathy. Allergic reactions of the GI tract are particularly intriguing, since, normally, upon oral ingestion of a potential allergen an anti-inflammatory TGF-β-mediated response develops, a mechanism described as oral tolerance. In contrast, parenteral administration of the same antigen provokes a marked T cell-driven inflammatory response. Therefore, it was suggested that a defect in or a loss of anti-inflammatory control mechanisms might be a key step in the development of food allergy [20]. The number of TGF-β-producing T cells, presumably regulatory T cells, was reported to be reduced in the duodenal mucosa of children with food allergy [26]. That regulatory T cells play an important role in food allergy is largely supported by the observation of allergic symptoms including food allergy in patients with the IPEX syndrome. The commensal intestinal flora was proposed as an environmental factor involved in the stimulation of the mucosal immune system. It was suggested that changes in the composition of the intestinal microflora early in life may result in an insufficient stimulation of innate immune response contributing to impaired development of regulatory T cells [27].

Additional factors, potentially affecting the function of the intestinal barrier, also seem to play a key role in the onset of food allergy-induced enteropathy. Increased intestinal permeability and increased uptake of allergens were described in children with cow's milk protein allergy [20]. The molecular basis of the pathological transport of allergens via intact enterocytes was recently revealed [28] with an IL-4-induced upregulation of CD23, a low-affinity IgE type II transmembrane glycoprotein, on IEC. This causes an exaggerated IgE-CD23-mediated endosomal uptake of allergens, which are subsequently released at the basolateral side of enterocytes. Eosinophils, basophils, monocytes, mast and T cells recruited to the lamina propria release upon interaction with this allergen large amounts of prostaglandins, leukotrienes, histamine, tryptase and various cytokines. In the resulting acute phase, inflammatory reactions provoke GI (vomiting, diarrhea, bleeding) and systemic symptoms (fever, anaphylaxis, etc.). Th2 cytokines, such as IL-4, IL-5 and IL-13, are responsible for an Ig switch to IgE, chemoattraction and accumulation of inflammatory cells such as eosinophils and basophils and T cells within the intestinal mucosa. On histological examination, villous atrophy along with an intense polymorph inflammatory infiltrate of the lamina propria and an enhanced number of intraepithelial T cells is seen in food-allergic enteropathy. Theoretically, food allergy is cured by an avoidance diet; however, this is not always so easy and a high degree of morbidity can be caused by this disorder.

Conclusions

The clinical stereotype presentation of abundant watery, sometimes mucous diarrhea within the first days or weeks of life can be related to a large variety of different diseases. According to the clinical characteristics, date of onset, persistence on complete bowel rest, fecal electrolyte concentration, presence of inflammatory elements or a protein-losing enteropathy, the diagnosis can be rapidly made. For early-onset constitutive enterocyte disorders a genetic background is suspected; however, no candidate genes have yet been identified. These constitutive enterocyte disorders can be related to intrinsic enterocyte defects or a defective anchoring mechanism of enterocytes. No causal or curative therapy is available; therefore, most of these children are on long-term parenteral nutrition or treated by intestinal transplantation.

Immunoallergic, inflammatory or autoimmune conditions include a second clearly distinct group of chronic enteropathies with onset early in life. Major advance were made in the role and understanding of the retrocontrol via regulatory T cells within the intestinal mucosa indicating new pathogenetic and therapeutic strategies for these disorders.

References

1 Avery GB, Villacivencio O, Lilly JR, Randolph JG: Intractable diarrhea in early infancy. Pediatrics 1968;41:712–722.
2 Schmitz J, Ginies JL, Arnaud-Battandier F, et al: Congenital microvillous atrophy, a rare cause of neonatal intractable diarrhea. Pediatr Res 1982;16:1041.
3 Cutz E, Rhoads JM, Drumm B, et al: Microvillus inclusion disease: an inherited defect of brush-border assembly and differentiation. N Engl J Med 1989;320:646–651.
4 Phillips AD, Schmitz J: Familial microvillous atrophy: a clinicopathological survey of 23 cases. J Pediatr Gastroenterol Nutr 1992;14:380–396.
5 Ruemmele FM, Jan D, Lacaille F, et al: New perspectives for children with microvillous inclusion disease: early small bowel transplantation. Transplantation 2004;77:1024–1028.
6 Reifen RM, Cutz E, Griffiths AM, et al: Tufting enteropathy a newly recognized clinicopathological entity associated with refractory diarrhea in infants. J Pediatr Gastroenterol Nutr 1994;18:379–385.
7 Goulet O, Kedinger M, Brousse N, et al: Intractable diarrhea of infancy: a new entity with epithelial and basement membrane abnormalities. J Pediatr 1995;127:212–219.
8 Giraut D, Goulet O, Ledeist F, et al: Intractable diarrhea syndrome associated with phenotypic abnormalities and immune deficiency. J Pediatr 1994;125:36–42.
9 Carruthers L, Dourmaskhin R, Phillips A: Disorders of the cytoskeleton of the enterocyte. Clin Gastroenterol 1986;15:5–20.
10 Michail S, Collins JF, Xu H, et al: Abnormal expression of brushborder membrane transporters in the duodenal mucosa of two patients with microvillous inclusion disease. J Pediatr Gastroenterol Nutr 1998;27:536–542.
11 Phillips A, Fransen J, Haari HP, Sterchi E: The constitutive exocytotic pathway in microvillous atrophy. J Pediatr Gastroenterol Nutr 1993;17:239–246.
12 Phillips AD, Brown A, Hicks S, et al: Acetylated sialic acid residues and blood group antigens localise within the epithelium in microvillous atrophy indicating internal accumulation of the glycocalyx. Gut 2004;53:1764–1771.
13 Patey N, Scoazec JY, Cuenod-Jabri B, et al: Distribution of cell adhesion molecules in infants with intestinal epithelial dysplasia (tufting enteropathy). Gastroenterology 1997;113: 833–843.
14 Ay NG, Waring P, Ristevski S, et al: Inactivation of the transcription factor Elf3 in mice results in dysmorphogenesis and altered differentiation of intestinal epithelium. Gastroenterology 2002;122:1455–1466.
15 Ruemmele FM, Brousse N, Goulet O: Autoimmune enteropathy – molecular concepts. Curr Opin Gastroenterol 2004;20:587–591.
16 Kapel N, Roman C, Caldari D, et al: Fecal TNFα and calprotectin as differential diagnostic markers for severe diarrhea of small infants. J Pediatr Gastroenterol Nutr 2005;41: 396–400.
17 Wildin RS, Smyk-Pearson S, Filipovich AH: Clinical and molecular features of the immunodysregulation, polyendocrinopathy, enteropathy, X-linked (IPEX) syndrome. J Med Genet 2002;39:537–545.
18 Gambineri E, Torgerson T, Ochs HD: Immune dysregulation, polyendocrinopathy, enteropathy, and X-linked inheritance (IPEX), a syndrome of systemic autoimmunity caused by mutations of FOXP3, a critical regulator of T-cell homeostasis. Curr Opin Rheumatol 2003;15: 430–435.
19 Bindl L, Torgerson T, Perroni L, et al: Successful use of the new immune-suppressor sirolimus in IPEX (immune dysregulation, polyendocrinopathy, enteropathy, X-linked syndrome). J Pediatr 2005;147:256–259.

20 Heine RG: Pathophysiology, diagnosis and treatment of food protein-induced gastrointestinal disease. Curr Opin Allergy Clin Immunol 2004;4:221–229.
21 Wildin RS, Ramsdell F, Peake J, et al: X-linked neonatal diabetes mellitus, enteropathy and endocrinopathy syndrome is the human equivalent of mouse scurfy. Nat Genet 2001;27: 18–20.
22 Bennett CL, Christie J, Ramsdell F, et al: The immune dysregulation, polyendocrinopathy, enteropathy X-linked syndrome (IPEX) is caused by mutations of FOXP3. Nat Genet 2001;27: 20–21.
23 Schubert LA, Jeffery E, Zhang Y, et al: Scurfin (FOXP3) acts as a repressor of transcription and regulates T cell activation. J Biol Chem 2001;276:37672–37679.
24 Bennett CL, Brunkow ME, Ramsdell F, et al: A rare polyadenylation signal mutation of the FOXP3 gene leads to the IPEX syndrome. Immunogenetics 2001;53:435–439.
25 Owen CJ, Jennings CE, Imrie H, et al: Mutational analysis of the FOXP3 gene and evidence for genetic heterogeneity in the immunodysregulation, polyendocrinopathy, enteropathy syndrome. J Clin Endocrinol Metab 2003;88:6034–6039.
26 Perez-Machado MA, Ashwood P, Thomson MA, et al: Reduced transforming growth factor beta 1-producing T cells in the duodenal mucosa of children with food allergy. Eur J Immunol 2003;33:2307–2315.
27 Karlsson H, Hessle C, Rudin A: Innate immune response of human neonatal cells to bacteria from the normal gastrointestinal flora. Infect Immun 2002;70:6688–6696.
28 Tu Y, Salim S, Bourgeois J, et al: CD23 mediated IgE transport across human intestinal epithelium: inhibition by blocking sites of translation of binding. Gastroenterology 2005;129: 928–940.

Discussion

Dr. Milla: I would not be quite so pessimistic about bone marrow transplantation for autoimmune enteropathy. We have now transplanted something like 10 patients in the UK; the first 5 rather like yours were horrendous, and they took a long time to recover. With rather better conditioning regimes things got somewhat easier and the last 3 or 4 have come through relatively well. So I am quite clear in my mind this is the way to treat them because immunosuppression is extremely toxic if you want to control a severe disease like IPEX. I don't believe we are any closer to understanding microvillous atrophy or microvillous inclusion disease, call it what you will. Whether there are really inclusions or whether it is just the apical surface thrown up into all sorts of convolutions so when you section it you appear to have an inclusion, I don't know. But what I would like you to speculate on is why do the majority of these patients die from hepatic failure?

Dr. Ruemmele: I am aware of your good data on bone marrow transplantation in IPEX patients. After multiple discussions with our immunologists, we feel that bone marrow transplantation for IPEX is perhaps most difficult, but it is hopefully the future for these patients. To your question on microvillous atrophy, in fact it is not clear how these inclusions that we see on electron microscopy really develop. To date, we can only speculate on the molecular mechanisms. With regard to your questions how do children with microvillous atrophy develop hepatic failure: these children are very unstable, and most difficult to handle and to stabilize. They often have hypovolemic shock which is very difficult to explain. I have to admit that we were able to stabilize a couple of patients without hepatic involvement, who are scheduled for isolated small bowel transplantation. This indicates that not all children necessarily develop hepatic failure, so it is perhaps the management more than the disease.

Dr. Imanzadeh: What are the definition and scientific criteria for intestinal failure?

Dr. Ruemmele: Intestinal failure can be defined as the critical reduction of functional gut mass below the minimal amount necessary for adequate digestion and absorption to satisfy body nutrient and fluid requirements, resulting in dependency on parenteral nutrition [1]. I am not sure if there is a real validated definition. In our hands it is a dependency on parenteral nutrition.

Dr. Davidson: You mentioned that the incidence of microvillous inclusion disease seems to be restricted to certain population groups, but in my experience that may not be the case. The first families that I saw with this condition were in Melbourne, Australia and they were of European Caucasian origin with two children dying in each family. Similarly in Toronto there were several Caucasian families [2]. I think this condition is not restricted to particular population groups even though it may be more common in certain groups such as the Navajo American Indian population.

Dr. Ruemmele: I completely agree with you; most of the patients we saw are of Turkish or Arab origin, but we have also French or Italian families. There are different phenotypes of the disease and, perhaps I have to add this to the question of Dr. Milla, some children have very itchy pruritus indicating perhaps a hepatic involvement for some of them. We never saw a particular genetic background.

Dr. Davidson: With regard to hepatic failure, many of these children are on long-term parenteral nutrition and this may be a contributing factor.

Dr. Milla: We are very skilled at parenteral nutrition; we know how to stop patients getting hepatic failure. But it is almost as if they are following a time table once you have kept them alive long enough, and now we have quite a large group of these patients. They almost inevitably develop hepatic failure, especially if they are those who present in the first week or so of life. It is something about their disease; I just don't believe it is parenteral nutrition, it is an acquired thing.

Dr. Saavedra: Our experience at John Hopkins is rather limited; most people have anecdotal cases more than series and hopefully we can put a large series together. We have had children with microvillous inclusion disease, a total of 3 for more than a year, who have been on parenteral nutrition without any problem, and in one case up to 3 years without liver disease. I don't know if it may or may not be geographic. The one child with liver disease had on biopsy the features of what we would consider parenteral nutrition-associated cholestasis. Intestinal failure, or what we prefer calling intestinal dysfunction, which is persistent to the point that the patient requires transplantation, we typically call failure, so there are varying degrees of dysfunction as we would call them. The dysfunction persists to the point of getting liver disease or occasionally running of central line sites, which is the other excuse for transplantation, at the point that we would typically call it failure, otherwise it is a prolonged intestinal dysfunction. You did discuss the digestive potentials of chronic illnesses that present early in life, certainly the absorptive group. But there is this large group of children with motility problems and digestive absorptive motility and barrier. Would you comment briefly on where we are with myopathies and neuropathies at the molecular level if you had to compare them to where we are with microvillous inclusion.

Dr. Ruemmele: When I presented my data I started with diarrhea and I did it this way because enteropathy is a large topic and it is very difficult to cover all aspects. If you start with the general problem and definition of intestinal failure this topic would be completely different, you have to talk about short bowel syndrome which is partially caused by intestinal failure, motility disorders and constitutive enterocyte disorders that I presented today. On intestinal failure the pathologies must be grouped differently but this is not really the point I wanted to make. A lot is known about motility disorders, such as Hirschsprung disease, there are a lot of hypotheses. Regarding mitochondrial disorders or neurological-muscular disorders, only very few data exist. I am not really able to answer all aspects of your question.

Dr. Lack: Your speculation that this might be a good model for food allergy is fascinating. One of the main differences that I see though is that this is a generic regulatory T cell defect, so it presumably would be evidence of multiple food allergies, whereas in food allergy there are 1 or 2 or 3 food allergens. First is the polyconal IgE elevated; do you actually find antigen-specific IgE on RAST testing, and do these children have positive skin prick tests?

Dr. Ruemmele: These children have the highest IgE levels you ever saw. In our institution, we normally see IgE levels lower than 40 kU during the first year of life. However IPEX boys often have several thousands, up to 70,000 kU, and if you perform RAST testing they are all positive. We did not go further to test if these IgE levels are really functional. It is not very surprising when you have 10,000 times the normal level, you find cross-reaction.

Dr. Lack: Do they have immediate hypersensitivity when you give them foods?

Dr. Ruemmele: They show both. They have immediate and also delayed symptoms. They never have pulmonary symptoms. In our institution we followed 12 patients and none of them developed pulmonary symptoms. I am not sure if this is part of this entity. IPEX boys never wheeze; they only have skin and GI symptoms, both immediate and delayed type.

Dr. S. Koletzko: Did you or anybody in the audience also see mild cases of IPEX syndrome or are they always severe? If we intervene with bone marrow transplantation it should be done early before the toxic effect of the therapy comes on. Or is there any mild form?

Dr. Ruemmele: There are very few data in the literature. Powell et al. [3] described a family with 18 male members who have a very mild form. They have survived until adult age and have minimal immunosuppression. The genetic defect in this family does not affect the FOXP3 gene but it does affect the polyacids just before the gene. It is incomplete regulation of the gene. With Michael Lentze we had a patient in Bonn who presented with the first symptoms at the age of 7 years. He had been treated for severe food allergy, which was not as severe as IPEX. His disease worsened and at the age of 15 years we made the diagnosis on a genetic basis revealing a substitution of one single amino acid in the FOXP3 gene. So yes, mild forms or atypical forms exist, and it is worth testing all patients we suspect to have a form of autoimmune enteropathy on FOXP3 mutations.

Dr. Milla: I guess it also depends on what you mean by autoimmune enteropathy because IPEX is not the only form of autoimmune enteropathy. There are at least 4 different syndromes and if you call autoimmune enteropathy the ability of an enterocyte to produce an autoantibody or the ability of the immunocytes to produce an autoantibody against enterocyte components, then there are probably a lot of different syndromes. If you look at the early literature that describes autoimmune enteropathy there are quite a few patients who do not fit into the IPEX phenotype. Many of them are girls and they often have rather mild disease, and respond just to food elimination. The last part of Dr. Ruemmele's talk about barrier function is very interesting because of the consequences of the loss of barrier function and the way in which the gut-associated lymphoid tissue responds to that. Surely one possibility is that it responds by producing autoantibodies and maybe not in very severe IPEX-like phenotype. At least that is what is in the literature.

Dr. Ruemmele: I completely agree, I emphasized IPEX because we know the molecular basis; however other forms of autoimmune enteropathy exist. Girls do not develop IPEX, at least it has never been described, but we know some little girls with autoimmune GI diseases. For me, the definition of autoimmune enteropathy is the production of autoimmune antibodies directed against the gut combined with the clinical picture of a protein-losing enteropathy. IPEX is a particular form, very severe, in a subgroup of patients.

Dr. Sorensen: Do girls really never develop it? In many immune deficiency diseases, in situations of extreme lionization, female carriers can express a form of the disease.

Dr. Ruemmele: You are right and in fact there are some patients who you think have IPEX but it cannot be proven on a molecular basis. All the publications, except one, a very curious publication, checked the girls and the family members. I showed you over 4 generations with 22 female carriers who do not have a single symptom; they are not atopic, they have nothing. So it is very unlikely but I have never heard of this kind of pathology.

Dr. Lentze: I talked to one of my Dutch colleagues today because children in the Netherlands start to eat peanut butter very early and he told me they don't have peanut allergies in the Netherlands. So perhaps Dr. Kneepkens can say something. Is that true?

Dr. Kneepkens: Of course we have peanut allergy in the Netherlands but not to the extent that you see it in England or in the US. Maybe that is the point, maybe we are more like Israel.

References

1   Goulet O, Ruemmele F: Causes and management of intestinal failure in children. Gastroenterology. 2006;130(suppl 1):S16–S28.
2   Davidson GP, Cutz E, Hamilton JR, Gall GD: Familial enteropathy: a syndrome of protracted diarrhea from birth, failure to thrive, and hypoplastic villous atrophy. Gastroenterology 1978;75:783–790.
3   Powell BR, Buist NRM, Stenzel P: An X-linked syndrome of diarrhea, polyendocrinopathy, and fatal infection in infancy. J Pediatr 1982;100:731–737.

Cooke RJ, Vandenplas Y, Wahn U (eds): Nutrition Support for Infants and Children at Risk.
Nestlé Nutr Workshop Ser Pediatr Program, vol 59, pp 89–104,
Nestec Ltd., Vevey/S. Karger AG, Basel, © 2007.

Chronic Enteropathy: Clinical Aspects

Troy Gibbons, George J. Fuchs

University of Arkansas for Medical Sciences, Arkansas Children's Hospital,
Little Rock, AR, USA

Abstract

Diarrheal disease is a major cause of childhood morbidity and mortality worldwide.
Chronic enteropathy with subsequent persistent diarrhea and associated vicious
cycles of malnutrition, increased gut permeability and secondary immunodeficiency
are particularly devastating in the childhood population. The major causes of chronic
enteropathy differ significantly between developed countries and developing countries. In developed countries, infectious and postinfectious diarrhea as well as abnormalities in immune response including celiac disease, food-induced allergic enteropathy
and idiopathic inflammatory bowel disease account for most cases of chronic
enteropathy. In developing countries, syndromic persistent diarrhea associated with
malnutrition and secondary immunodeficiency due to human immunodeficiency virus
(HIV) infection predominate as the major causes of chronic enteropathy. These latter
two causes account for a disproportionate share of the more than 2.5 million deaths of
children under 5 years of age due to diarrhea each year worldwide. From a practical
perspective, diagnostic evaluation of chronic enteropathy in developing countries is
often limited to identifying potential causative enteropathogens and antimicrobial
treatment. Proper management with an emphasis on fluid homeostasis and proto-
colized nutritional therapy and rehabilitation is essential to successful treatment of
syndromic persistent diarrhea.

Copyright © 2007 Nestec Ltd., Vevey/S. Karger AG, Basel

Introduction

Diarrheal disease remains a major cause of all childhood morbidity and
mortality. Chronic enteropathy leading to persistent diarrhea is particularly
damaging, although the major causes differ between developed and developing countries with socioeconomic and nutritional status being the main determinants. From a global perspective, chronic enteropathy manifested as
syndromic persistent diarrhea accounts for a disproportionate share of the

more than 2.5 million deaths each year of children under 5 years of age due to all diarrheal illness.

Defining Chronic Enteropathy

For the present discussion, chronic enteropathy is defined as chronic functional derangement of the small bowel. The primary consequence of chronic enteropathy is persistent diarrhea which is loose or watery stools at least 3 times per day of more than 14 days' duration, with change in stool consistency more meaningful than stool frequency. Depending on the specific pathophysiology, other symptoms may dominate the clinical picture; for example, Crohn's disease may present with bloody stool or the child with celiac disease (CD) who, able to partially compensate for reduced absorptive capacity by increasing dietary intake, may present with stunting.

Infectious Enteropathy

Postinfectious persistent diarrhea occurs in infants and young children associated with a variety of enteric viral and bacterial pathogens that cause acute infectious diarrheal disease including rotavirus, enteric adenovirus, astrovirus, *Shigella*, and *Salmonella*, among others. Postinfectious diarrhea may follow a single severe episode of acute diarrhea or more commonly repeated distinct episodes of acute diarrhea by different pathogens, persisting well after the inciting infectious agent is no longer detectable. Secondary disaccharidase deficiency and sensitization to food antigens due to small bowel mucosal damage leading to disaccharide malabsorption as central mechanisms of postinfectious persistent diarrhea, while operative in some children, has been shown to be less prevalent than initially thought. When postinfectious persistent diarrhea occurs in the context of malnutrition, it is often referred to as syndromic persistent diarrhea because of stereotypical pathophysiologic derangements and treatment implications. In contrast, certain pathogens are associated with chronic enteric infection and chronic enteropathy resulting in prolonged watery diarrhea that is often profuse and with growth failure and malnutrition (table 1) [1]. *Giardia*, *Cryptosporidia*, and *Cyclospora* are common causes of persistent diarrhea and poor nutritional outcomes in both immunocompetent and immunocompromised children. Two diarrheagenic *Escherichia coli*, enteropathogenic *E. coli* (EPEC) and enteroaggregative *E. coli* (EaggEC), are the most important bacterial causes of persistent diarrhea in children. EPEC is a major pathogen in children less than 1 year and especially less than 6 months of age; compared to other pathogens, EPEC has been associated with more severe diarrhea and dehydration, cow's milk intolerance, and progression to persistent diarrhea [2].

Table 1. Causes of chronic enteropathy in children

	Comments
Enteric infection *Giardia lamblia* *Cryptosporidia parvum* *Cyclospora cayetanensis* EaggEC EPEC *Mycobacterium avium-intracellulare* complex *Isospora belli* *Microsporidia*	*Mycobacterium-avium intracellulare*, *Isospora*, and *Microsporidia* occur in inadequately treated HIV infection

Immune deficiency
 Primary immune deficiencies (enteric
  infection including small bowel
  overgrowth)
 Secondary immune deficiencies
   Protein energy and
   micronutrient malnutrition, HIV
	Primary immune deficiencies are uncommon causes; secondary immune deficiencies including due to HIV infection and malnutrition are major causes worldwide

Abnormal immune response
 CD
 Food-allergic enteropathy
 Autoimmune disorders
  Autoimmune enteropathy
  Graft versus host disease	

Idiopathic inflammatory bowel disease Crohn's disease	More common in developed countries

Congenital persistent diarrhea
 (structural defects?)
  Microvillus inclusion disease
  Tufting enteropathy
  Congenital chloride diarrhea
  Congenital disaccharidase (lactase,
  sucrase-isomaltase) deficiencies
  Congenital bile acid malabsorption
	Rare

Syndromic persistent diarrhea (associated with malnutrition)	Of greatest importance worldwide

EaggEC is the most common cause of persistent diarrhea and its nutritional sequelae in many children in developing countries [3].

Immune Deficiency Including Human Immunodeficiency Virus

The mucosal lining of the gastrointestinal tact is constantly exposed to an ever-changing environment rich in microbial pathogens, dietary antigens and

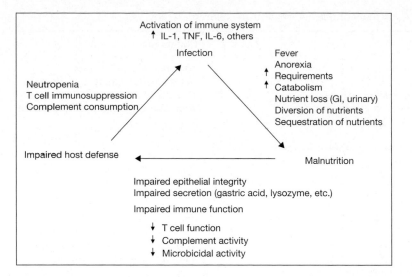

Fig. 1. The vicious cycle of infection, malnutrition, and immune dysfunction.

toxins. The immune system plays a pivotal role in ensuring homeostasis is maintained within the system. The immune-deficient child is susceptible to common gastrointestinal infections that can occur in the immune-competent host; however, chronic enteropathy in immunodeficiency is characterized by recurrent, persistent, severe unusual and opportunistic infections with subsequent secondary malabsorption and maldigestion states. The immune-deficient child with persistent diarrhea often rapidly spirals into a cycle of anorexia, inadequate dietary intake, catabolic losses to combat infection, and catabolic losses from the gastrointestinal tract (fig. 1). Micronutrient and general malnutrition are key risk factors for as well as consequences of many chronic enteropathies resulting in well-defined impairments of immunity. The combination of immunodeficiency, malnutrition, and chronic enteropathy and their mutually reinforcing properties is a major global cause of childhood morbidity and mortality (discussed in greater detail under the heading Syndromic Persistent Diarrhea below). Optimal management includes aggressive search and treatment of infectious etiologies for chronic enteropathy, fluid and electrolyte replacement, close monitoring of nutritional status, and nutritional rehabilitation.

Though generally rare, over 70 different primary immunodeficiencies have been described. Chronic enteropathy is commonly associated with many of these, although the precise abnormalities as well as risk for and type of enteric infection may differ depending on the specific aspect of the immune system that is abnormal. Treatment effects of primary immune deficiency can have a role in the development of chronic enteropathy, such as graft versus host disease involving the bowel following bone marrow transplantation.

From a global prospective, chronic enteropathies associated with secondary immunodeficiency states are perhaps the most consequential in terms of total numbers of children affected and morbidity and mortality. Primary malnutrition and human immunodeficiency virus (HIV)/acquired immunodeficiency syndrome (AIDS) constitute the majority of cases of secondary immunodeficiency. The World Health Organization AIDS Epidemic Update in December 2005 estimates that 40.3 million people are infected with HIV worldwide, 90% of whom live in resource-poor settings in Asia, Africa, and South America [4]. Secondary malnutrition and persistent diarrhea are the hallmarks of inadequately treated HIV. Children with HIV are susceptible to all of the pathogens causing persistent diarrhea in the immunocompetent child as well as to opportunistic pathogens that rarely make otherwise normal children ill. Chronic diarrhea and secondary malnutrition are nearly universal comorbidities in HIV-affected people living in developing countries [5]. Indeed, persistent diarrhea in HIV-infected children can be attributable to the HIV-induced malnutrition as an important associated risk factor [6]. *Cryptosporidia*, *Giardia*, and the opportunistic pathogens *Mycobacterium avium-intracellulare*, *Isospora*, and *Microsporidia* are associated with immune deficiency states and especially inadequately treated, advanced HIV infection and AIDS. Individuals with HIV/AIDS are not uncommonly infected with multiple pathogens. Immune recovery related to highly active antiretroviral therapy has led to resolution of persistent diarrhea due to opportunistic infections previously considered untreatable. However, since highly active antiretroviral therapy is not accessible by the great majority of HIV-infected children in developing countries, these pathogens remain important causes of morbidity and mortality in this population [7]. Not all cases of persistent diarrhea in advanced HIV/AIDS have an infectious etiology and in up to 45% of patients no enteric pathogen can be identified [8]. The enteropathy is characterized by reduced villous height and increased crypt depth, with severity of enteropathy often independent of infection but related to nutritional status and immune dysregulation [9, 10]. Other important causes of persistent diarrhea include side effects of protease inhibitors in up to 50% of patients, gastrointestinal malignancies of Kaposi sarcoma and lymphoma, and 'HIV enteropathy' [11, 12].

Abnormal Immune Response

Celiac Disease
CD is complex autoimmune enteropathy caused by a permanent sensitivity to gluten in genetically predisposed individuals. European and US studies indicate the prevalence of CD in children between 2.5 and 15 years is approximately 3–13 per 1,000 children [13]. Previously considered rare in children in developing

countries, more recent evidence challenges this view [14]. In some ways, CD also represents an important form of food-allergic enteropathy. Small bowel damage occurs following mucosal exposure to ingested wheat gluten and similar grains, most notably rye and barely. Unlike other food-allergic enteropathies, CD susceptibility is determined in part by a common HLA association, namely the major histocompatibility complex class II antigens HLA-DQ2 (86–100% patients) and HLA-DQ8 (5% patients) haplotypes. Gliadin, the main wheat protein, presented by HLA-DQ2 and/or HLA-DQ8 molecules to T cells stimulates production of proinflammatory cytokines that damage intestinal mucosa and activate plasma cells to produce antibodies to gliadin, tissue transglutaminase (TTG), and endomysium.

While symptoms can be protean and nongastrointestinal, the classical clinical expression of CD in children is a persistent malabsorptive enteropathy and diarrhea, malnutrition, abdominal pain, vomiting and abdominal distention. Nongastrointestinal symptoms may predominate and occur in the apparent absence or subtle gastrointestinal symptoms and include proximal muscle wasting, dermatitis herpetiformis, dental enamel hypoplasia of permanent teeth, osteoporosis, short stature, delayed puberty, iron deficiency anemia resistant to oral iron, among others. The risk of CD is much higher among first-degree than second-degree relatives and in children with certain chronic disease such as type-1 diabetes mellitus (2–5%) and autoimmune disorders, IgA deficiency (10%), Down's syndrome (10%), Turner's syndrome, and Williams syndrome.

Diagnosis of CD is defined by characteristic changes seen on small intestinal histology: villous atrophy, crypt hyperplasia and increased intraepithelial lymphocytes. With the advent of accurate serologic markers and in cases where there is full clinical remission with gluten withdrawal from diet, it is no longer considered necessary to confirm the diagnosis by gluten challenge and repeat biopsy. Of available serological tests, neither IgG nor IgA antigliadin antibody test is routinely recommended due to variable sensitivity and specificity. Measurement of IgA antibody to human recombinant TTG is recommended and is highly sensitive and specific; IgA antibody to endomysium is as accurate as TTG but observer dependent and hence subject to error. In patients with features suggestive of CD concomitant assessment for IgA deficiency is helpful since IgA deficiency is associated with CD and a low TTG IgA in this context is not reassuring. In such a case, TTG IgG levels should be determined. Once the diagnosis is confirmed, the only treatment is lifelong use of a gluten-free diet. Compliance in children and especially the adolescent is always a problem. TTG level may be used to monitor dietary adherence.

Food-Induced Allergic Enteropathy

There are three clinically distinct food protein-induced gastrointestinal disorders that can involve the small bowel and cause persistent diarrhea: enterocolitis syndrome, enteropathy, and eosinophilic gastroenteritis. Food protein enterocolitis syndrome is a cell-mediated hypersensitivity disorder that typically occurs in infants within the first 3 months of life, most commonly in reaction to ingested dairy or soy protein [15]. The disease process is often restricted to the distal colon and is the most common cause of bloody stool in infants in developed countries following enteric *Salmonella* infection. Involvement of the small bowel as well as colon typically manifests as watery or bloody diarrhea, vomiting, and failure to thrive if diagnosis is delayed. Food protein-induced enteropathy (excluding CD) is an uncommon condition that occurs within the first several months of life and is manifested by persistent diarrhea and malabsorption; clinical presentation is the same as classical CD but usually with vomiting. Histological changes can be very similar to that found in CD, but less severe [16]. There is patchy distribution of mucosal damage, some degree of villous atrophy, crypt hyperplasia, and increased intraepithelial lymphocytes. As with dietary protein enterocolitis, dairy and soy protein are the typical offending antigens. The underlying immune dysregulation shares many of the features of CD; its relationship, if any, to the dietary protein enterocolitis syndrome is unknown. Eosinophilic gastroenteritis is a rare, incompletely understood disorder that at times but not always is associated with an identifiable dietary antigen. It is IgE and/or cell-mediated and can occur at any age. Clinical presentation depends on the anatomic site of gastrointestinal involvement and depth of eosinophilic infiltration; when manifested as an enteropathy, diarrhea, iron deficiency anemia, and protein-losing enteropathy are characteristic. In contrast to food protein-induced enteropathy, eosinophilic inflammation is the distinguishing histological finding. The double-blind, placebo-controlled oral food challenge remains the gold standard for diagnosis of food-induced allergic disorders especially for cell-mediated sensitivities, but there are often practical limitations to its use. Diagnosis therefore often depends heavily on the medical history, attempting to determine if a food reaction is a possible cause, the specific food implicated, and whether the condition likely represents a cell-mediated or IgE reaction. Skin prick tests are useful in screening for IgE-mediated food sensitivity, with a larger size wheal increasing the specificity. The greatest value of skin testing is a negative test, which confirms the absence of an IgE-mediated dietary allergy. However a positive skin test combined with an unequivocal history implicating a specific food is considered diagnostic by many. RAST testing provides similar qualitative diagnostic information but is increasingly being replaced by quantitative food-specific serum IgE which has greater positive predictive value. Intestinal biopsy has a particular complementary role in diagnosis of food allergic enteropathy.

Autoimmune Enteropathy

Autoimmune enteropathy is a rare disorder that usually results in death in early infancy or childhood. Its hallmarks are severe, protracted diarrhea and antienterocyte antibodies along the apex and basolateral enterocyte border

95

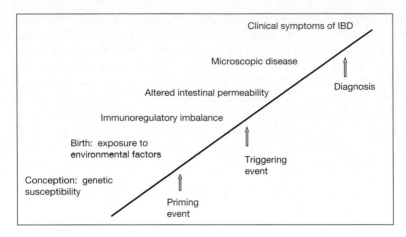

Fig. 2. Conceptual framework of Crohn's disease etiology. IBD = Inflammatory bowel disease.

[17]. It is frequently associated with extraintestinal disease including diabetes mellitus, glomerulopathy, and hemolytic disease as well as immunodeficiency such as IPEX (immunodysregulation, polyendocrinopathy and enteropathy, X-linked) syndrome.

Idiopathic Inflammatory Bowel Disease: Crohn's Disease

Crohn's disease is a chronic inflammatory disorder that can affect any part of the gastrointestinal tract; involvement of the small bowel may be referred to as Crohn's enteritis. Crohn's disease is comparatively more common in North America and Europe which have the highest incidence; the disease is relatively rare elsewhere, particularly in developing countries. To put it in context of all causes of enteropathy, recent data suggests the incidence of all childhood and adolescent Crohn's disease in northern hemisphere countries is estimated to be 2–3.7 cases per 100,000. The cause of Crohn's disease has not been defined, although the pathogenesis is complex involving an interrelation between genetic predisposition and environmental factors (fig. 2). The intestinal manifestations reflect the anatomic site of involvement, with Crohn's enteritis manifested in various combinations as diarrhea, fever, occult or gross blood in the stool, abdominal pain, aphthous ulcers, weight loss and malnutrition. Numerous extraintestinal manifestations can be associated including joint involvement (arthritis, ankylosing spondylitis and arthralgia), eye involvement (uveitis, episcleritis and orbital myositis), liver (primary sclerosing cholangitis) and skin (erythema nodosum and pyoderma gangrenosum). Management is focused on treating acute presenting disease or exacerbation and, once controlled, maintaining remission while ensuring adequate nutritional status. A variety of anti-inflammatory and immune-modulating agents are used depending on severity and site of disease activity. The more recent introduction of biological agents targeting specific host immune components such as tumor necrosis factor-α represents a new class of agents that improve the ability to reach treatment goals; however, there are no long-term studies of the use of these drugs in the pediatric population.

Congenital Persistent Diarrhea

These quite rare, severe chronic enteropathies include microvillus inclusion disease, tufting enteropathy, congenital chloride diarrhea, and congenital disaccharidase deficiencies [18]. These are conditions of defects in epithelial structure or gut transport mechanisms and present within hours to days of birth (table 1). Except for the disaccharidase deficiencies, the diarrhea is predominantly secretory and may lead to life-threatening electrolyte abnormalities and malnutrition. In the case of congenital diarrhea due to ultrastructural abnormalities, total parental nutrition with subsequent intestinal transplant is the likely route of management. A subset of early onset protracted diarrhea involves the primary maldigestion and malabsorption disorders. Though quite rare, secondary maldigestion and malabsorption form an integral part of almost all chronic enteropathies. Primary maldigestion arising from the intestinal tract is rare and includes congenital enterokinase deficiency which results in abnormal stool and failure to thrive from birth. The diagnosis is suspected when exogenous enterokinase restores proteolytic activity in duodenal juice and can be confirmed by direct measurement of enterokinase activity in the duodenal mucosa. Congenital sucrase-isomaltase deficiency and the extremely rare congenital lactase deficiency with corresponding disaccharide malabsorption are characterized by loose or liquid stool often with low stool pH due to fermentation. Congenital disaccharidase deficiency may be determined by a breath hydrogen test using the suspected sugar; however, intestinal biopsy with quantification of disaccharidase activity is the reference standard diagnostic test.

Syndromic Persistent Diarrhea

Syndromic persistent diarrhea in context of the current discussion refers to a condition of chronic enteropathy and diarrhea in infants and young children in developing countries, typically associated with malnutrition often in a vicious cycle, downward spiral relationship (fig. 3). While persistent diarrhea constitutes less than 10% of all diarrheal episodes in developing countries, it

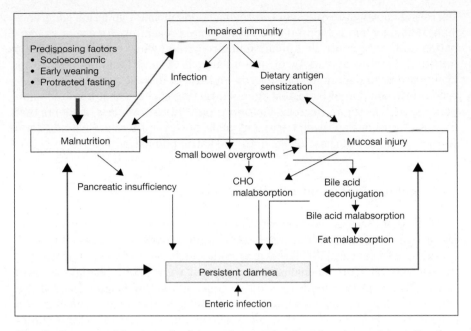

Fig. 3. Conceptual framework of the pathogenesis of syndromic persistent diarrhea.
CHO = Carbohydrate.

accounts for 30–50% of all diarrheal deaths. Risk factors include antecedent
general malnutrition, vitamin A or zinc micronutrient deficiency, and nonexclusive breastfeeding in early infancy. The pathogenesis is undeniably complex and multifactorial; however, prolonged small bowel damage is a final
common pathway [19]. Infectious and food-sensitive enteropathies have been
proposed as distinct and sometimes concomitant mechanisms contributing
to development of syndromic persistent diarrhea, although their relative
importance is not fully defined. Persistence of diarrhea may follow a single
episode of infectious diarrhea in a malnourished child or repeated distinct
episodes of acute diarrhea by different pathogens leading to malnutrition and
persisting well after the inciting enteropathogen is no longer detectable. This
is discussed in more detail in a preceding section, Infectious Enteropathy.
Evidence also implicates dietary antigen sensitization due to increased intestinal permeability caused by acute or chronic diarrhea and that leads to allergic enteropathy, usually dairy soy, in the vulnerable patient.

Protein energy as well as micronutrient malnutrition promote persistent
diarrhea by structural and functional abnormalities including alterations in
host defense, immune dysfunction, mucosal injury, and impaired intestinal
repair [20]. Gastric acid output is decreased in malnourished children, leading to a compromised gastric barrier against oral bacteria and important

pH-sensitive enteropathogens, notably *Shigella* and *Vibrio cholerae*. Abnormalities of the small intestine are variable, but typically include chronic cell-mediated enteropathy with crypt hyperplasia, villous atrophy, and marked increase in intraepithelial lymphocytes. Mucosal profile indicates an imbalance that favors proinflammatory overregulatory cytokines and a poorly controlled Th1 cell-mediated proinflammatory response that accounts for many of the histological changes. Several factors in combination explain the observed pathology in syndromic persistent diarrhea including small bowel bacterial overgrowth and subsequent bile acid deconjugation, impaired motility, reduced pancreatic and biliary secretions, and abnormal intestinal immunity and especially reduced secretory IgA. Protein energy malnutrition and/or micronutrient deficiencies such as zinc, copper, selenium, iron, vitamin A, vitamin C, and vitamin E result in consequential immune dysfunction. Disruption of mucosal surfaces and increased intestinal permeability integrity lead to nutrient and bile acid malabsorption, fluid and electrolyte losses, and translocation of endotoxin and dietary allergen with pathologic sequelae including sepsis [21]. Even the 'healthy undernourished' child has increased intestinal permeability and mucosal cellular immune changes that can affect long-term growth and may be the underlying cause of tropical enteropathy in malnutrition [22].

From a practical clinical perspective, diagnostic studies are limited to testing of stool for enteric pathogens amenable to specific antimicrobial therapy. Because certain fundamental abnormalities are stereotypical while others vary at any given point in time, costly testing to document abnormalities such as small bowel overgrowth, disaccharide or fat malabsorption, among others does not lead to a change in management and therefore are not routinely necessary. In resource-constrained developing countries, this is especially important. Proper management, essential to achieve recovery and reduce mortality, is focused on fluid and electrolyte homeostasis and systematic enteral nutritional rehabilitation. Fluid and electrolyte replacement is best achieved using a reduced osmolarity oral rehydration solution [23]. The addition of soluble fiber to the oral rehydration solution promotes rehydration and recovery through its property as a short chain fatty acid precursor that uniquely promotes colonic as well as small bowel recovery [24, 25]. Algorithmic dietary management using locally available foods and simple clinical guidelines is effective in most children [26]. Breast milk feeding should be continued for children who are not weaned in addition to the therapeutic diets described in the algorithm. Lactose malabsorption, previously considered a common limiting factor in recovery, is problematic in a relatively small proportion of children; lactose-free diets therefore are reserved for the few children who fail diets containing modest amounts of lactose. Micronutrients have a key role in the treatment and prevention of persistent diarrhea; zinc supplementation of children with persistent diarrhea promotes earlier recovery and may prevent death while combined zinc and vitamin A supplementation synergistically prevent persistent diarrhea [27, 28]. Severe malnutrition, common in children with persistent diarrhea, treated using a malnutrition management protocol significantly increases the likelihood of survival and includes diets described above but with additional nutritional interventions, avoidance of intravenous fluids, anticipatory antibiotic therapy, and prevention or prompt management of hypothermia and hypoglycemia [29].

Approach to Defining Cause of Chronic Enteropathy

There are numerous causes for chronic enteropathy in children and all methods of categorizing have their advantages and deficiencies. The majority of the worldwide burden of chronic enteropathy is due to malnutrition and secondary immune deficiency and should be readily diagnosed if in the associated context; most other forms of chronic enteropathy are rare. Regardless, a detailed and careful history is of primary importance in determining the potential causes of chronic enteropathy in the individual child and avoiding unnecessary and costly investigations. Clues to early onset enteropathy may be contained in the prenatal history such as a mother's infectious status including exposure to HIV. In environments where antenatal ultrasonography is routine, fetal fluid-filled dilated loops of intestine and polyhydramnios may be an early indication of congenital enteropathy syndrome such as congenital chloride-losing diarrhea. A careful history of the age and time of onset of symptoms should be obtained. An association with feeding type, feeding modifications including early introduction of complementary feeding, and extraintestinal manifestations such as recurrent pneumonias, neutropenia, arthritis, mouth ulcers and a family history of similar illness may all provide clues to the underlying pathology.

References

1 Ochoa TJ, Salazar-Lindo E, Cleary TG: Management of children with infection-associated persistent diarrhea. Semin Pediatr Infect Dis 2004;15:229–236.
2 Fagundes-Neto U, Scaletsky IC: The gut at war: the consequences of enteropathogenic *Escherichia coli* infection as factor of diarrhea and malnutrition. Sao Paulo Med J 2000;118: 21–29.
3 Steiner TS, Lima AA, Nataro JP, Guerrant RL: Enteroaggregative *Escherichia coli* produce intestinal inflammation and growth impairment and cause interleukin-8 release from intestinal epithelial cells. J Infect Dis 1998;177:88–96.
4 AIDS epidemic: update December 2005: Joint United Nations Programme on HIV/AIDS (UNAIDS) and World Health Organization (WHO), 2005.
5 Monkemuller KE, Wilcox CM: Investigation of diarrhea in AIDS. Can J Gastroenterol 2000;14: 933–940.
6 Johnson S, Hendson W, Crew-Brown H, et al: Effect of human immunodeficiency virus infection on episodes of diarrhea among children in South Africa. Pediatr Infect Dis J 2000;19: 972–979.
7 Rosen S, Sanne I, Collier A, Simon JL: Hard choices: rationing antiretroviral therapy for HIV/AIDS in Africa. Lancet 2005;365:354–356.

8 Cárcamo C, Hooton T, Wener MH, et al: Etiologies and manifestations of persistent diarrhea in adults with HIV-1 infection: a case-control study in Lima, Peru. J Infect Dis 2005;191:11–19.
9 Kelly P, Davies SE, Mandanda B, et al: Enteropathy in Zambians with HIV related diarrhoea: regression modeling of potential determinants of mucosal damage. Gut 1997;41:811–816.
10 Brink AK, Mahé C, Watera C, et al: Diarrhoea, CD4 counts and enteric infections in a community-based cohort of HIV-infected adults in Uganda. J Infect 2002;45:99–106.
11 Kartalija M, Sande MA: Diarrhea and AIDS in the era of highly active antiretroviral therapy. Clin Infect Dis 1999;28:701–707.
12 Kotler DP: HIV infection and the gastrointestinal tract. AIDS 2005;19:107–117.
13 Hill ID, Dirks MH, Liptak GS, et al: Guidelines for the diagnosis and treatment of celiac disease in children: recommendations of the North American Society for Pediatric Gastroenterology, Hepatology, and Nutrition. J Pediatr Gastroenterol Nutr 2005;40:1–19.
14 Bhatnagar S, Gupta SD, Mathur M, et al: Celiac disease with mild to moderate histologic changes is a common cause of chronic diarrhea in Indian children. J Pediatr Gastroenterol Nutr 2005;41:204–209.
15 Sampson HA: Update on food allergy. J Allergy Clin Immunol 2004;113:805–819.
16 Savilahti E: Food-induced malabsorption syndromes. J Pediatr Gastroenterol Nutr 2000;30 (suppl):S61–S66.
17 Russo P, Brochu P, Seidman EG, Roy CC: Autoimmune enteropathy. Pediatr Dev Pathol 1999;2:65–71.
18 Murch SH: Toward a molecular understanding of complex childhood enteropathies. J Pediatr Gastroenterol Nutr 2002;34:S4–S10.
19 Sullivan PB: Studies of the small intestine in persistent diarrhea and malnutrition: the Gambian experience. J Pediatr Gastroenterol Nutr 2002;34:S11–S13.
20 Cunningham-Rundles S, McNeeley DF, Moon A: Mechanisms of nutrient modulation of the immune response. J Allergy Clin Immunol 2005;115:1119–1128.
21 Lunn PG, Northrop-Clewes CA, Downes RM: Recent developments in the nutritional management of diarrhoea. 2. Chronic diarrhoea and malnutrition in The Gambia: studies on intestinal permeability. Trans R Soc Trop Med Hyg 1991;85:8–11.
22 Campbell DI, Lunn PG, Elia M: Age-related association of small intestinal mucosal enteropathy with nutritional status in rural Gambian children. Br J Nutr 2002;88:499–505.
23 Sarker SA, Mahalanabis D, Alam NH, et al: Reduced osmolarity oral rehydration solution in severe persistent diarrhoea in infants: a randomized controlled clinical trial. J Pediatr 2001;138: 532–538.
24 Rabbani GH, Teka T, Zaman B, et al: Clinical studies in persistent diarrhea: dietary management with green banana or pectin in Bangladeshi children. Gastroenterology 2001;121: 554–560.
25 Alam NH, Meier R, Sarker SA, et al: Partially hydrolysed guar gum supplemented comminuted chicken diet in persistent diarrhoea: a randomized controlled trial. Arch Dis Child 2005;90: 195–199.
26 International Working Group on Persistent Diarrhea: Evaluation of an algorithm for the treatment of persistent diarrhea: a multicentre study. Bull WHO 1996;74:479–489.
27 Bhutta ZA, Bird SM, Black RE, et al: Therapeutic effects of oral zinc in acute and persistent diarrhea in children in developing countries: pooled analysis of randomized controlled trials. Am J Clin Nutr 2000;72:1516–1522.
28 Rahman MM, Vermund SH, Wahed MA, et al: Simultaneous zinc and vitamin A supplementation in Bangladeshi children: randomized double blind controlled trial. BMJ 2001;323: 314–318.
29 Ahmed T, Ali M, Ullah MM, et al: Reduced mortality among severely malnourished children with diarrhoea through the use of a standardized management protocol. Lancet 1999;353: 1919–1922.

Discussion

Dr. Chubarova: Could you please tell us the distinguishing criteria between hypertrophy of the mucosa, normal mucosa and atrophy, I mean villus-crypt relation or maybe the height of the villus?

Dr. Fuchs: I am not sure I fully understand your question but typically what happens is that crypt cell hypertrophy is relative to the villus, which reflects increased secretion by the crypt cell and decreased absorption by the apical cell.

Dr. Chubarova: It seems absolutely clear in your figures and when we take a biopsy we want to know the figures. How many micrometers is normal?

Dr. Fuchs: I have to apologize; I don't know the specific cutoff value.

Dr. Chubarova: Maybe for LH that we are talking about?

Dr. Fuchs: Does anybody else want to comment on that?

Dr. Milla: Most of us used to look at the villus-crypt ratio as a means of determining the normality of the mucosa and it varies at different ages. In adults you would expect the villus to be at least 3 maybe 4 times as long as a crypt; this is a simple way of determining whether the mucosa is normal or not. In younger children you would probably use a range of 2.5–3 as the villus-crypt ratio. The thing that you look at rather than measuring the length of the villus in micrometers is the relationship of the villus to the crypt. When the crypt becomes longer than the villus you start talking about crypt hypertrophy. But there are other signs of crypt hypertrophy as well insofar as you have to have an increased turnover of cells before looking to see if there is increased mitosis in the crypt; in other words the crypt contains too many dividing cells.

Dr. Balanag: Do you have any data showing what would happen in a patient with chronic diarrhea treated with probiotics, and then it is found that the patient has HIV?

Dr. Fuchs: The data on probiotics which I am familiar with are not convincing. There are some encouraging data but I have not seen anything that suggests that we should routinely recommend probiotics. Of course there are great differences in types of probiotic bacteria and dose amount. But of course the concern in any immune-deficient individual given probiotics is the potential for infection by these organisms that, based on a few case reports coupled with the lack of defined efficacy, make it hard to recommend them at this point.

Dr. Saavedra: You showed a couple slides relative to the frequency of pathogens in different geographic areas, and in one of them it is obvious that in many developing countries there is a very low percentage of rotavirus diarrhea. Is the percentage low because there are so many other pathogens and not because there is little rotavirus diarrhea? The point being that rotavirus diarrhea is probably there, it is just overwhelmed by the frequency of other bacterial pathogens. I do think rotavirus has a practical relevance to this vicious cycle of diarrhea and malnutrition in developing countries. Ultimately we need to rehabilitate the patient nutritionally because that is how they will recover from whatever the original pathogen was. What should we do for prevention? Would therapies that might prevent rotavirus diarrhea in developing countries make a difference?

Dr. Fuchs: I was showing the prevalence of pathogens associated with persistent diarrhea and, in this regard, we think of rotavirus as generally being associated with acute diarrhea. I know you have done quite a bit of work with probiotics in the prevention of rotavirus. The encouraging data are primarily from developed countries where use may be more feasible. I don't know if developing countries are in a position to apply probiotics for no other reason than cost. Expenditure on health care in developing countries averages USD 12–15 or less per child per year for all health care including immunizations, micronutrient supplementation, etc. So one has to prioritize which interventions to implement. You are right that we must consider not only the type of bacteria but the dose of the bacteria as well. I and my colleagues have studied different probiotic preparations of the same bacteria from different manufacturers and have seen positive effects by some but not others; the dosing and concentration of organisms were different not the type.

Dr. Rivera: I have to disagree with the data presented on rotavirus and persistent diarrhea. In the *New England Journal of Medicine* we published a paper on the efficacy of a new rotavirus vaccine [1]. Our epidemiological data showed that 63% of acute diarrhea was due to rotavirus vaccine. Furthermore we found that up to 10% of those cases of rotavirus had persistent diarrhea rather than the 5% that you reported.

Dr. Fuchs: Again this was persistent diarrhea, and you are absolutely right there are all sorts of explanations for the variation in rates. For example, it might reflect a different time in the year of the study, seasonality of an epidemic. There is no question that if the same study is done in different areas the rates may be different. In fact my slide showed that in the studies in Peru and Bangladesh the rates are not exactly the same. There is variation, so I suggest it is not a reason to be unsettled if it is 10% in that particular series and 5% in another.

Dr. Kamenwa: We have started a program on rotavirus surveillance in my country and we will be able to answer some of the questions that have been asked here in the next 1 or 2 years. How long do you recommend zinc supplementation for a child who has recurrent episodes of diarrhea given that when supplemented during a diarrheal episode it is probably protective for about 2–3 months? What is the pathophysiology of constipation and food allergy because you alluded to constipation being a phenotype of food allergy?

Dr. Fuchs: The recommendation for acute diarrhea is to supplement zinc at approximately twice the RDA for about 2 weeks (20 mg/day for children and 10 mg/day for infants <6 months for 10–14 days) [2]. The question of periodic supplementation of zinc analogous to periodic vitamin A supplementation programs is a very interesting one. Periodic zinc supplementation in otherwise normal children at high risk of diarrheal disease would be expected to be beneficial, but to my knowledge periodic zinc supplementation on an ongoing basis over several years has not been studied. It is a very interesting question to which we still don't have an answer.

Dr. Sorensen: When you talked about immunity, you mentioned T cells, neutrophils, complement. The only immunological intervention that I know of that has reversed chronic infectious diarrhea is the use of oral Ig preparations. I have used them in chronic rotavirus infection, in clostridium infection and in microsporidia. All those patients have T cell deficiencies; we cure them basically with IgG. We have to reevaluate the role of IgG-mediated immunity in these diseases too.

Dr. Fuchs: There is evidence that the immune system is more broadly involved and may differ for different specific infections. Good correlation has been shown for skin test reactivity to standard antigens and the risk of diarrhea and infection; quite clearly T cell immunity is involved. But the primary focus in an international health context regarding reconstitution of immune function has been on the particularly important role of micronutrients. There has been a lot of work on zinc and its positive effects on a variety of aspects of immune function and persistent diarrhea outcome. This and other micronutrients such as vitamin A also effect epithelial cell repair, for example. If you concentrate too much on one area of host defense you run the risk of overfocusing when it has a broader spectrum.

Dr. Imanzadeh: How long do you give the diet? As you mentioned chronic infection and bile acid conjugation may induce or activate persistent diarrhea. Oral gentamicin and cholestyramine can be used in the treatment of persistent diarrhea.

Dr. Fuchs: I don't recall the duration of the studies, but the diet should be given for 3 or 4 days and concern should arise if there is no effect in a positive direction. At this point you start having trouble maintaining electrolyte status. There are some reports from South Africa using gentamicin for persistent diarrhea, and cholestyramine can bind bile acids. On a case by case basis there may be a role in specific situations, but there are problems in broadly administering those agents. With regard to antibiotic therapy, if you look at all the data, it does not really have a consistent impact on recovery from persistent diarrhea. Cholestyramine again is treating the symptom rather than the cause, so it may have a cosmetic effect but it is not going to actually lead to recovery very quickly.

References

1   Ruiz-Palacios GM, Perez-Schael I, Velazquez FR, et al; Human Rotavirus Study Group: Safety and efficacy of an attenuated vaccine against severe rotavirus gastroenteritis. N Engl J Med 2006;354:11–22.
2   WHO: Implementing the New Recommendations on the Clinical Management of Diarrhoea. Geneva, WHO, 2006.

Cooke RJ, Vandenplas Y, Wahn U (eds): Nutrition Support for Infants and Children at Risk.
Nestlé Nutr Workshop Ser Pediatr Program, vol 59, pp 105–114,
Nestec Ltd., Vevey/S. Karger AG, Basel, © 2007.

Transition from Parenteral to Enteral Nutrition

Peter J. Milla

Gastroenterology and Autoimmunity Unit, UCL Institute of Child Health, London, UK

Abstract

Children are unique as their food intake must provide sufficient nutrients not only for the maintenance of body tissues but also for growth. Improvements in techniques for nutritional support has resulted in very long term parenteral nutrition being available for those with chronic intestinal failure in addition to those who require short term parenteral feeding either following surgery or whilst treatment for an underlying enteric disease becomes effective. Parenteral nutrition is required whenever insufficient nutrients cannot be provided enterally to prevent or correct malnutrition or to sustain appropriate growth. Somatic growth is fastest in infancy and puberty but other organs such as the brain may only grow and differentiate at one particular time. When a period of more liberal feeding intervenes catch-up of growth and function occurs. In adolescence the risk is of not achieving growth potential. Timing and methods of weaning from parenteral to normal nutrition remain controversial. In infants and children it is essential to consider carefully whether gastrointestinal function is sufficient for enteral nutrition to adequately support them. Thus the time when the infant and child can be weaned from parenteral nutrition will depend both on the activity of the underlying disease and the age and size of the infant or child.

Copyright © 2007 Nestec Ltd., Vevey/S. Karger AG, Basel

Introduction

Children are unique as optimal growth is of paramount importance to them and their food intake must provide sufficient nutrients not only for the maintenance of body tissues but also for growth. During infancy and adolescence children grow extremely rapidly. At these times children are particularly sensitive to energy restriction because of high basal and anabolic requirements. The ability to provide sufficient nutrients parenterally to sustain growth in infants and children suffering from intestinal failure or severe functional intestinal immaturity represents one of the most important therapeutic advances in pediatrics over the last three decades [1]. Improvements in techniques for nutritional support has resulted in very long-term parenteral nutrition being available for a cohort of patients with very chronic intestinal failure in addition to those who require short-term parenteral feeding in hospital either following surgery or whilst treatment for an underlying enteric disease becomes effective. Children with prolonged intestinal failure have the potential to grow and develop normally and to enjoy a good quality of life within the constraints of their underlying disease [2].

Whilst advances in knowledge of nutrient requirements, improved methods of nutrient delivery and understanding of the prevention and management of complications ensure that parenteral nutrition [3] can be delivered safely and effectively there nevertheless remain areas of uncertainty particularly with regard to weaning from parenteral to normal nutrition. In considering when and how to wean a child back to enteral feeding a number of general factors as well as specific gastrointestinal states need to be considered.

In general parenteral nutrition is required whenever sufficient nutrients cannot be provided enterally to prevent or correct malnutrition or to sustain appropriate growth. Malnutrition in children, in addition to the general effects of impaired tissue function, immunosuppression, defective muscle function and reduced respiratory and cardiac reserve also results in impaired growth and nutrition.

Whilst somatic growth exhibits a bimodal pattern being fastest in infancy, then dropping off and receiving a further spurt around puberty other organs of the body may grow and differentiate only at one particular time. This is particularly true of the brain for which the majority of growth occurs in the last trimester of pregnancy and in the first 2 years of life. Poor nutrition at critical periods of growth results in slowing and stunting of growth which may later exhibit catch-up when a period of more liberal feeding occurs. In adolescence there is a risk of not achieving growth potential if severe and continuous disease occurs and adequate provision is not made for their nutritional needs. The sick child is at the greatest risk of growth failure and nutritional disorder [4].

Neonates and very small infants because of small energy reserves are at a considerable disadvantage compared with older children and adolescents when weaning from parenteral nutrition [1]. In these small infants it is essential to consider carefully whether gastrointestinal function is sufficient for enteral nutrition to adequately support the infant. Thus the time when the infant and child can be weaned from parenteral nutrition will depend both on individual circumstances and the age and size of the infant or child. Some patients will have only required short-term parenteral nutrition following major intestinal surgery, chemotherapy, severe acute pancreatitis, or multiorgan failure in extensive trauma, burns and prematurity. Others will have needed long-term parenteral nutrition when they suffered prolonged episodes of intestinal failure most often caused by protracted diarrhea of infancy, short bowel syndrome, gastroschisis or chronic intestinal pseudoobstruction.

Weaning from Parenteral Nutrition

General Considerations

Parenteral nutrition is a potentially life-threatening form of nutritional support; the overriding priority is to wean the child off parenteral nutrition as soon as is possible. Infants and children who have an acute episode of severe intestinal failure with a previously normal gut, e.g. after surgery or during a course of chemotherapy, may when gut function has recovered tolerate the rapid reintroduction of a normal diet. On the other hand, children with primary gut disease will often need the introduction of enteral feed tailored according to the nature and activity of the underlying disease.

In all children the following factors are critical to the success of introducing enteral nutrition:

- Appropriate minimal enteral feeds should be given wherever possible to prevent gut atrophy [5]
- Encourage adaptation and treat aggressively underlying gastrointestinal disease [6–9]
- Reduction of the risk of parenteral nutrition-associated liver disease [2, 10]

The following practical points may ensure success:

- Involve an experienced dietitian and nutrition support team
- Only make one change in treatment at a time to assess tolerance, e.g., when the volume of enteral nutrition is increased, the concentration of the nutrition solution should remain constant
- Maintain central venous access until the child is fully enterally fed
- In those with severe intestinal failure feed volumes should be increased slowly according to tolerance

Methods of Feeding

Some children can be weaned straight on to bolus feeds, in others continuous feeding may be required. In these as soon as enteral nutrition can be introduced a liquid enteral feed infused as continuous enteral nutrition over 4- to 24-hour periods, using a dedicated feeding pump and enteral feeding system, should be started. The main advantage of a continuous feed is that the feed can be more easily controlled and adjusted to the guts' absorptive capacity. The feed should be prepared carefully under hygienic conditions and should not be kept at room temperature longer than 8 h. Some children will not tolerate bolus feeds and in these children it may be necessary to use continuous feeding long-term. Although cumbersome this is preferable to long-term parenteral nutrition as the mortality and morbidity are markedly lower.

Liquid enteral feeds can also be given as bolus or sip feeds either orally or via a gastrostomy or feeding tube. It may be necessary to give the bolus feeds as frequently as 2-hourly while the child is awake and continuously at night. If bolus feeds are needed more frequently, a continuous feed is more practical and should be commenced. Whenever possible bolus feeds should be offered by mouth. Smaller infants should not be woken up to give oral feeds to avoid fatigue. If gastric feeds are poorly tolerated (vomiting/large amounts of feed aspirated) feeding into the jejunum should be undertaken with the help of an expert gastroenterology or nutrition support team, as this is a high risk technique.

Children who rapidly recover intestinal function may be weaned straight on to normal food. Every possible attempt is made to encourage children to eat normally. Spoon feeding should be introduced at the normal age, that means around 6 months of age, even if only small amounts can be offered. Some mothers will find it difficult to accept that their child ceases to eat voluntarily when an adequate amount of enteral feed is infused via an artificial feeding device. Some children may develop severe oral hypersensitivity or have delayed oromotor development which may be associated with gastro-esophageal reflux. Injudicious increases in feed volume or texture often result in a deterioration of their feeding problem [11].

Types of Feed

In newborn infants with a short but normal gut expressed breast milk is the preferred form of nutrition to optimize adaptation. Mother's own milk should be given pasteurized when continuous feeding is used but fresh if oral or tube bolus feeds are given.

Children with gastrointestinal disease causing intestinal failure usually require a specially formulated pediatric enteral feed when weaning. Elemental, hydrolyzed protein or whole protein feeds are selected according to the child's ability to tolerate the feed constituents or availability in the case of expressed breast milk. If there is any possibility of persistent intestinal inflammation an appropriate protein hydrolysate or amino acid-based formula should be used [12]. In neonates with short gut syndrome the outcome is improved with breast milk [10] or an amino acid-based formula feed [13, 14]. In both these situations diet may need to be adjusted as there appears to be a high incidence of cow's milk or soy protein intolerance. If at all possible a commercially available complete feed that provides the child's entire nutritional requirements should be used. This reduces the risk of providing an unbalanced diet and the risk of infectious complications.

Modular feeds should only be used when complete feeds appropriate for the individual have not been tolerated. The advantage of a modular feed is that protein, carbohydrate and fat (medium- vs. long-chain triglycerides) can each be gradually introduced as tolerated. Electrolytes, vitamins and minerals must all be added according to requirements. Thus the feed is tailored for the individual child. Modular feeds are generally not recommended due to the risk of bacterial contamination; the possibility of accidentally omitting essential nutrients, preparation at home can be complicated, and there may be settling out of the feed constituents when the feed is administered continuously. However, in children with ultrashort bowel syndrome modular feeds may enable improved enteral energy intake and tolerance.

Timing of Weaning

Reduction in the amount of parenteral nutrition may be attempted as soon as the child is stabilized, i.e. intestinal losses from vomiting and diarrhea have been minimized and an optimal nutritional state reached. The underlying intestinal failure should be investigated and treated in a specialist pediatric gastroenterological unit. All children on parenteral nutrition should continue to have a minimal amount of enteral feed to maintain enterohepatic circulation and possibly gut integrity [10, 15, 16] whenever possible. As soon as a small volume of the desired feed is tolerated at low rate, the volume should be increased. The feed should be given at normal concentrations and not diluted, otherwise the child will achieve normal fluid intake without adequate nutrition. The aim should be to maintain a good nutritional intake by decreasing the parenteral feed and increasing the enteral feed by similar amounts. This is best achieved by reducing the parenteral feed slightly faster than the rate the enteral feed is increased. Enteral tolerance is more likely to be achieved by avoiding excessive fluid intake. In children with more severe intestinal failure, enteral feeds may need to be introduced and increased as slowly as 1 ml/kg per 24 h. Parenteral nutrition might be reduced by 5 ml/kg per 24 h every few days. If a chosen weaning strategy fails it is worth trying again, but at a slower pace, e.g. with smaller rate or volume increments.

In children who are stable and thriving on parenteral nutrition at home the quality of life for the family can be vastly improved by removing one parenteral nutrition infusion per week allowing them a night of normal life [17]. If tolerated, further reductions can be made by reducing parenteral nutrition one night at a time over several weeks or months. Weaning can be facilitated by reducing/halving the parenteral nutrition given one night a week and seeing how well the child is the following day. If fluid and electrolyte loss becomes an issue nocturnal provision of an oral rehydration solution via a nasogastric tube may be a solution. In infancy and childhood a night off parenteral nutrition would, usually, only be tried when at least 50% of nutrients are tolerated enterally. The ability to tolerate a night off parenteral nutrition varies according to the underlying disease. A night off is usually well tolerated by children with short bowel syndrome who are stable with improving intestinal function. In children with short bowel, weaning is prolonged in the presence of bacterial overgrowth and associated enteritis [12]. In children with chronic intestinal pseudoobstruction, especially with ileostomy and major fecal losses, removing one night of parenteral nutrition often leads to a rapid increase in oral fluid and feed intake due to thirst and hunger leading to aggravation of symptoms.

The child's ability to tolerate the reduction in parenteral nutrition is assessed by checking hydration, weight gain, growth, and blood indices.

Problems that can arise when weaning is not tolerated include D-lactic acidosis due to lactate production from fermentation of nutrients dumped in the colon and distal ileum by the bacterial flora due to the increased intake of enteral nutrition exceeding the absorptive capacity of the small intestine. Although some studies have indicated that bacterial fermentation is more of a problem in the absence of the ileocecal valve [18], this does not always seem to be the case [12]. Such complications may be prevented by manipulating the colonic flora with a low fiber diet, bicarbonates and, sometimes, anaerobic antibiotics (metronidazole) plus probiotics [12]. However in order for this problem not to occur the enteral intake needs to be matched to the ability of the child to digest and absorb the enteral load. Sometimes it may be necessary to reduce the intestinal load and increase parenteral nutrition again whilst treating the underlying disease more effectively or waiting for intestinal adaptation to improve allowing for recommencement or continuation of the weaning process.

Avoiding Feeding Problems

Whenever possible it is important to maintain small volumes of oral feeds and monitor the adequacy of feeding skills, even if the infant or child is established on continuous feeds.

Solids should be started at the usual recommended age for healthy infants when possible. It is best to limit these initially to a few foods that are least likely to have an allergenic effect (especially in intestinal inflammation), e.g. rice, chicken or carrot, and which will be suitable for the underlying gastrointestinal disease, e.g. low sucrose/low in long-chain triglyceride fat or low fiber in short bowel and/or extensive colon resection.

When food is introduced, the aim is to encourage normal textures for age [11]. Even if the amount and range of foods are limited, introducing normal food will promote normal feeding behavior. Encouraging oral feeding will help to prevent feeding problems which can continue for many months or even years.

Even in younger infants, bolus feeds may have beneficial psychological and social effects. For example, the mother will feel that she is doing something to help her sick child. Maternal bonding may be improved by the close contact between mother and child. Feeding by mouth should be a pleasurable event for both mother and child.

References

1 Heird WC, Driscoll JM, Schullinger IN, et al: Intravenous alimentation in paediatric patients. J Pediatr 1972;80:351–372.
2 Larchar V, Shepherd R, Francis D, Harries JT: Protracted diarrhoea in infants. Arch Dis Child 1997;52:597–605.
3 Beath SV, Booth IW, Murphy MS, et al: Nutritional care and candidates for small bowel transplantation. Arch Dis Child 1995;73:348–350.
4 Milla PJ: Paediatric nutritional requirements; in Payne-James J, Grimble G, Silk D (eds): Artificial Nutrition Support in Clinical Practice. London, Arnold, 1995, pp 167–174.
5 Williamson RC: Intestinal adaptation (first of two parts). Structural, functional and cytokinetic changes. N Engl J Med 1978;298:1393–1402.
6 Levine GM, Deren JJ, Steiger E, et al: Role of oral intake in maintenance of gut mass and disaccharide activity. Gastroenterology 1974;67:975–982.
7 Greene HL, McCabe DR, Merenstein GB: Protracted diarrhea and malnutrition in infancy: changes in intestinal morphology and disaccharidase activities during treatment with total intravenous nutrition or oral elemental diets. J Pediatr 1975;87:695–704.
8 Johnson LR, Copeland EM, Dudrick SI, et al: Structural and hormonal alterations in the gastrointestinal tract of parenterally fed rats. Gastroenterology 1975;68:1177–1183.
9 Feldman EJ, Dowling RH, McNaughton J, et al: Effects of oral versus intravenous nutrition on intestinal adaptation after small bowel resection in the dog. Gastroenterology 1976;70: 712–719.
10 Andorsky DJ, Lund DP, Lillehei CW, et al: Nutritional and other postoperative management of neonates with short bowel syndrome correlates with clinical outcomes. J Pediatr 2001;139: 27–33.
11 Strudwick S: Gastro-oesophageal reflux and feeding: the speech and language therapist's perspective. Int J Pediatr Otorhinolaryngol 2003;67:S101–S102.
12 Kaufman SS, Loseke CA, Lupo JV, et al: Influence of bacterial overgrowth and intestinal inflammation on duration of parenteral nutrition in children with short bowel syndrome. J Pediatr 1997;131:356–361.
13 Vanderhoof JA, Murray ND, Kaufman SS, et al: Intolerance to protein hydrolysate infant formulas: an underrecognized cause of gastrointestinal symptoms in infants. J Pediatr 1997;131: 741–744.
14 Bines J, Francis D, Hill D: Reducing parenteral requirement in children with short bowel syndrome: impact of an amino acid-based complete infant formula. J Pediatr Gastroenterol Nutr 1998;26:123–128.
15 Fisher RL: Hepatobiliary abnormalities associated with total parenteral nutrition. Gastroenterol Clin North Am 1989;18:645–666.
16 McClure RJ, Newell SI: Randomised controlled trial of trophic feeding and gut motility. Arch Dis Child Fetal Neonatal Ed 1999;80:F54–F58.
17 Bisset WM, Stapleford P, Long S, et al: Home parenteral nutrition in chronic intestinal failure. Arch Dis Child 1992;67:109–114.
18 Goulet OJ, Revillon Y, Jan D, et al: Neonatal short bowel syndrome. J Pediatr 1991;119:18–23.

Discussion

Dr. Fakhraee: Most neonatologists are concerned with necrotizing enterocolitis in premature babies. What is the incidence of necrotizing enterocolitis with minimal enteral feeding; is it decreased or increased or is there no change in the incidence of necrotizing enterocolitis?

Dr. Milla: Clearly necrotizing enterocolitis is a problem in premature infants. I am not aware of formal studies addressing the point that you have made. If you look at series of patients with necrotizing enterocolitis it is clear that it started as soon as nutrients were introduced into the bowel. I can't answer your question as to what the figures are, but the advantages of minimal enteral nutrition outweigh the disadvantages.

Dr. Jochum: You did not touch on the point of nonnutritive sucking in neonates. Could you comment on the use of probiotics in neonatal nutrition?

Dr. Milla: As far as nonnutritive sucking is concerned there is certainly evidence to show that where you use nonnutritive sucking in a premature infant you will be able to introduce feeds sooner than if you don't give them that practice. It has more to do with gut motility than the ability of the gut to absorb food. Nonnutritive sucking is useful in neonates in terms of trying to get them to tolerate particularly oral feeds. As far as probiotics are concerned I am not a neonatologist, I don't have any experience of that. These are rather severe diseases that result in the need of parenteral nutrition. Probiotics have some effect but not a major effect, and they have never enabled us to get them off parenteral nutrition and to wean them onto enteral feeds.

Dr. Balanag: Can you elaborate on the use of occult blood as a screening method for starting enteral feeding?

Dr. Milla: If you use occult blood in most patients who have an enteropathy it would be found to be positive a lot of the time. I am not a great fan of occult blood tests because I think most of them are far too sensitive. Many patients with inflammatory enteropathy bleed. I don't use occult blood because it is not going to tell me anything which is going to alter my management of that individual. On the other hand if there is obvious blood in the stool then that is a significant amount. The majority of patients who have this sort of disease lose more blood from the investigations than the disease. I have never found this test helpful.

Dr. Ruemmele: It is a difficult topic and your experience is helpful in developing a strategy to wean these patients from parenteral nutrition. Could you comment on the role of bacterial flora in this context? I am not talking about prebiotics but the commensal bacteria of the flora. For instance bacterial overgrowth is seen in children with short bowel; once these children are off parenteral nutrition the situation can be very dangerous. The simple use of antibiotics for a bacterial infection may cause a loss of intestinal autonomy and parenteral nutrition must be restarted. Could you comment on that?

You introduced your topic saying that the major function of the small bowel is absorptive. I would add, and this is my personal view, that the small bowel is also a major immune organ. I would not just reduce it to its absorptive function.

Dr. Milla: The gut is the major immune organ of the body and the reason for this is that it has to be permeable to let all these nutrients through. Because of this it will let through a lot of other things which are very injurious. Bacteria are a problem and there are at least 3 situations in which they are particularly important. If there is a short gut and anastomosis has occurred or adaptation has taken place, if there is a stricture to the anastomosis then subacute obstruction can occur. If there is excessive adaptation and the bowel is largely dilated then motor activity results in ineffective transit and bacterial overgrowth occurs. This is one of the reasons tapering enteroplasty or stricture resection can be extremely helpful in these patients. There are other conditions in which bacterial overgrowth occurs because the immune system is defective in some way, and in patients who have primary immunodeficiency as well as AIDS patients, it may be that this is the cause of the bacterial overgrowth, and it needs to be treated in a variety of ways. Antibiotics are one way, and Dr. Sorensen told us about oral immunoglobulin, which is frequently used in patients with neuromuscular disease and functional obstruction to try to clear their bowel. The biggest problem with these patients is that muscle disease may worsen the functional obstruction. The inflammatory process that caused the bacterial overgrowth results in alterations of muscle cell function. They start to participate as amateur antigen-presenting cells in the inflammatory process. Two things which appear to be contradictory need to be done: treat the bacterial overgrowth and treat the inflammation.

Dr. Hendarto: We have a few cases of functional intestinal obstruction. How long should the patient be on parenteral nutrition before giving hypoallergenic formula?

Dr. Milla: Severe neuromuscular disease that causes functional obstruction is not easy to manage and if obstruction continues then sufficient nutrition to support them becomes difficult. Parenteral nutrition is the only practical way of getting many of these patients over these prolonged episodes of ileus. On the other hand in some of the milder diseases, the episodes of functional obstruction are not very long lasting. As soon as stomach emptying becomes more normal, my practice is to start introducing feed when the nasogastric aspirates drop below 150 ml/day. As soon as this occurs they start passing wind, which is the time to introduce a continuous whey protein hydrolysate. There is very good experimental data showing that whey proteins are emptied from the stomach faster than all other whole proteins with the exception of human breast milk. It is emptied at about the same rate as human breast milk, so we use whey proteins in preference to any other form of hydrolysate for this purpose.

Dr. Rivera: Regarding the issue of feeding methods for premature babies, the ability to suck and some of their reflexes are very important for them to feed. An alternative to nipple feeding is a small cup which enables us to feed babies up to 27 weeks of gestational age. We are very successful with the use of this small cup, and we don't have any extra loss of calories.

Dr. Shaaban: In the procedure of adaptation, when changing from parenteral to enteral nutrition, what form of the nutrient do you deliver, liquid, semisolid or solid food? If you take into consideration the gastric emptying time and the density of the nutrients, would you still chose the continuous method of delivery or would you prefer bolus feeding at a longer interval?

Dr. Milla: Over the years we have found continuous liquid feed to be most successful, which is why I was suggesting that. All of the other things that you suggest depend entirely upon there being virtually normal motor activity, particularly in the stomach and duodenum. The problem with most of these patients, particularly if they have inflammatory enteropathy, is that motor activity won't be normal and stomach emptying will not be sufficiently smooth. Coordinating gastric with duodenal activity will enable the supply of sufficient nutrients but once the ability to empty the stomach is exceeded then the stomach distends and vomiting starts. I am very convinced that using continuous liquid feeds is the simplest, safest and best way to get the most calories into an infant. Parents in particular think because their child is being given a liquid that they are not having food, which is not the case, and they must be convinced that it is the best way forward.

Dr. Bojadzieva: My question is whether partial parenteral nutrition and partial enteral nutrition will perhaps reduce bacterial translocation, especially for premature babies and very low birth weight babies?

Dr. Milla: If I was being very provocative I would say forget about bacterial translocation because the evidence that it occurs is not very good. If you think about the structure of the gut and its immune system and the lymphatic drain into the gut, you would realize that the notion of flooding the vasculature with bacteria is probably not a sustainable idea. There is some evidence to suggest that it might take place. I haven't really found it to be a major problem and we send home a lot of patients on parenteral nutrition. They all have active disease. The one thing that marks them out is that they don't get sepsis. One of our patients had the same line in for 10 years without infection. It has all to do with how the lines are looked after and I don't worry about things like bacterial translocation. Sometimes you need to do both parenteral and enteral feeding and there is no doubt that if you have a patient who requires long-term parenteral nutrition and you can get them onto at least 30% of the calories enterally, they are a lot easier to manage. The majority of our patients are treated with a mix of parenteral and enteral feeding. I try to avoid total parenteral nutrition, because it is bad news long term.

Dr. Fakhraee: Regarding Dr. Rivera's comment on cup feeding; this is recommended by WHO and UNICEF to feed premature babies because bottle feeding causes a phenomenon called 'nipple confusion'. Babies who are only bottle fed may not be able to breastfeed, and because of that WHO recommends cup feeding. We also have experience with cup feeding in very small premature babies and I think it is a good practice.

Dr. Milla: If you want premature infants to grow to their potential I doubt that using a normal formula supplies babies with sufficient calories to survive. But what is the appropriate standard? All the work that people like Dr. Lucas have done would suggest that the standards we have for the growth of premature infants are probably not right, and a lot more thought needs to be put toward how this is done. Survival is one thing, growth to their potential is another thing.

Dr. S. Koletzko: I have a question with respect to your study with the new formula. You said they were young children with inflammatory enteropathy. Could you please tell us more about their diagnoses; did you also include patients with short gut syndrome?

Dr. Milla: There were some short gut patients but basically they were all patients who had a small intestinal inflammatory enteropathy. The enteropathy could have had many different causes. Some had mild autoimmune disease; we excluded patients who required immunosuppression.

Dr. S. Koletzko: Also patients with long-term diarrhea?

Dr. Milla: They all had long-term diarrhea otherwise they would never have come to us. These were patients who would have been treated in a district general hospital.

Cooke RJ, Vandenplas Y, Wahn U (eds): Nutrition Support for Infants and Children at Risk.
Nestlé Nutr Workshop Ser Pediatr Program, vol 59, pp 115–131,
Nestec Ltd., Vevey/S. Karger AG, Basel, © 2007.

Chronic Enteropathy and Feeding

Silvia Salvatore[a], *Bruno Hauser*[b], *Yvan Vandenplas*[b]

[a]Clinica Pediatrica di Varese, Università dell'Insubria, Varese, Italy; [b]Academisch Ziekenhuis Kinderen, Vrije Universiteit Brussel, Brussels, Belgium

Abstract

Enteropathy defines abnormalities of the small intestinal mucosa, visible with the light microscope, of various etiologies, that can be separated into acute versus chronic conditions. This review focuses on these areas in which recent progress has been made. Severe infections increase mucosal permeability and induce local expression of co-stimulatory molecules allowing antigen penetration in the mucosa, T cell activation and possible disruption of oral tolerance. Biotherapeutics are of importance in the prevention and treatment of (chronic) enteropathy of infectious origin. Celiac disease and cow's milk protein allergy are key examples of chronic enteropathy. The dietary approach to allergy has evolved to include active stimulation of the immature immune system in order to support the establishment of tolerance. Supplementation with probiotics may provide maturational signals for the lymphoid tissue and improve the balance of pro- and anti-inflammatory cytokines. Enteral polymeric feeding is effective in Crohn's disease. Dietary nucleotides may improve growth and immunity, optimize maturation, recovery and function of rapidly dividing tissue. Adequate dietary lipids are important not just for caloric value but also for immune-modulatory effects. Lipids may prevent allergic sensitization by downregulating inflammatory response (n-3 but not n-6 fatty acids) whilst protecting the epithelial barrier, regulating immune function and modifying the adherence of microbes to the mucosa, thereby contributing to host-microbe interactions.

Copyright © 2007 Nestec Ltd., Vevey/S. Karger AG, Basel

Introduction

Enteropathy defines abnormalities of the small intestinal mucosa visible with the light microscope [1]. Clinical entities in children include infection, food hypersensitivity, immune dysregulation, or primary abnormalities of the enterocytes. The overall prevalence of chronic enteropathy in children is difficult to estimate because of the large spectrum of etiologies, patient selection, and other factors. Herein we will discuss some selected enteropathies focusing on either the causal or the therapeutic role of feeding.

Infection

Acute and chronic infections play a key role in the occurrence of enteropathy. Enteropathogenic *Escherichia coli*, rotavirus, *Salmonella*, *Giardia lamblia* and *Cryptosporidium* are pathogens more frequently responsible for persistent small bowel damage with increased severity in case of inadequate initial nutrition and realimentation [2]. Optimal nutritional rehabilitation is consequently considered as the cornerstone of management of (persistent) diarrhea [2]. Malnutrition not only increases the severity of a gastrointestinal infection due to an impaired immunological response but also impairs the recovering of damaged mucosa with secondary intestinal and pancreatic enzymatic reduction [2].

Severe infections increase mucosal permeability and induce local expression of co-stimulatory molecules allowing antigen penetration in the mucosa, T cell activation and possible disruption of oral tolerance. In the last decades, rapid realimentation in acute gastroenteritis has reduced the incidence of postenteritis syndrome with food intolerance and persistent diarrhea. Complex carbohydrates, probiotics and prebiotics, such as maize, green banana fibers and pectin, have been hypothesized to enhance epithelial gut repair and absorption. L-Glutamine, the 'fuel' for the intestine, nucleotides, causing proliferation of enterocytes, growth factor(s) with trophic effects on the intestinal mucosa, bovine colostrum and bovine serum concentrate have also been evaluated, without evidence of any substantial benefit [2].

Probiotics, such as some specific lactobacilli (e.g. *Lactobacillus casei* DN-114 001, *Lactobacillus plantarum* 299v) or yeast *(Saccharomyces boulardii)* reduce the invasiveness of intestinal pathogens and beneficially affect the increased intestinal permeability caused by selected bacterial pathogens [3–5]. But not all the literature is in agreement: administration of *Lactobacillus* GG (LGG) during 30 days showed no effect on the intestinal integrity of 3- to 5-year-old Malawian children with tropical enteropathy [6].

Much research has highlighted the possible role of zinc supplementation in reducing both the severity and the duration of diarrhea in immunocompetent and immunocompromised patients [7, 8].

Enteropathy Caused by Food Hypersensitivity

Celiac Disease

The incidence of celiac disease (CD) is increasing worldwide, with a prevalence as high as 1:300 and even 1:80 children [9]. One of the major reasons for the increase in prevalence is improved serological screening in subjects without overt gastrointestinal complaints. However, regional differences are emerging. The incidence of histological abnormalities suggestive of CD is lower than 1/250 children undergoing upper endoscopy for various indications (pers. data). Wheat, rye and barley are the predominant grains containing gluten peptides, very rich in proline and glutamine and resistant to digestive enzymes, known to cause CD. Variability exists in the age of onset of symptoms, in extraintestinal and autoimmune manifestations, in serological positivity, and in severity of histological involvement and no clear explanation has emerged despite major advances in the identification of toxic peptides, immune cascade and genetic susceptibility. The incidence of CD in mothers giving birth to preterm or immature babies is higher than in a control population (pers. data); in other words, undiagnosed CD in pregnant women challenges the outcome of pregnancy, and subsequently the nutritional status of the newborn. The variable histological findings of CD include increased intraepithelial lymphocytes (>30 lymphocytes per 100 enterocytes, with a mitotic index >0.2%), inflammatory infiltration into the lamina propria and crypt hyperplasia, decreased height of the epithelial cells (changes from columnar to cuboid to flat epithelium) and decreased villous/crypt ratio, and partial to total villous atrophy. Modern histological (Marsh) classification consists of 4 CD types ranging from a normal preinfiltrative stage (type 0), to infiltrative lesions with increased intraepithelial lymphocytes (type 1), hyperplastic lesions (type 2: type 1 + hyperplastic crypts), destructive lesions (type 3: type 2 + variable degree of villous atrophy), and hypoplastic lesions with total villous atrophy and crypt hypoplasia (type 4). Marsh type 3 was subsequently modified into type 3a (partial villous atrophy), type 3b (subtotal villous atrophy) and type 3c (total villous atrophy). In Marsh type 1 and type 2 lesions, positive celiac antibodies and clinical and serological response to a gluten-free diet support the diagnosis of CD [9]. After diagnosis of CD, a life-long gluten-free diet results in the disappearance of clinical manifestations, mucosal healing and reduction of CD-related complications. However the importance of dietetic compliance in asymptomatic patients, the real risk of complications in patients with only subtle mucosal involvement (Marsh type 1), the individual threshold of gluten sensitivity and the clinical significance of seropositivity in the absence of enteropathy require further clarification [10]. The role of prolonged breastfeeding, timing of introduction and dosing of gluten-containing food especially in subjects with a high genetic risk is under evaluation.

Future therapeutic strategies include peptidase supplementation (from experimental bacterial sources) which cleaves residues next to proline to facilitate proteolysis of immunogenic peptides, transgenic wheat without antigenic peptides, modulation of permeability (by control of the immune cascade and zonulin release) and block of innate and acquired immunity triggered by gluten in celiac patients [10]. Further efforts are needed to clarify and standardize the definition of a gluten-free diet, to simplify the labeling of ingredients in food products, to improve and support the social life of celiac patients and to increase early identification of celiac patients [10].

Food Allergy

Cow's milk protein (CMP), soy, wheat, oats, rice, eggs and fish have all been reported to cause enteropathy in selected children [11, 12]. A 30-kD protein in soy cross-reacts with casein [13] and may favor a concomitant soy and cow's milk hypersensitivity especially in infants with (IgE-negative) CMP enteropathy or enterocolitis. In the last decades an increased number of children has been reported to be sensitized to multiple food antigens, especially (or even) during exclusive breastfeeding, with allergic manifestations early in life due to an impaired development of oral tolerance. In selected infants, acute gastroenteritis increasing permeability and contact of antigens in the lamina propria may provoke sensitization to dietary antigens.

Chronic diarrhea, malabsorption, edema and failure to thrive are the most common clinical manifestations of food-related enteropathy. Other gastrointestinal (abdominal pain, frequent regurgitation or vomiting, constipation, refusal to feed, protein-losing enteropathy), dermatological (atopic dermatitis, napkin rash, swelling of the lips or eye lids), respiratory (runny nose, chronic cough or wheezing, laryngeal edema), and general (persistent distress, colic) manifestations may be additional features. In many patients, the nongastrointesinal manifestations are predominant. Especially regarding CMP, most children will tolerate the offending allergen after the age of 1 year although food enteropathy may persist longer in a minority of them [14].

In food allergy, duodenal, ileal and colonic lymphonodular hyperplasia may be detected [15] as a consequence of immune activation. Histological abnormalities are variable: from total to patchy or even absent villous atrophy, mild to moderately increased intraepithelial CD8 cells, lymphoid follicles, activated lamina propria CD4 cells (with increased IFN-γ with or without IL-4 or TNF-α) and decreased regulatory cytokines (especially TGF-β) [16].

Different from CD, enteropathy caused by food allergy presents a thin mucosa, a prominent patchy distribution, only moderate crypt hyperplasia and less intraepithelial lymphocyte infiltration. The infiltration of eosinophils and mast cells is frequent and related to antigen-induced dysmotility and enteric neural dysfunction. The mucosal lesions may cause reduction in brush border disaccharidase expression and secondary exocrine pancreatic impairment, caused by decreased duodenal CCK production, with mild-to-moderate steatorrhea and reduced fecal elastase [17].

As food-related enteropathy is mostly cellular mediated, total and specific serum IgE and skin prick tests are often negative. PATCH tests seem a promising diagnostic tool for T cell (late) response to dietary antigen. Fecal calprotectin has recently been proposed as an (unspecific) noninvasive marker of enteropathy.

Mechanisms inducing oral tolerance are in general not complete at birth but develop postnatally, mainly in response or intimate relation to the gut flora and to activation of specific Toll-like receptors on regulatory T cells [1, 18]. The key role of the luminal bacteria is highlighted by the impaired tolerance in germfree mice [1], by the different intestinal flora in populations that will develop atopy, by the immune-modulatory properties of specific probiotics and by the promising results of interventional studies. Allergic infants showed, even before the appearance of symptoms, a significantly higher prevalence of clostridia, coliforms and *Staphylococcus aureus* versus lactobacilli and *Bifidobacterium (bifidum)*. Manipulation of the gut flora as early as in the first days or months of life may influence through microenvironment modification and competition subsequent colonization and expression of regulatory cytokines. Specific probiotics including LGG may induce anti-inflammatory IL-10 and TGF-β [19] and possibly exert a tolerogenic effect before sensitization occurs. According to 2 trials using supplementation of LGG and *E. coli* in the perinatal period, in particular non-IgE-mediated allergies are reduced [19, 20]. Maternal supplementation with LGG during pregnancy and 6 months after delivery increases the concentration of TGF-β in the breast milk of at-risk mothers and confers protection against atopy.

Supplementation of a cow's milk-based formula with prebiotics has the ability to manipulate the intestinal flora with a bifidogenic effect, but a beneficial prospective effect on food allergy has not been demonstrated so far with prebiotic supplementation. Comparing symptoms suggesting atopic sensitization at the age of 3–4 years in 27 exclusively breastfed babies during 6 months, in 16 infants on oligosaccharide-supplemented formula and in 17 infants on standard infant formula, the incidence was similar in breastfed and standard formula-fed infants (59 vs. 58%) and decreased by 50% in the supplemented formula group (31%) (pers. data).

Prenatal prevention is complex and multifactorial and dietetic intervention during pregnancy is not currently substantiated by scientific evidence [21]. Postnatally, dietetic prevention is actually recommended in high-risk infants only and is based on the promotion of breastfeeding (with no conclusive evidence of inconsistently proposed exclusion of peanuts and nuts), hypoallergenic formulas for bottle-fed infants and late introduction of solid foods. Compared to extensive hydrolysate formulas (eHFs), partial hydrolyzed formulas offer economical and taste advantages and a theoretical benefit in inducing oral tolerance to CMP as they still have enough residual allergenicity to induce tolerance but too low allergenicity to induce allergic reactions.

Up to now, for the treatment of food allergies, guidelines worldwide recommend exclusion of the causative antigen. For the infant who is sensitized while being breastfed, maternal exclusion of the more relevant antigens (CMP, egg white, (pea)nut) is advised. In cow's milk-sensitive enteropathy, eHF or, in those refusing to drink eHF or those not responding to the elimination diet, amino acid formulas are recommended. Infants and children with multiple food allergy have often more severe symptoms with possible reactions even to a small quantity of antigens (like those present in breast milk), are unresponsive to eHFs, and have late acquisition of tolerance. The maintenance of a nutritionally adequate diet is not easy especially in the case of compromised absorption or multiple allergies but is mandatory for each child. It is fortunate that manufacturers continue to make efforts to be able to offer new formulas with improved hydrolyzation, amino acid profile, additional beneficial components such as prebiotics, probiotics, nucleotides, medium-chain triglycerides (MCT) and long-chain polyunsaturated fatty acids, and last but not least cost and taste.

Immune Dysregulation

Different immune deficiencies have been related to an (often patchy) enteropathy, caused by the primary immune disorder and/or by the increased occurrence of (common and opportunistic) infections.

In a-γ- and hypo-γ-globulinemia, the plasma cells in the lamina propria are absent or reduced, respectively, with an increased rate of intestinal infections and malabsorption. In isolated IgA deficiency, enteropathy may be primary or secondary to (increased coexistence of) CD, food allergy and giardiasis. Reduced plasma cells, nodular hyperplasia and giardiasis have also been described in common variable immunodeficiency. Intractable (even fatal) diarrhea due to autoimmune inflammation and chronic pathogen infections is frequent in severe combined immunodeficiency. AIDS is an important cause of (a variable degree of) enteropathy.

In HIV infection, intestinal biopsy is characterized by increased intraepithelial lymphocytes, proinflammatory cytokines (TNF-α, IL-1β and IFN-γ), and lamina propria mononuclear cells with decreased CD4 cells, villous atrophy, and crypt hyperplasia [22]. In immunodeficiency, infections of common or opportunistic pathogens are frequent and discrimination between primary and secondary enteropathy is often difficult. Nutritional support exerts a positive effect on the immune function with a reduction of serum cytokine levels, a decrease of (opportunistic) infections and HIV replication [22]. Especially micronutrients, including vitamins, antioxidants and trace elements (particularly zinc), play an important role in immunomodulation. Supply of fat and carbohydrate is necessary to satisfy the energy requirements (increased up to 150% of the recommended daily intake) but maldigestion and malabsorption should be closely monitored to avoid further malnutrition [22].

T cell activation defects with a failure of tolerance and/or impaired apoptosis represent the basis of autoimmune enteropathy. Intestinal biopsies are characterized by (variable) villous atrophy, crypt hyperplasia and a marked infiltration of activated T cells into the lamina propria without a significant increase of intraepithelial lymphocytes. Patients present positive serum antibodies against enterocytes, frequent extraintestinal manifestations of autoimmunity, and diarrhea starting after the first 8 weeks of life with clinical response to potent immune suppression.

Defective central (thymic) or peripheral (i.e. gut) tolerance is also responsible for other rare immune disorders with multiorgan involvement and frequent enteropathy. In the APECED (autoimmune polyendocrinopathy, candidiasis, ectodermal dystrophy) and Omenn's syndrome there is an abnormal expression of the AIRE thymic factor which is crucial for central deletion of autoreactive T cells. Mutation of the transcription factor Foxp3 which is the pivot molecule in the generation of (peripheral) regulatory lymphocytes induces a specific severe multifocal disease, the IPEX syndrome, which includes immune dysregulation with severe autoimmune enteropathy, polyendocrinopathy, and X-linked inheritance.

Enteral tolerance is present in a minority of patients but most of severe enteropathies require long-term parenteral nutrition. Bone marrow or, more recently, stem cell transplants have recently been suggested for these patients.

In addition to the 'classic' immune disorders, more subtle immune dysregulations have been reported both in food-sensitive and in inflammatory bowel disease (see specific paragraphs).

Eosinophilic Gastroenteropathy

Eosinophilic enteropathies are rare conditions with eosinophil-rich inflammation in the absence of known causes for eosinophilia (e.g., drug reactions, parasitic infections and malignancy) that may affect part or all of the gut (esophagus, stomach, small and large bowel) and different layers of the intestine, such as the mucosa, submucosa, muscular layer or serosa. The disease often has patchy involvement and normal macroscopic appearance, necessitating the analysis of multiple biopsy specimens and quantification of eosinophil infiltration from each intestinal segment. Clinical manifestations are variable, including vomiting, dysphagia, abdominal pain, diarrhea, blood stools, iron deficiency anemia, malabsorption, protein-losing enteropathy, failure to thrive, obstructive symptoms, and even ascites in the serosal form. A trial of specific food antigen and aeroallergen avoidance is often indicated and in selected cases, an elemental formula is necessary. Glucocorticoids (systemic or topical) have also shown beneficial results, especially in eosinophilic esophagitis. Other treatments, such as cromoglycate, montelukast, ketotifen, suplatast tosilate, mycophenolate mofetil, 'alternative Chinese medicines', anti-IL-5, the tyrosine kinase inhibitor imatinib mesylate, CCR3 antagonists, and IL-4/IL-13 inhibitors, have all been used in the attempt to decrease eosinophilic infiltration but without clear evidence. The primary pathogenic role of eosinophils and of food and inhalant allergens remains to be established [23].

Crohn's Disease

Crohn's disease may affect any part of the gut (most commonly the ileum and colon) with patchy mucosal ulceration and transmural inflammation due to excess (Th1 and macrophages) immune activation, increased free radicals and overexpression of matrix metalloproteinases. Crohn's disease results from a complex interaction among immune, genetic and environmental factors producing a dysregulated immune response to the gut flora. Tolerance to autologous flora appears to be lost and thus the luminal 'content' represents a persistent driving factor of the cell-mediated inflammatory process further stimulated by a possible defective response to (selected?) pathogens. The concept that the enteric flora is of profound importance in the development of Crohn's disease is supported by the absence of disease in germ-free conditions, by the recognition that a specific disease-associated gene such as Nod-2 encodes an intracellular molecule important in the inflammatory response to bacterial peptidoglycans and by the production of IFN-γ induced in these patients by extracts of their own commensal flora. Furthermore recent studies showed reduced defensin expression, defective activation of NF-$\kappa\beta$ and IL-8 secretion and enhanced IL-12 production (due to a failed inhibition of TLR2 signaling). Thus, interaction between the luminal antigens (from dietary products and microorganisms) and the immune system is crucial and beneficial manipulation of diet and selected probiotic supplementation is intriguing. Many diet trials (i.e. with fibers, carbohydrate restriction or PUFA supplementation) have been tried without significant benefit. Conversely, enteral nutrition (EN) with a polymeric formula has a proven therapeutic effect for inducing (clinical and histological) remission in pediatric Crohn's disease, improves weight gain, and reverses growth failure and nutrient deficiencies. Some progress has been made in understanding the mechanisms by which EN exerts its beneficial influence in Crohn's disease. Nutritional restitution, modulation of enteric flora and inflammatory cytokines and alteration of the expression of specific genes (with immune effects) within the epithelium have all been considered. A recent report pointed out that the efficacy of EN is significantly dependent on ileal involvement [24]. A profound modification of the fecal microflora after EN (Modulen IBD, Nestlé) has been demonstrated [25] although the mechanisms of the interaction between the formula used and the gut flora still need to be clarified. Selected probiotics could, in theory, restore the luminal balance and exert regulatory or anti-inflammatory effects. However, a recent randomized, placebo-controlled trial of LGG supplements added to standard therapy did not prolong remission in 39 children with Crohn's disease [26].

Primary Enterocyte Abnormalities

Intestinal Epithelial Dysplasia (Tufting Enteropathy)

Intestinal epithelial dysplasia presents at neonatal age with chronic watery diarrhea, impaired growth and possible facial dysmorphisms. Small bowel biopsies reveal variable villous atrophy, crypt hyperplasia and slightly increased inflammatory activation in the lamina propria without a marked increase of intraepithelial lymphocytes. The characteristic feature of tufting enteropathy is the presence of focal epithelial 'tufts' composed of closely packed enterocytes with rounding of the apical plasma membrane which results in a teardrop configuration of the affected epithelial cell likely due to a defect in the basement membrane and in the expression of cellular adhesion molecules. Parenteral nutrition is necessary in most affected patients.

Microvillous Inclusion Disease

Microvillous inclusion disease is a rare (often fatal) enteropathy with severe watery diarrhea starting in the first days of life. Variable villous atrophy with mild crypt hyperplasia, and an absence of marked inflammatory infiltrate in the lamina propria are present in the biopsies. On higher magnification, the surface enterocytes are disorganized, with extensive vacuolization and positive staining for periodic acid-Schiff, alkaline phosphatase and CD10 (a leukemia antigen normally expressed in the brush border of enterocytes) of the apical cytoplasms indicating an internalization or a defective exocytosis of the glycocalyx. On transmission electron microscopy, intracytoplasmic microvillous inclusions and apical secretory granules in surface epithelial are pathognomonic of microvillous inclusion disease. The severity of the secretory diarrhea and the concomitant different alterations of brush-border membrane transport cause the need of long-term parenteral nutrition and eventual intestinal transplant.

Small Intestinal Lymphangiectasia

Small intestinal lymphangiectasia is a rare disease characterized by obstruction of the small bowel lymph drainage with dilated lymphatic vessels and patchy villous distortions and mucosal involvement. Lymphangiectasia may be caused by a congenital malformation or by a secondary lymphatic block (such as in abdominal or retroperitoneal tumors or fibrosis, mesenteric tuberculosis, intestinal malrotation, congestive heart failure, and constrictive pericarditis). Due to lymph stasis an excess loss of protein into the intestinal lumen may occur and peripheral edema (related to hypoalbuminemia) and malnutrition may manifest. Steatorrhea due to malabsorption of chylomicrons and fat-soluble vitamins (T-cells), lymphocytopenia and hypogammaglobulinemia are additional findings. On endoscopy scattered white opaque spots or plaques in the duodenal mucosa represent the dilated enteric lymphatic vessels detected on the biopsies. The mainstay of dietary treatment is a low-fat, high-protein MCT diet with additional calcium salt and water-soluble forms of fat-soluble vitamins required in selected patients. EN (with elemental diet or polymeric diet containing MCT) appears to have a similar efficacy to total parenteral nutrition.

A-β-Lipoproteinemia

In a-β-lipoproteinemia chylomicron formation is impaired (related to mutations in the MTP gene) and the absorbed dietary fats (chylomicrons, VLDL, LDL) are absent from the plasma and are accumulated, as vacuoles, in the cytoplasm of the enterocytes. Steatorrhea and failure to thrive may be associated with retinitis pigmentosa, progressive neurological manifestations (absent deep tendon reflexes, ataxia, tremors, impaired position and vibration sensitivity), and acanthocytes related to vitamin E deficiency. Large supplements of fat-soluble vitamins and reduced long-chain fat intake replaced by MCT are required.

Protein-Losing Enteropathy

Protein-losing enteropathy is a broad term including all the conditions that cause an abnormal loss of plasma proteins from the gut. Three main mechanisms are responsible for protein-losing enteropathy: enhanced mucosal permeability to proteins (as in eosinophilic gastroenteritis and Menetrier's disease), mucosal erosions or ulceration (as in erosive gastritis and inflammatory bowel disease), and lymphatic obstruction (congenital or secondary). Enteric loss of protein may be revealed noninvasively by an increased stool concentration of α_1-antitrypsin or, more expensively, by radioactive methods (intravenous administration of ^{51}Cr albumin or chloride).

Specific Dietary Interventions

Nucleotides

Dietary nucleotides build blocks of RNA, DNA, ATP, and therefore a supplemented formula may improve growth and immunity, optimize the maturation, recovery and function of rapidly dividing tissue, such as the gastrointestinal tract mucosa. Infant studies have shown that the addition of nucleotides decreases the incidence of diarrhea and upper (but not lower) respiratory tract infections, affects NK cell activity, increases serum IgA, T cell maturation and antibody level after *Haemophilus influenzae* type B (but not hepatitis B) vaccination [27, 28]. 'Most' dietary nucleotides are rapidly metabolized and excreted. However, 'some' are incorporated in tissue, probably depending on many factors such as age at supplementation. In infants with severe intrauterine growth retardation nucleotides enhance catch-up growth. The supplementation of nucleotides in infant feeding can be regarded as very safe; therefore the cost/benefit ratio is of major importance. As a consequence, the addition of nucleotides in infant feeding should be considered in 'at risk' infants such as the preterm and immature infant, or after severe intestinal injury.

Glutamine

Glutamine supplementation is reported as safe, and tends to be associated with less infectious morbidity and mortality. However, glutamine-enriched EN did not improve feeding tolerance or short-term outcome in very low birth weight infants and the available data from good quality randomized controlled trials suggest that preterm infants do not clinically significantly benefit from glutamine supplementation [29].

Lipids

Increasing evidence has demonstrated that adequate dietary lipids are extremely important not just for their caloric value but also for their immune-modulatory effects. Lipids may prevent allergic sensitization by downregulating inflammatory response (n-3 but not n-6 long-chain fatty acids) whilst protecting the epithelial barrier, regulate immune function and modify the adherence of microbes to the mucosa, thereby contributing to host-microbe interactions. Medium-chain (8–12 carbons) fatty acids (MCT) seem to have more strongly antiviral and antibacterial properties (against Rous sarcoma virus, herpes simplex virus, *H. influenzae* and group B streptococcus) than long-chain triglycerides [30]. According to a recent Cochrane review, there is no evidence of differences between MCT and long-chain triglycerides in short-term growth, gastrointestinal intolerance, or necrotizing enterocolitis [31].

References

1 Walker-Smith JA, Murch SH: Diseases of the Small Intestine in Childhood, ed 4. Oxford, Isis Medical Media, 1999.
2 Parassol N, Freitas M, Thoreux K, et al: *Lactobacillus casei* DN-114 001 inhibits the increase in paracellular permeability of enteropathogenic *Escherichia coli*-infected T84 cells. Res Microbiol 2005;156:256–262.
3 Bhutta ZA, Ghishan F, Lindley K, et al: Persistent and chronic diarrhea and malabsorption: Working Group Report of the Second World Congress of Pediatric Gastroenterology, Hepatology, and Nutrition. J Pediatr Gastroenterol Nutr 2004;39:S711–S716.
4 Dahan S, Dalmasso G, Imbert V, et al: *Saccharomyces boulardii* interferes with enterohemorrhagic *Escherichia coli*-induced signalling pathways in T84 cells. Infect Immun 2003;71: 766–773.
5 Altwegg M: Influence of *Saccharomyces boulardii* on cell invasions of *Salmonella typhimurium* and *Yersinia enterocolitica*. Microb Ecol Health Dis 1999;11:158–162.
6 Galpin L, Manary MJ, Fleming K, et al: Effect of *Lactobacillus* GG on intestinal integrity in Malawian children at risk of tropical enteropathy. Am J Clin Nutr 2005;82:1040–1045.
7 Bhutta ZA, Bird SM, Black RE, et al: Therapeutic effects of oral zinc in acute and persistent diarrhea in children in developing countries: pooled analysis of randomized controlled trials. Am J Clin Nutr 2000;72:1516–1522.
8 Bobat R, Coovadia H, Stephen C, et al: Safety and efficacy of zinc supplementation for children with HIV-1 infection in South Africa: a randomised double-blind placebo-controlled trial. Lancet 2005;366:1862–1867.

9 Hill DI, Dirks MH, Liptak GS, et al: Guideline for the diagnosis and treatment of celiac disease in children: recommendations of the North American Society for Pediatric Gastroenterology, Hepatology and Nutrition. J Pediatr Gastroenterol Nutr 2005;40:1–19.
10 Troncone R, Bhatnagar S, Butzner D, et al: Celiac disease and other immunoloically mediated disorders of the gastrointestinal tract: Working Group Report of the Second World Congress of Pediatric Gastroenterology, Hepatology, and Nutrition. J Pediatr Gastroenterol Nutr 2004;39:S601–S610.
11 Vitoria JC, Camarero C, Sojo A, et al: Enteropathy related to fish, rice, and chicken. Arch Dis Child 1982;57:44–48.
12 Nowak-Wegrzyn A, Sampson HA, Wood RA, Sicherer SH: Food protein-induced enterocolitis syndrome caused by solid food proteins. Pediatrics 2003;111:829–835.
13 Rozenfeld P, Docena GH, Anon MC, Fossati CA: Detection and identification of a soy protein component that cross-reacts with caseins from cow's milk. Clin Exp Immunol 2002;130:49–58.
14 Kokkonen J, Haapalahti M, Laurila K, et al: Cow's milk protein sensitive enteropathy at school age. J Pediatr 2001;139:797–803.
15 Kokkonen J, Tikkanen S, Karttunen TJ, Savilahti E: A similar high level of immunoglobulin A and immunoglobulin G class milk antibodies and increment of local lymphoid tissue on the duodenal mucosa in subjects with cow's milk allergy and recurrent abdominal pains. Pediatr Allergy Immunol 2002;13:129–136.
16 Pérez-Machado MA, Ashwood P, Thomson MA, et al: Reduced transforming growth factor-beta1 producing T cells in the duodenal mucosa of children with food allergy. Eur J Immunol 2003;33:2307–2315.
17 Schappi MG, Smith VV, Cubitt D, et al: Faecal elastase 1 concentration is a marker of duodenal enteropathy. Arch Dis Child 2002;86:50–53.
18 Caramalho I, Lopes-Carvalho T, Ostler D, et al: Regulatory T cells selectively express toll-like receptors and are activated by lipopolysaccharide. J Exp Med 2003;197:403–411.
19 Kalliomaki M, Salminen S, Poussa T, et al: Probiotics and prevention of atopic disease: 4-year follow-up of a randomised placebo-controlled trial. Lancet 2003;361:1869–1871.
20 Lodinova-Zadnikova R, Cukrowska B, Tlaskalova-Hogenova H: Oral administration of probiotic *Escherichia coli* after birth reduces frequency of allergies and repeated infections later in life (after 10 and 20 years). Int Arch Allergy Immunol 2003;131:209–211.
21 Salvatore S, Keymolen K, Hauser B, Vandenplas Y: Intervention during pregnancy and allergic disease in the offspring. Pediatr Allergy Immunol 2005;16:558–566.
22 Wittenberg D, Benitez CV, Canani RB, et al: HIV infection: Working Group Report of the Second World Congress of Pediatric Gastroenterology, Hepatology, and Nutrition. J Pediatr Gastroenterol Nutr 2004;39:S640–S646.
23 Rothenberg ME: Eosinophilic gastrointestinal disorders. J Allergy Clin Immunol 2004;113:11–28.
24 Afzal NA, Davies S, Paintin M, et al: Colonic Crohn's disease in children does not respond well to treatment with enteral nutrition if the ileum is not involved. Dig Dis Sci 2005;50:1471–1475.
25 Lionetti P, Callegari ML, Ferrari S, et al: Enteral nutrition and microflora in pediatric Crohn's disease. J Parenter Enteral Nutr 2005;29(suppl 4):S173–175.
26 Bousvaros A, Guandalini S, Baldassano RN, et al: A randomized, double-blind trial of *Lactobacillus* GG versus placebo in addition to standard maintenance therapy for children with Crohn's disease. Inflamm Bowel Dis 2005;11:833–839.
27 Buck RH, Thomas DL, Winship TR, et al: Effect of dietary ribonucleotides on infant immune status. 2. Immune cell development. Pediatr Res 2004;56:891–900.
28 Yau KI: Effect of nucleotides on diarrhea and immune responses in healthy term infants in Taiwan. J Pediatr Gastroenterol Nutr 2003;36:37–43.
29 Tubman TR, Thompson SW, McGuire W: Glutamine supplementation to prevent morbidity and mortality in preterm infants. Cochrane Database Syst Rev 2005;1:CD001457.
30 Isaacs CE: Antimicrobial activity of lipids added to human milk, infant formula, and bovine milk. J Nutr Biochem 1995;6:362–366.
31 Klenoff-Brumberg HL, Genen LH: High versus low medium chain triglyceride content of formula for promoting short term growth of preterm infants. Cochrane Database Syst Rev 2003;1:CD002777.

Discussion

Dr. Rivera: This morning I glanced at the *European Journal of Nutrition* and I saw a very interesting topic on the use of probiotics in pancreatitis with apparent good results [1]. I wonder if you have any comments or if you have heard about this study or any particular experience that you may have had with pancreatitis?

Dr. Vandenplas: I am not aware of clinical studies on probiotics in human patients with pancreatitis. However, probiotics have been demonstrated to equilibrate the gastrointestinal ecosystem. Also, they have been shown to be beneficial in different infectious diseases, even outside the gastrointestinal tract, such as urinary tract infections and vaginitis. Therefore, it could be possible that probiotics may also have a role in pancreatitis.

Dr. B. Koletzko: You cited the paper by Yau et al. [2] from Taiwan who supplemented nucleotides; you interpreted their data as showing a reduction in respiratory disease and respiratory infections with added nucleotides. I think there was a mistake; in fact these authors reported that nucleotide supplementation, at a relatively high level exceeding 10 mg/100 kcal, increased rather than decreased the rate of respiratory infection. Thus this is one of the studies that actually raise the question whether higher levels of nucleotides in infant formulae are appropriate.

Dr. Saavedra: When we look specifically at 'probiotics' we should use the term as a concept. But when we get to recommendations we should not use the word as a concept, we should use the specific strains that we are talking about. This is a common mistake. In any recommendation paper, not a conceptual paper, that is making recommendations, when we use the word 'probiotics' relative to safety or efficacy it is naïve or simplistic to say that antibiotics are safe or efficacious. In the future, if we stick to recommendations regarding the safety or efficacy of these agents, we should talk about the specific agent being studied.

My question refers to the use of some of these microorganisms early in life. Most breastfed babies get nonsterile formula, i.e. breastfeeding, and get it in the least allergenic way (human proteins). What we have done with 'modern' formula is to give sterile formula in the most allergenic form we know (cow proteins). What does the inclusion of microorganisms in the diet of babies in early life have to do with regular or constant bacterial stimulation? That is, do you have to keep giving these organisms or is it enough to inoculate a child with potential microorganisms to establish the flora which leads to less necrotizing enterocolitis or diarrhea.

Dr. Vandenplas: I fully agree with the proposed definition of probiotics. Recommendations should be strain specific. Probiotics should be separated into groups referred to as 'food supplements' and 'medications'. Whether you call these probiotics simply 'medication' or 'biotherapeutic' is a question of making agreements and reaching a consensus. Food supplements are clearly different.

It is true that on the one hand we sterilize the formulas for the preterm infants and then we add microbes to it. I do not know if that is good or not. The idea of adding prebiotics to starter formula to develop the infant's own gastrointestinal flora is also a possibility. In the future we may learn that prebiotics are a good concept for healthy term-born infants, whereas probiotics are a better concept for sick infants. Today, we have no information on this, and every statement is speculation. Most of the time the preterm infant is born by cesarean section and lives in a sterile environment; it gets antibiotics, but may be better off with probiotics. We do not have information on this today.

Dr. Fuchs: My question has to do with Modulen and the evidence that suggests it would be advantageous. What is your view of the evidence or just your personal opinion on where Modulen might fit in our treatment approach?

Dr. Vandenplas: Up to now, there is to my knowledge no consensus where exactly Modulen fits into the treatment. Some centers first focus on nutrition and use Modulen almost as first-line treatment. Other centers use Modulen after failure of 'classic' medical treatment. Opinions do differ. In our center, we first try medical treatment with corticoids, 5-ASA and Imuran. If this fails, we try nutritional therapy. But whether this is a better approach than starting with nutrition, I do not know. There are not enough randomized data to allow conclusions.

Dr. Fuchs: Specifically as it relates to Modulen, not just any formula, is there a potential role for Modulen as opposed to another elemental or semi-elemental formula?

Dr. Vandenplas: Yes, there are data suggesting that Modulen is effective. It tastes quite good, so most children succeed in drinking it as their only food for a couple of weeks or even months. This is a big advantage. In general tube feeding is very poorly accepted by adolescents, and causes psychological and emotional problems. If patients drink the formula, at least the psychological problem is solved.

Dr. Milla: As Dr. Fuchs said yesterday eosinophilic gastroenteropathy is probably a heterogeneous group of different conditions and mucosal eosinophilic gastroenteropathy seems to be quite different to transmural and serosal eosinophilic gastroenteropathy. Mucosal eosinophilic gastroenteropathy is becoming much more common in Europe and we may catch up with the east coast of the US. There was a paper in *Gut* showing that Montelukast, a chemokine antagonist, is helpful in mucosal eosinophilic gastroenteropathy but does not seem to help the other two [3]. Could you comment on the place of oats and oat withdrawal in gluten-induced enteropathy and the management of gluten-free resistant celiac disease.

Dr. Vandenplas: Regarding your comment, I fully agree with your statements. The short answer to your question would be no. Although there is no real consensus today on the question if the glutens present in oat are really not toxic or if they have a reduced toxicity compared to the glutens from the 3 other sources. The first thing to do in patients who do not improve on a gluten-free diet would be to reconsider the diagnosis. If the patient does not respond to a gluten-free diet, it is likely not celiac disease.

Dr. Ruemmele: Perhaps I can address some points regarding the question from Dr. Milla. We [4] and also Marti et al. [5] tracked down different peptides in glutens involved in celiac disease, there are immunostimulatory peptides and there are toxic peptides. Therefore, we have to consider different gliadin antigens involved in the pathogenesis of celiac disease. The improved understanding of these antigens may help to explain the varying clinical presentation of celiac disease. Once the immune process is stimulated, and it can be self-perpetuated by cytokines, such as IL-15, these patients no longer respond to glutens so this is the true mechanism on the way to lymphoma. We never saw this in pediatrics but in adult patients it is well known.

In the intestine we know that on one hand there are enterocytes, the epithelium, the mucosal immune system, and on the other hand in the lumen there are antigenic structures and bacteria, which were largely neglected in the past. We are wondering whether Modulen IBD in Crohn's disease patients is not one of those drugs that is very selective in improving this interplay. We know about its anti-inflammatory effects but perhaps this is related to a major impact on the intestinal flora. With the help of Nestlé we are addressing this in a study with Crohn's disease patients using Modulen IBD. There are preliminary data by Paolo Lionetti from Italy who observed a certain degree of change in the intestinal flora in these patients and we want to address this question in a systematic manner. By modifying the diet not only are the nutritional elements changed; the flora might be one of the major aspects modifying Crohn's disease.

Dr. Vandenplas: I would like to add that every one is so focused on gastrointestinal flora that it is now brought in relation to every condition. Many researchers have shown that the gastrointestinal flora is very important in immune system development and immune response. But it is also likely that the gastrointestinal flora is not the only factor influencing the immune development and response.

Dr. Picaud: As a neonatologist I would like to talk about probiotics in prematurity because it is rarely discussed and it could be interesting because we need something new to improve nutrition in preterm infants. There are some data from Japan showing that there is an improved feeding tolerance with these probiotics. On the other hand the benefits have been clearly shown in areas where there is a high incidence of necrotizing enterocolitis. More than 1,000 infants have been included in this type of study, and there is no problem with safety. Regarding safety, the balance between risks and benefits should be integrated. Indeed, the theoretical risk is bacterial translocation but there are some data showing that the translocation, at least in animals, decreases when probiotics are provided. Furthermore, when there is suspected late-onset sepsis in neonates, antibiotics are used. There could be a benefit from using probiotics in this clinical setting, and there are recent data showing that it is better when two probiotics are given rather than one.

Dr. Vandenplas: This is an interesting area that needs further research. There is laboratory research showing that it should be safe. On the other hand, the clinical studies that have been performed still have a limited number of children. Much more data are needed in sick newborns before we can be really sure that in 'daily life' the administration of probiotics is really safe. Side effects, such as septicemia, have been reported in preterms with short bowel. The effect of the introduction of probiotics from the very first day of life on the development of permanent gastrointestinal flora should also be further investigated. It is well known that when given later in life, probiotics do not colonize the gastrointestinal tract. They disappear from the flora a couple of days or weeks after the administration has stopped. But this natural evolution might be different when the probiotic is introduced at birth, because then it is part of the very first flora that will develop. It might be that colonization in this condition with the probiotic becomes more permanent. We do not know. As a consequence, we certainly do not know whether this might be beneficial or potentially dangerous.

Dr. Heine: Could you speculate on the mechanism of *Lactobacillus* GG that might be detrimental in Crohn's disease?

Dr. Vandenplas: I would not like the take-home message to be that probiotics in Crohn's disease are detrimental because the data available are very limited, and for the study I showed the difference was not significant. There was a trend towards more relapses in the group with *Lactobacilli*. However, several studies in adults with Crohn's disease did show some benefit from probiotics, especially in pouchitis. Presently the evidence that probiotics in Crohn's disease are really helpful is weak, except for pouchitis.

Dr. Jacobson: You spoke a little bit about Crohn's disease and enteral nutrition support, and you indicated that the polymeric diet is as efficacious as the elemental diet. Can you provide us with some thoughts as to why you think the polymeric is equally efficacious given that the theory behind the efficacy of the elemental diet is related to the reduced antigenic load.

Dr. Vandenplas: I do not have enough personal experience with the comparison of different feedings. It can be supposed that an elemental or normal polymeric diet probably approaches different mechanisms involved in Crohn's disease. One mechanism may be that a sick mucosa has an increased permeability. Elemental feeding would the be a logical choice. Another mechanism might be that with normal feeding there is a more balanced effect on gastrointestinal flora. We do not know why both seem to work. I also don't know of any study showing that elemental feeding is successful after failure of polymeric feeding.

Dr. Nowak-Wegrzyn: We followed a number of children with mucosal eosinophilic gastroenteritis in whom protein-losing gastroenteropathy was seen and on biopsies the only place where eosinophilic infiltrate was found is the stomach [6]. Have you had any patients like that? In your experience, is the stomach a common site for protein loss or have we missed the intestinal eosinophilic infiltrates, which are patchy in nature, or can't they be detected in the ileum?

Dr. Fuchs: I find it difficult to believe that all your protein loss is just from the stomach with that sort of histology. There are cases with protein loss just from the stomach, but my suspicion is that it probably reflects protein loss further down the small bowel.

Dr. S. Koletzko: The distribution can be very patchy. I have followed a child who has a severe eosenophilic enteropathy for several years and was endoscoped many times. On each occasion the distribution of the lesions was different; at one point the stomach and the next time the colon or the small bowel. So the lesions are probably patchy and that may be misleading in your case.

Dr. Vandenplas: Then you need a capsule which can take multiple biopsies in the small bowel.

Dr. Lentze: You and others have touched upon probiotics. Why do they work, how do they work and where do they work?

Dr. Vandenplas: There is quite a lot of in vitro laboratory research on the mechanisms of action of different microorganisms. Whether you can transpose those mechanisms to the clinical situation is another question. One of the mechanisms may be an increased secretion of IgA at the intestinal mucosa level. This may explain why the duration of diarrhea is shortened, even if dead microorganisms are administered. Maybe this is also the reason why there is less re-infection 1 month later as suggested in an open trial. But you are right, more research in clinical settings is needed on the mechanisms of action.

Dr. Saavedra: I think your question is very valid because it underlines what Dr. Vandenplas was saying earlier, we should not just say 'probiotics work', we have to say what we mean by 'they work'. In other words, maybe this is a bad analogy but it is like saying this particular diet works – it works for certain patients; similarly for probiotics, a particular probiotic has been shown to be safe and efficacious for a specific application. So of course we could say there are many *Lactobacilli* and they are all excellent for lactose digestion. It has been very well demonstrated and shown mechanically that they improve lactose tolerance in patients with lactose malabsorption [7]. This is very different than saying probiotics may improve or decrease the chances for rotaviral infection [8], or that they can increase specific anti-rotaviral IgA [9]. When we talk about these benefits we need to point out specific agents such as a specific *Bidifobacteria* for specific purposes, and not say that probiotics in general have this or that effect. We cannot generalize benefits or adverse effects to all probiotics, because we will never come to a conclusion.

References

1   Walker WA, Goulet O, Morelli L, Antoine JM: Progress in the science of probiotics: from cellular microbiology and applied immunology to clinical nutrition. Eur J Nutr 2006;45(suppl 9): 1–18.
2   Yau KI, Huang CB, Chen W, et al: Effect of nucleotides on diarrhea and immune responses in healthy term infants in Taiwan. J Pediatr Gastroenterol Nutr 2003;36:37–43.
3   Attwood SE, Lewis CJ, Bronder CS, et al: Eosinophilic oesophagitis: a novel treatment using Montelukast. Gut 2003;52:181–185.

4 Mention JJ, Ben Ahmed M, Begue B, et al: Interleukin 15: a key to disrupted intraepithelial lymphocyte homeostasis and lymphomagenesis in celiac disease. Gastroenterology 2003;125: 730–745.
5 Marti T, Molberg O, Li Q, et al: Prolyl endopeptidase-mediated destruction of T cell epitopes in whole gluten: chemical and immunological characterization. J Pharmacol Exp Ther 2005;312: 19–26.
6 Chehade M, Magid MS, Mofidi S, et al: Allergic eosinophilic gastroenteritis with protein-losing enteropathy: intestinal pathology, clinical course, and long-term follow-up. J Pediatr Gastroenterol Nutr 2006;42:516–521.
7 Shermak MA, Saavedra JM, Jackson TL, et al: Effect of yogurt on symptoms and hydrogen production in lactose-malabsorbing children. Am J Clin Nutr 1995;62:1003–1006.
8 Fukushima Y, Kawata Y, Hara H, et al: Effect of a probiotic formula on intestinal immunoglobulin A production in healthy children. Int J Food Microbiol 1998;42:39–44.
9 Saavedra JM, Bauman NA, Oung I, et al: Feeding of B. bifidum and S. thermophilus for prevention of diarrhea and shedding of rotavirus. Lancet 1994;344:1046–1049.

Cooke RJ, Vandenplas Y, Wahn U (eds): Nutrition Support for Infants and Children at Risk.
Nestlé Nutr Workshop Ser Pediatr Program, vol 59, pp 133–146,
Nestec Ltd., Vevey/S. Karger AG, Basel, © 2007.

Stressed Mucosa

Geoffrey Davidson, Stamatiki Kritas, Ross Butler

Centre for Paediatric and Adolescent Gastroenterology, Women's and Children's Hospital,
North Adelaide, Australia

Abstract

Stress has been defined as an acute threat to the homeostasis of the organism. The mucosal lining of the gastrointestinal tract, a single layer of epithelial cells held together by tight junctions, provides a barrier between the external environment and the body's internal milieu. Any mechanism that breaches the tight junction exposes the body to foreign material be it protein, microorganisms or toxins. Stresses include physiological (exercise), psychological, disease-related or drug-induced factors. Stress associated gastrointestinal disorders include functional dyspepsia irritable bowel syndrome (IBS), gastroesophageal reflux disease peptic ulcer disease, and inflammatory bowel disease (IBD). Some disease states disrupt gastrointestinal barrier function, e.g. infectious diarrhea, IBD, or celiac disease, whilst in others such as eczema it can be indirectly related to antigenic disruption of the barrier. Drugs, e.g. chemotherapy agents and nonsteroidal anti-inflammatory drugs, also disrupt barrier function. Malnutrition and nutritional deficiencies (zinc, folic acid, vitamin A) also predispose to mucosal damage. Assessment of gastrointestinal mucosal health has proved problematic as invasive techniques, whilst useful, provide limited data and no functional assessment. Noninvasive tests particularly breath tests do provide functional assessment and many can be used together as biomarkers to improve our ability to define a stressed mucosa. Therapeutic options include pharmacotherapies, immunomodulation or immunotherapy.

Copyright © 2007 Nestec Ltd., Vevey/S. Karger AG, Basel

Introduction

Stress can be defined as any threat to an organism's homeostasis. The function of the stress response is to maintain homeostasis [1]. The mucosal lining is a single layer of epithelial cells providing a barrier between the external environment, the luminal contents and the body's internal milieu. The epithelial cells are joined by tight junctions which if breached become permeable

Table 1. Factors contributing to a stressed mucosa

Stress	Conditions
Physiological stress	Elite athletes
Psychological stress	IBS
Disease states	IBD
	Infectious diarrhea
	Atopic diseases
	CD
Nutrient deficiencies	Malnutrition
	Micronutrient deficiency, e.g. Zn, folic acid, vitamin A
Drugs	Nonsteroidal anti-inflammatory drugs
	Chemotherapy agents

allowing the passage of undesirable luminal solutes, microorganisms, antigens or foreign proteins to enter the circulation [2].

There are many factors that contribute to barrier function including the mucous layer, mucosal enzymes, microflora as well as the tight junctions. The tight junctions do not only have a barrier function but also regulate paracellular transport, acting as a fence by maintaining separate apical and basolateral domains and have a signaling function during stress. The body has a number of mechanisms that allow it to protect this barrier from stress. For example the acidification of the stomach provides a barrier against infectious agents passing into the small intestine. However, if this acid is refluxed into the esophagus then it can act as a stressor causing esophageal mucosal damage. Gastrointestinal motility and the mucosal immune system are other mechanisms that provide protection for the gastrointestinal mucosa. The gut mucosa faces many potential stressors and the aim of this dissertation is to discuss some of these and where possible highlight the mechanisms and consequences of this stress.

One of the limitations to our understanding the effect of stress on the gastrointestinal mucosa is the lack of simple, safe, noninvasive diagnostic techniques. The ideal would be the ability to sample tissue at various levels of the gut but even then the biopsy may not inform on the whole of the intestine. Alternative safe, noninvasive tests that inform on the total gut function or regions of the gut individually such as stomach, small intestine or colon function, in health and disease, are being developed and will also be discussed.

Table 1 highlights possible contributors to a stressed mucosa and some of these factors including physiological and psychological stress, inflammation, infection, nutrient deficiencies, and drugs will be discussed below in more detail.

Physiological Stress

The gastrointestinal tract can be stressed by physical exertion such as long distance running producing symptoms of abdominal pain, diarrhea and flatulence [3]. The symptoms do not appear to correlate with either the intensity or duration of the exercise. Studies of the gastrointestinal tract have shown a high incidence of mucosal erosions with hemorrhagic and ischemic colitis [4, 5]. Oktedalen et al. [3] have also shown increased intestinal permeability in symptomatic athletes whereas others have shown similar changes but without gastrointestinal symptoms [6, 7]. There is also a correlation between the intensity of running and loss of barrier function expressed as permeability.

A recent study has shown that in recreational runners small intestinal permeability increased before and after an 8-week exercise program. The severity of the disturbance to barrier function in recreational runners was similar to that seen in patients with IBD in remission [8].

It has been suggested that gastrointestinal mucosal ischemia is the major stress leading to gastrointestinal damage [8]. Other factors such as dehydration and changes in body temperature may also contribute. It is also possible that the increased susceptibility of individual athletes to illness may be related to changes in intestinal permeability.

Attempts have been made to reduce the mucosal damage in athletes during training. Bovine colostrum has been shown to improve athletic performance, reduce infections and reduce intestinal permeability caused by administration of nonsteroidal anti-inflammatory drugs. A recent study in athletes during running training showed that bovine colostrum increased intestinal permeability [10]. It was postulated that this may have allowed absorption of bioactive components from the colostrum that enhanced athletic performance and immunity.

Psychological Stress

Several recent reviews [10, 11] have discussed the role of psychological stress in the pathophysiology of gastrointestinal disease. The stress response is complex and involves a number of regions in the brain and brain stem together with somatic and visceral afferents and the endocrine system (fig. 1).

The release of corticotrophin-releasing factor (CRF), an important mediator of the central stress response, triggers a cascade of events via the anterior pituitary gland, the adrenal gland and the autonomic nervous system reaching the enteric nervous system which contains a network of approximately 100 million neurons. The enteric nervous system in turn influences gut motility, exocrine and endocrine functions, and the microcirculation. Together with this there also appears to be an effect of chronic stress leading

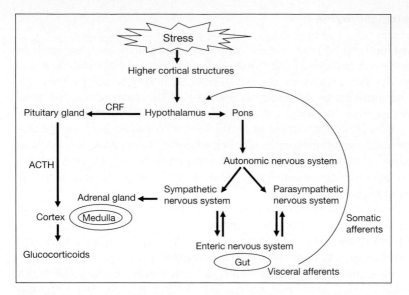

Fig. 1. Stress-induced pathways affecting the gastrointestinal tract. ACTH = Adrenocorticotrophic hormone.

Table 2. Stress-associated gastrointestinal disorders

Gastroesophageal reflux disease
Functional dyspepsia
Peptic ulcer disease
IBD
IBS

to increased CRF synthesis affecting both the immune system and causing a prolonged inflammatory response. In a recent study of patients with irritable bowel syndrome (IBS), the use of a nonselective CRF inhibitor significantly improved gastrointestinal motility, visceral perception and negative mood in response to gut stimulation [12].

Stress has been associated with a number of gastrointestinal disorders (table 2) and can be associated with increased colonic motility, increased water, electrolyte and colonic mucous secretions and increased mast cell mediators. There are few studies in humans demonstrating the above changes in gut function but quite strong evidence in IBD that stress associated with adverse life events is associated with a higher rate of relapse [13].

IBS is a common condition affecting up to 15% of the adult population. Major stressful life events, bacterial gastroenteritis and sexual abuse seem to be important trigger factors. Recent studies suggest that a low grade inflammation characterizes this syndrome. This supraphysiological inflammatory condition may predispose to an increased intestinal permeability and potentially contribute to altered motility in different regions of the gastrointestinal tract. Surrogate markers including fecal calprotectin (a neutrophil-specific protein) and intestinal permeability have been suggested as discriminators of organic versus nonorganic disease [14]. Carbohydrate malabsorption, particularly fructose and lactose, are also prominent in IBS and may contribute to symptoms [15].

Inflammatory Bowel Disease

IBD including Crohn's disease and ulcerative colitis is usually diagnosed in children, adolescents or young adults and has a prevalence of about 20/100,000 people. Clinical assessment of disease activity has proved to be problematic particularly in children. Conventional laboratory markers of disease activity such as erythrocyte sedimentation rate and C-reactive protein may reflect disease activity but do not reflect intestinal function.

Increased intestinal permeability may play a significant role in the pathogenesis of IBD and can be measured using nonmetabolized sugar probes such as L-rhamnose, mannitol and lactulose. The urinary excretion ratios of these probes such as lactulose/L-rhamnose or lactulose/mannitol provide a simple, noninvasive and reproducible index of intestinal permeability [16]. Intestinal permeability can be increased not only in active disease but also in noninflamed mucosa and in first degree relatives of patients with IBD [17]. Increased intestinal permeability has also been noted in children with active ulcerative colitis but not in inactive disease [16].

Alkanes are major volatile hydrocarbons and indicate lipid peroxidation which may be an important pathogenic factor in IBD and a marker of a stressed mucosa. They can be measured in breath and have been used as markers of IBD activity [18]. Other tests such as fecal calprotectin have also been used to noninvasively determine intestinal inflammation correlating with clinical disease activity [14].

Infectious Diarrhea

There are two major mechanisms leading to diarrhea secondary to infection. The most common may be a secretory diarrhea, e.g. enterotoxigenic *Escherichia coli* or *Vibrio cholerae* where a bacterial toxin stimulates secretion. The other mechanism is mucosal injury leading to an osmotic or malabsorptive diarrhea, e.g. rotavirus or *Campylobacter jejuni*.

The stressors for secretory diarrhea are generally toxins whilst the stressor in infectious diarrhea is cell penetration and lysis leading to rapid cell turnover with blunting of villi and replacement of mature enterocytes by immature enterocytes [19].

In a recent review, Liu et al. [2] discussed the mechanisms whereby pathogenic, enteric microorganisms interact with tight junctions. This interaction and disruption are related to the effect of various toxins on zonula occlusion proteins altering occludin distribution [20]. There is also a suggestion that rotavirus infection may act in a similar way through its nonstructural NSP4 protein.

In communities in the developing world rotavirus is often the first gut infection occurring as early as at 3–4 months of age. This is a very damaging illness, where both a secretory and osmotic diarrhea may be present concurrently. Acute infectious diarrhea is often a precursor to recurrent diarrhea and malnutrition. This occurs because of the recurrent infections both gastrointestinal and extraintestinal that children in developing countries are exposed to due to environmental contamination aggravated by undernutrition. It is likely that all children living in developing communities, particularly in the tropics, have an abnormal small intestinal mucosal structure and function with villous blunting, increased cellular infiltrate in the lamina propria, increased intestinal permeability and disaccharidase deficiencies, mainly lactase. This setting has been labeled as tropical or environmental enteropathy [21].

Kukuruzovic and Brewster [22] have studied the enteropathy in rural and urban Aboriginal communities in the north of Australia presenting to hospital with diarrheal disease and malnutrition. Their aim was to show that the severity of the diarrheal disease was a consequence of small intestinal mucosal damage. They measured intestinal permeability using lactulose/L-rhamnose ratios in Aboriginal children with and without diarrhea and non-Aboriginal controls. Aboriginal children with and those without diarrhea had markedly elevated permeability compared to non-Aboriginal controls. In the same study, diarrheal complications such as acidosis, hypokalemia and osmotic diarrhea were associated with high lactulose/L-rhamnose ratios reflecting greater small intestinal damage.

Atopic Diseases

There is evidence that intestinal barrier function particularly intestinal permeability is altered in patients with atopic eczema and gastrointestinal allergic symptoms [22]. The permeable mucosa allows food antigens to reach the submucosal immune system and stimulate the production of cytokines and inflammatory mediators which in turn further disrupt the mucosal barrier.

Celiac Disease

Celiac disease (CD) can be considered as an autoimmune-like systemic disorder in genetically susceptible persons perpetuated by gluten-containing cereals, wheat, rye, barley and possibly oats. Intestinal mucosal damage in

CD is dependent on dietary exposure to prolamins. There is a genetic predisposition to CD related to the HLA-DQ2 and HLA-DQ8 molecules. These molecules stimulate proliferation of T cells and excretion of inflammatory cytokines. There is evidence to show an increase in intestinal permeability in CD, which seems to relate to gluten intake. There is also evidence of increased intestinal permeability in unaffected relatives of celiac patients compared to nonrelated controls. Cummins et al. [24] have shown that improvement in intestinal permeability precedes by many months the recovery in intestinal morphology.

Malnutrition and Nutrient Deficiencies

Malnutrition is a major issue in the developing world with significant consequences of increased infections, growth retardation and diarrheal disease which creates a vicious cycle if malnutrition is present from early infancy. This cycle is often the basis for the tropical or environmental enteropathy seen in many developing countries [21]. This condition is aggravated by micronutrient deficiencies particularly zinc, folate and vitamin A. As previously noted there is a significant increase in this setting.

Permeability testing has been used in Malawi, a developing country, to show the superiority of a milk-based diet over local cereals in rehabilitating children with kwashiorkor [25]. Not only was there a significant improvement in intestinal permeability but also reduced mortality, sepsis and weight gains.

Zinc deficiency is now known to be a major contributor to the incidence severity and duration of diarrhea. Diarrhea results in a significant increase in fecal losses of zinc. There are a number of similarities between the features of zinc deficiency and those of an enteropathy including growth-faltering diarrhea, intestinal mucosal damage and inflammation. A recent study from Bangladesh suggests that zinc may be a factor in the etiology of the enteropathy with supplementation reportedly leading to improved gut function [26].

Drugs

There are obviously many drugs that can affect gastrointestinal function and stress the mucosa. Antibiotic therapy can cause diarrhea, alter gut flora and predispose to colitis. Nonsteroidal anti-inflammatory drugs have been implicated as a cause of gastrointestinal ulceration and bleeding. The pathogenesis of this damage is not established but the drugs do affect mitochondrial function and decrease prostaglandin production. Bovine colostrum has been shown to reduce the rise in intestinal permeability caused by nonsteroidal anti-inflammatory drugs and may provide a novel approach to prevention of this damage [27].

Table 3. Noninvasive techniques to assess the stressed mucosa

Function	Test		
	breath	urine	feces
Gut motility	^{13}C lactose ureide Lactulose		Marker dye
Gut inflammation	Ethane/pentane		
Pancreatic function	^{13}C-mixed triglyceride $^{13/14}$C triolein		Elastase
Gastric function	^{13}C urea ^{13}C octanoate	Sucrose permeability	
Small intestinal function	Small bowel Bacterial overgrowth Carbohydrate malabsorption (H$_2$ breath tests)	Permeability (lactulose/ L-rhamnose/ mannitol)	Calprotectin
Large intestine	Fermentation patterns (methane/ hydrogen)	Sucralose permeability	Short-chain fatty acids

Chemotherapy drugs are also a major cause of gastrointestinal mucosal injury (mucositis) most commonly affecting the mouth, esophagus, stomach and small intestine. Small intestinal injury can often be difficult to detect but a recent animal study has shown that breath testing may be a useful tool [28].

Assessment of the Stressed Mucosa

Small intestinal health is pivotal to whole body health and the bioavailability of drugs but it is difficult to assess it in animals and humans. Current invasive techniques such as endoscopy and biopsy are painful, invasive, expensive and not necessarily representative of gastrointestinal function. The recent advance of wireless capsule endoscopy may change our ability to visualize the bowel but again not its functionality.

Accurate noninvasive repeatable tests involving breath, urine and feces, are safe and available for use in both health and disease. Table 3 shows some examples of how these tests can be used alone and together to describe function. Using these tests as biomarkers will improve our ability to define stressed mucosa and help to understand the causal mechanisms. Newer imaging techniques may also improve our ability to assess the stressed gut.

Therapeutic Interventions

Pharmacotherapies have obviously been used in disease states such as IBD to reduce inflammation and induce mucosal repair. Nonpharmacological therapies such as enteral nutrition with modular or polymeric formulas have also been shown to be effective in inducing remission and gut repair in IBD.

There may also be a role for immunomodulation in protecting or repairing a stressed mucosa. One oral approach has been the use of pre- and probiotics either separately or in combination. A recent study using this combined approach with a synbiotic (combined pre- and probiotic) in patients with active ulcerative colitis showed reductions in TNF-α and interleukin-1α [29]. Probiotics have also been shown to have benefit in the treatment of viral diarrhea [30].

Immunotherapy using products such as human immunoglobulin, colostrum, and hyperimmune colostrum has been shown to provide passive protection against a number of viral and bacterial pathogens [31].

Conclusion

Stress clearly plays a role in many gastrointestinal diseases but the extent of its contribution to the pathogenesis of many of these disorders is still unclear. Emerging functional diagnostic techniques are likely to provide a better understanding of the pathophysiology of the stressed gut and provide a simpler and more acceptable method to assess interventions.

References

1   Mawdsley JE, Rampton DS: Psychological stress in IBD: new insights into pathogenic and therapeutic implications. Gut 2005;54:1481–1491.
2   Liu Z, Li N, Neu J: Tight junctions, leaky intestines, and pediatric diseases. Acta Paediatr 2005;94:386–393.
3   Oktedalen O, Lunde OC, Opstad PK, et al: Changes in the gastrointestinal mucosa after long-distance running. Scand J Gastroenterol 1992;27:270–274.
4   Gaudin C, Zerath E, Guezennec CY: Gastric lesions secondary to long-distance running. Dig Dis Sci 1990;35:1239–1243.
5   Schwartz AE, Vanagunas A, Kamel PL: Endoscopy to evaluate gastrointestinal bleeding in marathon runners. Ann Intern Med 1990;113:632–633.
6   Pals KL, Chang RT, Ryan AJ, Gisolfi CV: Effect of running intensity on intestinal permeability. J Appl Physiol 1997;82:571–576.
7   Ryan AJ, Chang RT, Gisolfi CV: Gastrointestinal permeability following aspirin intake and prolonged running. Med Sci Sports Exerc 1996;28:698–705.
8   Southcott E: The Use of Probiotics in Intestinal Protection; PhD thesis, University of Adelaide, 2002.
9   Kolkman JJ, Groeneveld AB, van der Berg FG, Rauwerda JA, Meuwissen SG: Increased gastric PCO_2 during exercise is indicative of gastric ischaemia: a tonometric study. Gut 1999;44:163–167.

10 Buckley JD, Brinkworth GD, Southcott E, Butler RN: Bovine colostrum and whey protein supplementation during running training increase intestinal permeability. Asia Pac J Clin Nutr 2004;13(suppl):S81.
11 Bhatia V, Tandon RK: Stress and the gastrointestinal tract. J Gastroenterol Hepatol 2005;20: 332–339.
12 Sagami Y, Shimada Y, Tayama J, et al: Effect of a corticotropin releasing hormone receptor antagonist on colonic sensory and motor function in patients with irritable bowel syndrome. Gut 2004;53:958–964.
13 Bitton A, Sewitch MJ, Peppercorn MA, et al: Psychosocial determinants of relapse in ulcerative colitis: a longitudinal study. Am J Gastroenterol 2003;98:2203–2208.
14 Tibble JA, Sigthorsson G, Foster R, et al: Use of surrogate markers of inflammation and Rome criteria to distinguish organic from nonorganic intestinal disease. Gastroenterology 2002;123: 450–460.
15 Fernandez-Banares F, Rosinach M, Esteve M, et al: Sugar malabsorption in functional abdominal bloating: a pilot study on the long-term effect of dietary treatment. Clin Nutr, in press.
16 Miki K, Moore DJ, Butler RN, et al: The sugar permeability test reflects disease activity in children and adolescents with inflammatory bowel disease. J Pediatr 1998;133:750–754.
17 Peeters M, Geypens B, Claus D, et al: Clustering of increased small intestinal permeability in families with Crohn's disease. Gastroenterology 1997;113:802–807.
18 Pelli MA, Trovarelli G, Capodicasa E, et al: Breath alkanes determination in ulcerative colitis and Crohn's disease. Dis Colon Rectum 1999;42:71–76.
19 Davidson GP, Barnes GL: Structural and functional abnormalities of the small intestine in infants and young children with rotavirus enteritis. Acta Paediatr Scand 1979;68:181–186.
20 Nusrat A, von Eichel-Streiber C, Turner JR, et al: *Clostridium difficile* toxins disrupt epithelial barrier function by altering membrane microdomain localization of tight junction proteins. Infect Immun 2001;69:1329–1336.
21 Salazar-Lindo E, Allen S, Brewster DR, et al: Intestinal infections and environmental enteropathy: Working Group Report of the Second World Congress of Pediatric Gastroenterology, Hepatology, and Nutrition. J Pediatr Gastroenterol Nutr 2004;39(suppl 2):S662–S669.
22 Kukuruzovic RH, Brewster DR: Small bowel intestinal permeability in Australian aboriginal children. J Pediatr Gastroenterol Nutr 2002;35:206–212.
23 Jackson PG, Lessof MH, Baker RW, et al: Intestinal permeability in patients with eczema and food allergy. Lancet 1981;i:1285–1286.
24 Cummins AG, Thompson FM, Butler RN, et al: Improvement in intestinal permeability precedes morphometric recovery of the small intestine in coeliac disease. Clin Sci (Lond) 2001;100:379–386.
25 Brewster DR, Manary MJ, Menzies IS, et al: Comparison of milk and maize based diets in kwashiorkor. Arch Dis Child 1997;76:242–248.
26 Baqui AH, Black RE, El Arifeen S, et al: Effect of zinc supplementation started during diarrhoea on morbidity and mortality in Bangladeshi children: community randomised trial. BMJ 2002;325:1059.
27 Playford RJ, MacDonald CE, Calnan DP, et al: Co-administration of the health food supplement, bovine colostrum, reduces the acute non-steroidal anti-inflammatory drug-induced increase in intestinal permeability. Clin Sci (Lond) 2001;100:627–633.
28 Pelton NS, Tivey DR, Howarth GS, et al: A novel breath test for the non-invasive assessment of small intestinal mucosal injury following methotrexate administration in the rat. Scand J Gastroenterol 2004;39:1015–1016.
29 Furrie E, Macfarlane S, Kennedy A, et al: Synbiotic therapy (*Bifidobacterium longum/*Synergy1) initiates resolution of inflammation in patients with active ulcerative colitis: a randomized controlled pilot trial. Gut 2005;54:242–249.
30 Isolauri E, Salminen S: Probiotics, gut inflammation and barrier function. Gastroenterol Clin North Am 2005;31:437–450.
31 Davidson GP: Passive protection against diarrheal disease. J Pediatr Gastroenterol Nutr 1996;23:207–212.

Discussion

Dr. Aulestia: Can vitamins and iron produce damage in the mucosa of the normal child?

Dr. Davidson: I am not aware that vitamins and iron can damage the mucosa of normal children. The opposite can occur, however, where a deficiency such as folic acid leads to mucosal damage [1].

Dr. Puplampu: I found the use of folate in animals very interesting. What is the dosage and what have you used in humans?

Dr. Davidson: In the animal model we used calcium folinate, a metabolite and active form of folic acid at $10\,mg/m^2$ which approximates that used in humans for methotrexate 'rescue' [2]. In the study mentioned above the folic acid dose was 0.5 mg daily.

Dr. Puplampu: I have been using 5 mg/day for 10 days in the management of diarrhea, of course without zinc, and that is what I am very much interested in.

Dr. Davidson: Zinc has certainly been shown to have an important role in gut repair [3]. Two randomized controlled trials have however found no benefit from folic acid compared to placebo [4].

Dr. Nowak-Wegrzyn: Could you comment on the time course of the intestinal permeability change with exercise? How fast does it go back to baseline? There is a condition called food-dependent exercise-induced anaphylaxis that may be caused by increased absorption of food allergens following exercise. It would be very interesting to know what the time course of exercise-induced changes in intestinal permeability is.

Dr. Davidson: We haven't looked at that specifically. My assessment would be that if you look at those athletes who undergo moderate exercise their mucosal lining will be normal. The elite athletes we studied had an 8-week period of intensive exercise and whether their mucosa returned to normal or not would depend on whether they continued to exercise at a high level. During the time period when their training was less intensive they seemed predisposed to infections, but at that point in time we did not study their mucosa.

Dr. Bayhon: Can you comment on the role free radicals in the development or the pathophysiology of stress-induced enteropathies, and in terms of pharmaceutical therapy are prostaglandin E_2 inducers used at all in children as they are in other countries? The results are very promising especially in terms of prevention and quality of healing in induced enteropathies.

Dr. Davidson: I don't have any experience or expertise in that area. I am sure free radicals are produced, and this has certainly been documented, but we have not done any work on it.

Dr. Balanag: Obviously ventilated babies are very stressed. Are there any studies on the role of probiotics in babies who are ventilated?

Dr. Davidson: The role of probiotics in neonatology is attractive because of their safety record. There is some evidence to support their use in preventing necrotizing enterocolitis but I am not aware of studies in ventilated babies.

Dr. Rivera: You showed data on premature infants who are in the respirator. What was the response in terms of inflammation with carbon-13 and the other tests that you used? Were there reliable results with these particular tests. Have you any experience with probiotics in conditions like asphyxia and necrotizing enterocolitis in newborn babies?

Dr. Davidson: Breath can be collected from premature infants. We have in fact studied gastric emptying using the ^{13}C-octanoic breath test in this age group. We have not studied the inflammatory response in neonates.

Dr. Rivera: Have you any experience or any knowledge on the use of probiotics in conditions like asphyxia and necrotizing enterocolitis in newborn babies [5]?

Dr. Davidson: No, I don't have any experience but as referred to above there is some supportive evidence at least for necrotizing enterocolitis.

Dr. B. Koletzko: I am fascinated by the methodology of the sucrose breath test and the results you obtained. You expressed them as a cumulative percentage of recovery over 90 min, so I assume you measured that in the postabsorptive state, in the fasted state? Is this not somewhat limiting in some patients, particularly at a young age or with certain diseases where it is difficulty to perform the test in a fasted state? Have you ever considered applying the test in a nonfasting state?

Dr. Davidson: We have not looked at the nonfasting state. We have created a normal range looking at children and adults up to the age of 70 because we are also doing studies in irritable bowel syndrome. The normal range is relatively tight so it has enabled us to actually provide a cutoff but most of the children and adults we look at had a 6- to 8-hour fast.

Dr. B. Koletzko: My other question is related to the ethane breath test. I assume its results are more prone to variations in the patients' metabolic rate. Have you had a chance to look at its sensitivity and specificity in inflammatory states? One would assume that it is much less precise than a stable isotope breath test.

Dr. Davidson: I think it would be. We started a study on breath ethane in inflammatory bowel disease but unfortunately the machinery broke down. When you say that you are looking at the severe end of the spectrum in inflammatory bowel disease it still gives you a guide. I think it does have potential, not only in inflammatory bowel disease but in other conditions such as cystic fibrosis, rheumatoid arthritis and maybe chronic lung disease.

Dr. Milla: The gut is always exposed to lots of free radicals; bacteria in the lumen are constantly producing them. The most dominant antioxidant is vitamin E. It sits in the apical membrane of enterocytes very close to the lipid rafts that contain the functional proteins. We spent a long time trying to deplete enterocytes of vitamin E and to increase free radical attack on them but we failed miserably. We also looked at patients with a β- and hyper-β-lipoproteinemia that have incredibly low vitamin E levels. We could not detect any physiological abnormality in the membrane of their enterocytes. Trying to look at free radical attack on enterocytes is probably a nonstarter. Enterocytes have a beautiful protective mechanism with large amounts of vitamin E in the membranes. It mops up all the free radicals and has access to an enormous electron sink. I would not go down that avenue, I wasted a lot of time doing it. The question goes back to the ethane breath test. Many gastrointestinal inflammatory conditions are associated with respiratory inflammatory conditions, especially the allergic condition cystic fibrosis. What happens to the ethane breast test if there is an inflammatory response in the bronchial tree?

Dr. Davidson: I haven't seen any studies that have actually tried to differentiate where ethane or pentane may be coming from. Most of the studies have been done in inflammatory bowel disease. It would have an additive effect; therefore, you have a problem if you try to distinguish between the two sites, obviously it is easier if you just have one disease.

Dr. Fuchs: I would like to make a comment about folic acid and gastroenteritis. In your work did you use folate as a supplement in children who were receiving methotrexate?

Dr. Davidson: No, this was an animal model. Our oncologists use it in children who are receiving methotrexate, but we haven't actually studied this group of children.

Dr. Fuchs: One of my colleagues published a paper a few years ago. I was surprised at how little data there were, in fact none at that time, on folate supplementation in acute watery diarrhea. He looked at all types of acute watery diarrhea irrespective of the pathogen and did not see a beneficial effect with folate, at least with the doses he was using. Why did you use sucrase as your marker as opposed to something else such as lactase?

Dr. Davidson: As you know the level of lactase tends to decrease over time and probably 90% of the world's population have lactase deficiency as adults but not necessarily malabsorption or intolerance. In children who are genetically predisposed to have lactase deficiency as adults the lactase level is decreased from about 3 years of age and 90% are deficient by the time they reach age 10 or 11. Sucrase activity however is maintained at a relatively constant level throughout life. Because sucrase like lactase is close to the villous tips it is affected by any event that damages the gastrointestinal mucosa, so it is a good marker.

Dr. Vento: Could ethane or pentane be predictive of necrotizing enterocolitis since they are also predictive of bronchopulmonary dysplasia?

Dr. Davidson: I am not aware of any definitive study of breath ethane or pentane in necrotizing enterocolitis but it may be worth studying as I am sure lipid peroxidation would occur in the gut and alkanes produced.

Dr. Heine: I would like to come back to your data on eczema and permeability. I was surprised that you found no change in permeability in eczema patients. Was this perhaps due to patient selection in your study? What was the age mix in your group?

Dr. Davidson: We looked at older children assessing them with SCORAD. We studied the more severe end of the spectrum; they were a fairly standardized group of children, but the average age was about 7 or 8.

Dr. Heine: So it may be different in younger children?

Dr. Davidson: Yes, I think so.

Dr. Chubarova: Do you have any information about intestinal permeability in malnourished children or those with physical delay but without infection?

Dr. Davidson: There is a lot of information in developing communities where they have malnutrition and not necessarily infection. Studies carried out in Darwin by Kukuruzovic and Brewster [6] showed that Aboriginal children without symptoms at the time and who were failing to grow had enteropathy; they were able to show increased intestinal permeability compared to nonindigenous children.

Dr. S. Koletzko: I was impressed by the lactose-rhamnose ratio in your athletes and that it was comparable to levels in IBD patients. Are there any data on athletes after they stop excessive training? How long does it take until the levels normalize? Do athletes have any long-term consequences from this barrier dysfunction?

Dr. Davidson: We did not follow this group long term, so I can't answer that question, particularly if it does have any long-term effects in these athletes [7]. There have been several studies from Adelaide actually looking at the use of bovine colostrum in trying to prevent this problem. During the 2000 Olympic Games some athletes took colostrum on a regular basis because it had actually been shown to have a performance-enhancing effect. Why that is, is not really well understood but one of the things that it seems to do is to reduce the downtime so athletes are able to continue to train, repeat their training and even improve their training without actually becoming unwell. The performance enhancement really is that it allows athletes to train to a higher level than if they weren't taking it.

Dr. Milla: You concentrated on the epithelium and I was fascinated by these runners. How much changes in the epithelium, how much might be due to vascular changes, because I can imagine the blood shunting through the gut when there is a significant change in exercise, and how much might be neural?

Dr. Davidson: There have been studies that you are probably aware of in athletes showing damage related to mucosal ischemia. They have a significant transfer of blood

145

flow away from the splanchnic region to muscle during exercise. This may well be a contributing factor that interferes [5] with mucosal function and integrity and so they may be reflecting not only the stressed mucosa but also these other changes that occur. These were athletes who were training at a very high level.

References

1 Davidson GP, Townley RRW: Structural and functional abnormalities of the small intestine due to nutritional folic acid deficiency in infancy. J Pediatr 1977;90:590–594.
2 Clarke JM, Pelton NC, Bajka BH, et al: Use of the ^{13}C-sucrose breath test to assess chemotherapy-induced small intestinal mucositis in the rat. Cancer Biol Ther 2006;5:34–38.
3 Bhutta ZA, Bird SM, Black RE, et al: Therapeutic effects of oral zinc in acute and persistent diarrhoea in children in developing countries: pooled analysis of randomised controlled trials. Am J Clin Nutr 2000;72:1516–1522.
4 Mahalanabis D, Bhan MK: Micronutrients as adjunct therapy of acute illness in children: impact on episode outcome and policy implications of current findings. Br J Nutr 2001;85 (suppl 2):5151–5158.
5 Bin-Nun A, Bromiker R, Wilschanski M, et al: Oral probiotics prevent necrotizing enterocolitis in very low birth weight neonates. J Pediatr 2005;147:192–196.
6 Kukuruzovic R, Brewster D: Small bowel intestinal permeability in Australian aboriginal children. J Pediatr Gastroenterol Nutr 2002;35:206–212.
7 Kolkman JJ, Groeneveld AB, van der Berg FG, Rauwerda JA, Meuwissen SG: Increased gastric PCO$_2$ during exercise is indicative of gastric ischaemia: a tonometric study. Gut 1999;44: 163–167.

Cooke RJ, Vandenplas Y, Wahn U (eds): Nutrition Support for Infants and Children at Risk.
Nestlé Nutr Workshop Ser Pediatr Program, vol 59, pp 147–159,
Nestec Ltd., Vevey/S. Karger AG, Basel, © 2007.

Nutrition for Children with Cholestatic Liver Disease

E. Leonie Los, Sabina Lukovac, Anniek Werner,
Tietie Dijkstra, Henkjan J. Verkade, Edmond H.H.M. Rings

Pediatric Gastroenterology/Research Laboratory of Pediatrics, Department of Pediatrics,
University Medical Center Groningen, University of Groningen, Groningen, The Netherlands

Abstract

Cholestatic liver disease (CLD) in children negatively affects nutritional status, growth and development, which all lead to an increased risk of morbidity and mortality. This is illustrated by the fact that the clinical outcome of children with CLD awaiting a liver transplantation is in part predicted by their nutritional status, which is integrated in the pediatric end-stage liver disease model. Preservation of the nutritional status becomes more relevant as the number of patients waiting for liver transplantation increases and the waiting time for a donor organ becomes prolonged. Nutritional strategies are available to optimize feeding of children with CLD. Patients with CLD, however, form a heterogeneous group and the clinical manifestations of their disease vary. This makes a tailor-made approach for these children crucial. Not all aspects of nutrient metabolism and absorption in children with CLD are well understood and studied. Experiments with stable isotope-labeled triglycerides and fatty acids have provided essential information about fat absorption under physiological and cholestatic conditions in animal models and humans. We expect that in the future, tests using other isotope-labeled macronutrients, i.e. carbohydrates and proteins, can be used to further assess nutritional status of children with CLD, thereby creating tailor-made nutritional therapies.

Copyright © 2007 Nestec Ltd., Vevey/S. Karger AG, Basel

Cholestasis and Nutritional Status

Cholestatic liver disease (CLD) negatively affects nutritional status, growth and development, particularly in infancy, i.e. when growth rates are highest. The presence of malnutrition and growth retardation (failure to thrive) compromises the clinical outcome for children with end-stage liver disease. Cholestatic children with a poor nutritional status, who require liver transplantation, have an increased risk of morbidity and mortality [1, 2]. To illustrate this, the nutritional status is an important contributor to pediatric end-stage liver disease (PELD) score for children under 2 years of age. The PELD score is a reliable predictor of mortality in children with CLD on the waiting list for liver transplantation. The PELD model was implemented by the United Network of Organ Sharing (UNOS) in the United States in February 2002 as an improved algorithm for allocating livers among pediatric orthotopic liver transplant candidates, and will be adopted by the Eurotransplant society in January 2007. It has recently been shown that the PELD score also correlates with posttransplant survival [3]. Preservation of the nutritional status becomes more relevant as the number of patients waiting for liver transplantation increases and the waiting time for a donor organ becomes prolonged.

Nutrition for Cholestatic Children

Poor dietary intake is an important factor in the pathophysiological basis of malnutrition in children with CLD. Furthermore, their nutritional status may be further compromised by decreased absorption of macronutrients, including fat, carbohydrates and proteins [4]. At an early age, fat accounts for the most important dietary energy source (up to 50% of total ingested energy). Essential fatty acids (EFA) and long-chain polyunsaturated fatty acids (LCP-UFA) are indispensable for proper development and function of different organs, for example the central nervous system. Micronutrient absorption may also be affected in CLD, including absorption of fat-soluble vitamins A, D, E and K.

The dietary prevention or treatment of failure to thrive during CLD involves some general principles applicable to virtually all patients and some more individual tailor-made approaches. Nutrition in infancy consists predominantly of breast milk or formula. For children with CLD, the dietary energy intake is usually increased to levels of 120–150% of recommended daily energy intake (corrected for age and gender). The adaptation of the formula diet usually involves increasing the concentration and amount ingested. In addition, up to 60% of the fat components, particularly long-chain triglycerides, are substituted by medium-chain triglycerides (MCTs), whose absorption can occur relatively independently from the presence of bile components in the intestinal lumen. The carbohydrate content can be increased by supplementation of formula with maltodextrin. Breastfed children receive additional formula and MCT-rich oil, while for older children feeding with formula is often prolonged and energy-rich liquids are provided. Adequate absorption of fat-soluble vitamins during CLD can usually be obtained by considerably increasing the dosages administered daily, well above regular recommendations for the age groups. Serum levels of fat-soluble vitamins are regularly monitored, in order that dosages can be adapted. Adequate intake of EFA and LCPUFA is not frequently monitored in CLD patients, but should be reached when these fatty acids are provided in ample amounts in the diet. Nevertheless, we reported that ~70% of children with CLD requiring liver transplantation have biochemical indications of EFA and LCPUFA deficiency [5].

Reduced gastric volume, vomiting, ascites and hypoglycemia lead to limited absorption of the required dietary nutrients when administered in regular (bolus) feedings. Under these circumstances, continuous nasogastric drip feeding may be needed to guarantee maximal uptake of nutrients.

For some time now, a special formula for infants with CLD has been available. The composition of this formula aimed to accommodate the general aspects of nutritional support needed for infants with CLD. So far, however, no data have become available to substantiate its benefit, nor its advantage over conventional dietary treatment: supplementation of MCT-rich formulas with carbohydrates, fat-soluble vitamins and EFA. Clinical data are needed to determine the role that this formula can play in the dietary treatment of infants with CLD.

Biological Aspects of Nutrition for Cholestatic Children

Cholestatic Diseases in Children

CLD is characterized by decreased or absent hepatic secretion of bile into the intestine. The most common cause of CLD in children requiring liver transplantation is biliary atresia. Biliary atresia is a progressive disorder characterized by an inflammatory reaction towards the extrahepatic and intrahepatic bile ducts, leading to their destruction and subsequent replacement by fibrotic scar tissue. The etiology of biliary atresia remains unknown, although an inflammatory reaction to a detrimental stimulus seems to play an initiating role. Suggested initiating stimuli include specific perinatal viral infections, genetic factors, defects in immune response, as well as defects in morphogenesis. Another disease that can lead to end-stage liver disease in infancy is Alagille's syndrome, an autosomal dominantly inherited syndrome including bile duct hypoplasia, and congenital anatomical defects in other organs. Progressive familial intrahepatic cholestasis (PFIC) is also a genetically transmitted disorder, but is inherited in an autosomal recessive fashion. Three phenotypic forms of PFIC have been characterized and attributed to gene defects in three different genes (PFIC1–3). Another cause of CLD is nonsyndromic paucity of the intrahepatic bile ducts, which is suggested to be the result of various infections, chromosomal disorders or metabolic disorders. Finally, inborn errors in bile acid synthesis account for part of the children with CLD. Defects have been identified in enzymes catalyzing cholesterol catabolism and bile acid synthesis [6].

CLD in adolescents and young adults is often due to autoimmune hepatitis, primary biliary cirrhosis or primary sclerosing cholangitis [6, 7].

Although the causes and clinical manifestations of CLD may vary, it is often accompanied by liver damage. The obstruction or absence of bile ducts leads to accumulation of bile acids in hepatocytes, which results in liver damage. Because the enterohepatic circulation of bile acids is interrupted, the resulting absence of bile acids in the intestinal lumen leads to impaired micellization and therefore to strongly reduced absorption of fats and fat-soluble nutrients. Another feature of CLD is the high serum bile acid level, which can cause secondary tissue injury.

In biliary atresia, it is often attempted to correct the enterohepatic circulation of bile acids by performing a Kasai portoenterostomy. During this procedure the liver is directly connected to the proximal small intestine to optimize bile flow into the intestine as much as possible. However, Kasai portoenterostomy is frequently only a transient solution, due to the presence of intrahepatic bile duct damage and ongoing liver damage. Most patients with biliary atresia eventually need liver transplantation. As is pointed out above, the nutritional status of children with CLD is important for the clinical outcome of liver transplantation and for long-term survival after liver transplantation. Besides the obviously reduced absorption of fats and fat-soluble vitamins, chronic cholestasis also affects dietary intake, energy metabolism and metabolism of macronutrients as well as micronutrients.

Dietary Intake and Energy Expenditure

Dietary Intake

Reduced dietary intake is an important contributor to malnutrition in children with CLD. Fatigue, anorexia, nausea, vomiting, diarrhea, altered or reduced ability to taste, and early satiety may all contribute to decreased ingestion of food. Organomegaly and ascites can further compromise dietary intake by reducing gastric capacity. Additionally, many diet modifications, for example sodium, fluid or protein restrictions, make food even more unpalatable. These dietary restrictions are imposed on patients with relatively high risks of fluid overload and encephalopathy, which, when left untreated, can lead to serious irreversible defects [8].

Energy Metabolism

Energy expenditure is composed of the basal metabolic rate (BMR), the amount needed for growth and metabolism. Although clinical data are conflicting, some children with CLD have been shown to have an increased BMR. Shanbhogue et al. [9] reported a higher BMR, when related to lean tissue in patients with end-stage liver disease. In children with biliary atresia energy expenditure was 29% higher than healthy controls [10]. Also Shepherd [11] reported higher energy expenditure per unit body cell mass in children with biliary atresia. In contrast, Muller et al. [12] found that patients with cirrhosis showed a variable BMR, in the range from hypometabolic to hypermetabolic. Another study showed an unchanged BMR in children with Alagille syndrome [13]. A hypermetabolic state could be an important factor in the clinical outcome for CLD, because it further aggravates nutritional status.

Recently, Watanabe et al. [14] found that bile acids induce energy expenditure by promoting intracellular thyroid hormone activation. In this study, mice were fed a bile acid (cholic acid)-containing high fat diet. These mice showed subsequent reduction in weight gain, white adipose tissue weight and brown adipose tissue weight compared to mice on a high fat diet. In addition, animals fed a high fat diet containing cholic acid had higher CO_2 production and O_2 consumption, indicating a higher level of energy expenditure. Human skeletal muscle myocytes showed an increase in O_2 consumption after treatment with bile acids. It is presently unknown, however, whether bile acid accumulation in patients with CLD is partly responsible for increased energy expenditure.

Nutrient Metabolism

Apart from reduced intraluminal bile acid concentrations, other consequences of CLD, such as gastrointestinal bleeding, impaired digestive enzyme production and secretion, mucosal congestion, villous atrophy, bacterial overgrowth or pancreatic insufficiency, can lead to maldigestion and malaborption of nutrients. In addition, even certain medications can aggravate malabsorption. For example, cholestyramine binds to bile acids in the intestinal lumen and thereby further reduces absorption of fat-soluble nutrients. Also, reduced availability of specific nutrients involved in digestion and/or absorption of other nutrients, specifically vitamins and minerals, affects intestinal absorption [8]. In the remaining part of this article we will focus on metabolism of fat, carbohydrates, protein and micronutrients in CLD.

Fat Metabolism

CLD is characterized by malabsorption of fat. Especially long-chain triglycerides, which are digested to fatty acids and monoacylglycerols in the intestinal lumen, are poorly absorbed during cholestasis, due to their impaired micellization during bile deficiency.

The route that fat undertakes from the diet to the blood can be divided in four steps: emulsification, lipolysis (lipases), solubilization (bile) and translocation (mucosa). During lipolysis lipases catalyze the conversion of triglycerides to glycerol and fatty acids. The latter need to be solubilized by bile acids to be transported towards the vicinity of the mucosa. Here, at the unstirred water layer, the micelles disintegrate, after which fatty acids and monoacylglycerols are taken up across the apical membrane of the mucosal cells. Inside the enterocytes, the absorbed lipids are reacylated to triacylglycerols,

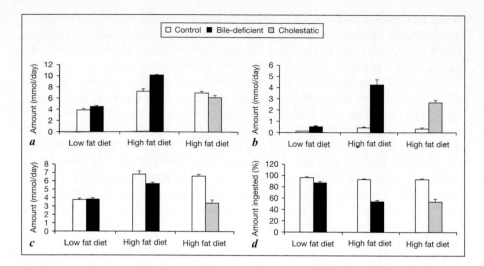

Fig. 1. Fat absorption in bile-deficient and cholestatic rats on a low fat and high fat diet, with fat intake (***a***), fecal fat excretion (***b***), net fat uptake (***c***), and dietary fat absorption as % of amount ingested (***d***) [adapted from 16 and 18].

assembled into chylomicrons, which are then secreted into lymph and subsequently appear in the circulation.

In our laboratory, Kalivianakis et al. [15] developed a stable isotope test to quantify lipolysis and absorption of long-chain fatty acids in rats. We determined absorption and appearance in plasma of ^{13}C-labeled palmitic acid in rats with malabsorption either due to chronic bile deficiency (permanent bile diversion as developed in our laboratory by Kuipers et al. [16]) or due to oral administration of the lipase inhibitor Orlistat. These models were used to discriminate between potential causes of fat malabsorption such as impaired intestinal lipolysis or reduced uptake of fatty acids. Rats were given a high fat diet (35% of total energy) compared to a low fat diet (14% of total energy) to potentiate the effect of fat malabsorption. Results were compared with the percentage absorption of ingested fat determined by fat balance. As expected, dietary fat absorption was significantly impaired in bile-deficient animals as compared to controls (fig. 1d). However, the net fat uptake (fig. 1c), defined as the difference between the amount of fat ingested (fig. 1a) and the amount of fat excreted ('lost') via the feces (fig. 1b) through fat malabsorption, was not significantly affected by the presence or absence of intestinal bile (control vs. chronic bile diversion), or the amount of fat in the diet (high fat vs. low fat). The percentage of total ingested fat absorbed in bile-deficient rats was only 87% with the low fat diet and 54% with the high fat diet (fig. 1d).

Apparently, bile deficieny (without cholestasis) increases the nutrient ingestion in rats, compensating sufficiently for the increased energy and fat loss via the feces. Bile deficiency due to bile diversion in rats led to a decreased concentration of plasma ^{13}C-palmitic acid, indicating impaired absorption of long-chain fatty acids. Control experiments showed that lipolysis was not affected in bile-deficient rats. Impairment of fat absorption due to Orlistat had no effect on plasma ^{13}C-palmitic acid, indicating the specificity of the test [15]. This test can also be utilized to generate clinical data as was demonstrated by Rings et al. [17]. Rings et al. showed that the absorption of free fatty acids, but not fat digestion was rate-limited in neonates, and developed to adult competence within 2 months after term age. Neonates are known to have a mild 'physiological' cholestasis during the first months of life, and this may be the mechanism underlying this observation.

EFA and LCPUFA are crucial for normal development and function. They cannot be synthesized endogenously and therefore must be provided by the diet. As is reviewed by Sealy et al. [5], the percentage of n-3 and n-6 fatty acids is reduced in pediatric cholestasis. This observation reflects the inability of CLD patients to absorb sufficient amounts of EFA and LCPUFA, due to absence of bile in the intestinal lumen in combination with frequently compromised dietary intake. An important consequence of this inability to acquire sufficient amounts of LCPUFA is EFA deficiency. The quantitatively most important EFAs are linoleic acid (LA) and α-LA, members of the n-6 and n-3 family of fatty acids. Linoleic and linolenic acid are precursors for LCPUFAs, including arachidonic acid (C20:4n-6), eicosapentaenoic acid (C22:5n-3), and docosahexaenoic acid (C22:6n-3), respectively.

Minich et al. [18] investigated fat malabsorption as a possible cause of EFA deficiency in rats that were intestinally bile deficient due to either permenant bile diversion or to bile duct ligation (cholestasis). Absorption of the EFA LA was quantified by fat balance and by measuring plasma concentrations of [^{13}C]-LA after its intraduodenal administration. Plasma concentration of [^{13}C]-LA was decreased in bile-diverted rats, while net absorption of LA from the intestine was unaffected. The fact that net absorption of fat and LA was not affected in bile-deficient rats corresponded with increased food intake (see above) in addition to relative preservation of EFA absorption under bile-deficient conditions, in comparison with nonessential saturated fatty acids, such as palmitic acid (C16:0) and stearic acid (C18:0). In cholestatic rats, however, both plasma concentration and net absorption of unlabeled or [^{13}C]-labeled LA were decreased. Metabolism of LA into arachidonic acid was not affected, indicating that LA deficiency in these rats is due to decreased net absorption. The compensatory increase in nutrient ingestion during intestinal bile deficiency on the basis of permanent bile diversion (see above) did apparently not occur in rats with intestinal bile deficiency on the basis of bile duct ligation. It is tempting to speculate that the accumulation of bile products during the latter cholestatic condition abolishes the compensatory mechanism of increased nutrient ingestion. This observation is in accordance with clinical experience that nutrient intake and appetite are compromised in children with CLD.

Children with CLD are sometimes given a fat-restricted diet, since effects such as steatorrhea/diarrhea are expected. According to the study of Kalivianakis et al. [15] the amount and fraction of dietary fat lost via the feces is indeed significantly less on a low fat than on a high fat diet (fig. 1b). However, net fat uptake from a high fat diet was almost 2-fold higher than that from a low fat diet (fig. 1c). The net absorption reflects the amount of nutrients (fat) that actually becomes available for energy and growth needs of CLD patients. This observation underlines a clinical strategy to increase, rather than to restrict the amount of fat intake in patients with CLD, even at the expense of steatorrhea, in order to maximize their nutritional condition.

Carbohydrate Metabolism

In children with CLD, carbohydrate homeostasis can be affected by hepatic failure itself, for example by a decreased capacity of gluconeogenesis. Frequently also peripheral utilization of glucose is reduced, which may decrease the risks of hypoglycemia. In CLD, hepatic degradation of insulin may also be decreased, which may be one of the causes for the 2-fold higher insulin response in CLD compared to control patients. Elevated plasma levels of insulin in combination with glucose tolerance imply insulin resistance, which could be further aggravated by increased circulating free fatty acids as seen in CLD [8].

Apart from the hepatic effects on glucose homeostasis, the intestinal carbohydrate absorption could also be affected by CLD. However, no data are yet available about carbohydrate absorption under cholestatic conditions. Recently our group has started to investigate intestinal carbohydrate absorption under cholestatic conditions in vitro and in vivo. The underlying hypothesis for this research is that cholestasis, i.e. high serum bile acid concentrations could alter intestinal function by affecting proliferation, differentiation and/or apoptotic cell death of the absorptive intestinal epithelium [19]. These effects of cholestatic bile acid concentrations on other cell types have been well delineated. For example, relatively low concentrations of bile acids induce apoptosis in hepatocytes [20].

Protein Metabolism

The catabolic reduction in total body protein as seen in CLD is mainly due to extensive liver damage. Tavill [21] and McCullough and Glamour [22] found no significantly changed protein turnover in CLD patients. Amino acid oxidation is normal or reduced in these patients, consistent with appropriate adaptation to reduced nutrient supplies. Due to hepatic insufficiency occurring in later stages of CLD, oxidation of aromatic amino acids is reduced as is the metabolism of branched-chain amino acids. Mager et al. [23] reported an increased dietary need for branched-chain amino acids in children with mild-to-moderate chronic

CLD, due to increased postabsorptive leucine oxidation. In general, amino acids seem to be conserved in CLD, probably due to the body's ability to increase protein synthesis and reduce amino acid oxidation. This increased protein synthesis is, however, at the cost of muscle proteolysis [21, 22]. Increased protein oxidation resulted in a virtually zero nitrogen balance in children with biliary atresia and even in oxidation of endogenous proteins [10]. Stable experimental conditions do not necessarily reflect the spectrum of clinical conditions frequently encountered, such as episodes of metabolic stress or infections that can increase protein turnover and catabolism [8]. Interestingly, Sokal et al. [24] found that branched chain amino acids improve body composition and nitrogen balance in a rat model of extrahepatic cholestasis.

Overall, addition of proteins, and especially specific amino acids such as branched chain amino acids, could improve nutritional status of children with CLD. However, care must be taken, because an excess of protein can negatively influence encephalopathy.

Micronutrient Metabolism

The absence of bile acids in the intestinal lumen as observed in cholestasis reduces absorption of fat-soluble vitamins A, D, E and K, as briefly described above. Calcium uptake is at risk as a result of formation of nonsoluble calcium fatty acid soaps during fat malabsorption. Hypovitaminosis D may increase renal loss of phosphate and hypovitaminosis A may induce zinc deficiency. Zinc deficiency has a negative impact on cognitive function, appetite and taste, immune function, wound healing and protein metabolism. In addition, zinc deficiency has frequently been associated with EFA deficiency [25]. Finally, uptake of selenium can be disturbed due to EFA deficiency and iron depletion is seen as a result of gastrointestinal bleeding, insufficient uptake, transport and handling of iron. In addition, liver dysfunction strongly reduces storage capacity of vitamins such as folate, riboflavin, nicotinamide, pantothenic acid, pyroxidine, vitamin B_{12}, thiamine and vitamin A. Hepatocellular injury in CLD also results in defects in vitamin activation, conversion, release and transport [8].

As described above, children with CLD receive higher dosages of fat-soluble vitamins. Furthermore, addition of zinc to the diet could counteract a part of the poor dietary intake.

Concluding Remarks

Influencing nutritional intake and metabolism is a critical aspect of the management of children with CLD. Patients with CLD form a heterogeneous group and the clinical manifestations of their disease vary. This makes a tailor-made approach for these children crucial. Not all aspects of nutrient metabolism and absorption in children with CLD are well understood and studied. Experiments with stable isotope-labeled triglycerides and fatty acids have provided essential information about fat absorption under physiological and cholestatic conditions in animal models and humans. We expect that in the future, tests using other isotope-labeled macronutrients, i.e. carbohydrates and proteins, can be used to further assess nutritional status of children with CLD, thereby creating tailor-made nutritional therapies.

Acknowledgements

The research described in this manuscript was in part supported by the Dutch Digestive Diseases Foundation (MLDS). Edmond H.H.M. Rings and Henkjan J. Verkade were supported by a fellowship of the Royal Netherlands Academy of Arts and Sciences.

References

1 Balistreri WF: Neonatal cholestasis. J Pediatr 1985;106:171–184.
2 Dick MC, Mowat AP: Hepatitis syndrome in infancy – an epidemiological survey with 10 year follow up. Arch Dis Child 1985;60:512–516.
3 Barshes NR, Lee TC, Udell IW, et al: The pediatric end-stage liver disease (PELD) model as a predictor of survival benefit and posttransplant survival in pediatric liver transplant recipients. Liver Transpl 2006;12:475–480.
4 Mattar RH, Azevedo RA, Speridiao PG, et al: Nutritional status and intestinal iron absorption in children with chronic hepatic disease with and without cholestasis. J Pediatr (Rio J) 2005;81:317–324.
5 Sealy MJ, Muskiet FAJ, Boersma ER, et al: Essential fatty acid deficiency in pediatric patients. Tijdschr Kindergeneeskd 1997;65:144–150.
6 Poupon R, Chazouilleres O, Poupon RE: Chronic cholestatic diseases. J Hepatol 2000;32 (suppl):129–140.
7 Narkewicz MR: Biliary atresia: an update on our understanding of the disorder. Curr Opin Pediatr 2001;13:435–440.
8 Matos C, Porayko MK, Francisco-Ziller N, DiCecco S: Nutrition and chronic liver disease. J Clin Gastroenterol 2002;35:391–397.
9 Shanbhogue RL, Bistrian BR, Jenkins RL, et al: Resting energy expenditure in patients with end-stage liver disease and in normal population. JPEN J Parenter Enteral Nutr 1987;11:305–308.
10 Pierro A, Koletzko B, Carnielli V, et al: Resting energy expenditure is increased in infants and children with extrahepatic biliary atresia. J Pediatr Surg 1989;24:534–538.
11 Shepherd R: Energy expenditure in infants in health and disease. Can J Gastroenterol 1997;11:101–104.
12 Muller MJ, Lautz HU, Plogmann B, et al: Energy expenditure and substrate oxidation in patients with cirrhosis: the impact of cause, clinical staging and nutritional state. Hepatology 1992;15:782–794.
13 Wasserman D, Zemel BS, Mulberg AE, et al: Growth, nutritional status, body composition, and energy expenditure in prepubertal children with Alagille syndrome. J Pediatr 1999;134:172–177.
14 Watanabe M, Houten SM, Mataki C, et al: Bile acids induce energy expenditure by promoting intracellular thyroid hormone activation. Nature 2006;439:484–489.
15 Kalivianakis M, Minich DM, Havinga R, et al: Detection of impaired intestinal absorption of long-chain fatty acids: validation studies of a novel test in a rat model of fat malabsorption. Am J Clin Nutr 2000;72:174–180.
16 Kuipers F, Havinga R, Bosschieter H, et al: Enterohepatic circulation in the rat. Gastroenterology 1985;88:403–411.

17 Rings EH, Minich DM, Vonk RJ, et al: Functional development of fat absorption in term and preterm neonates strongly correlates with ability to absorb long-chain fatty acids from intestinal lumen. Pediatr Res 2002;51:57–63.
18 Minich DM, Havinga R, Stellaard F, et al: Intestinal absorption and postabsorptive metabolism of linoleic acid in rats with short-term bile duct ligation. Am J Physiol Gastrointest Liver Physiol 2000;279:G1242–G1248.
19 Los EL, Wolters H, Suh E, et al: Bile salts induce prolonged mitogenic signaling in proliferating intestinal epithelial cells. Digestive Disease Week and the 106th Annual Meeting of the American Gastroenterological Association. May 14–19, 2005, Chicago, Illinois, USA (abstracts). Gastroenterology 2005;128(suppl 2):A1–A821.
20 Faubion WA, Guicciardi ME, Miyoshi H, et al: Toxic bile salts induce rodent hepatocyte apoptosis via direct activation of Fas. J Clin Invest 1999;103:137–145.
21 Tavill AS: The synthesis and degradation of liver-produced proteins. Gut 1972;13:225–241.
22 McCullough AJ, Glamour T: Differences in amino acid kinetics in cirrhosis. Gastroenterology 1993;104:1858–1865.
23 Mager DR, Wykes LJ, Roberts EA, et al: Branched-chain amino acid needs in children with mild-to-moderate chronic cholestatic liver disease. J Nutr 2006;136:133–139.
24 Sokal EM, Baudoux MC, Collette E, et al: Branched chain amino acids improve body composition and nitrogen balance in a rat model of extra hepatic biliary atresia. Pediatr Res 1996;40:66–71.
25 Chin SE, Shepherd RW, Thomas BJ, et al: The nature of malnutrition in children with end-stage liver disease awaiting orthotopic liver transplantation. Am J Clin Nutr 1992;56:164–168.

Discussion

Dr. Chubarova: It is well known that polyunsaturated fatty acids are absorbed better than saturated acids. Have you used high amounts of these fatty acids to improve the absorption of fat? Is there any situation, not only during cholestasis, when medium-chain fatty acids are not absorbed well enough? Unsaturated fatty acids are usually absorbed less well than polyunsaturated acids. Have you used a high level of linoleic acid in the diet to improve absorption?

Dr. Rings: We know that it is difficult to achieve. I think most children are depleted of linoleic acid. We try to improve absorption by giving specific oils in which it is available. The second question concerns the medium-chain fatty acids. There are also reasons that they are not absorbed that well, for instance when the length of the bowel is reduced. In children with cholestasis, we have no indication that that is a problem. We will not go over 50%. I think we have no reason for that.

Dr. Heine: Regarding the mechanisms of fat malabsorption you showed different mechanisms for cystic fibrosis and pancreatic insufficiency. Isn't fat malabsorption in cystic fibrosis patients due to pancreatic insufficiency?

Dr. Rings: I think you are right; there is a combination of these mechanisms. Using stable isotope-labeled fat we could see that the lipolytic events are really impaired. This is the major cause, but then the reduced bile flow into the intestine will also have the effect that you see with respect to fat absorption.

Dr. Heine: Have you decreased the lipid content in the formula that you use?

Dr. Rings: Yes, not the total amount because the formula is designed in a way that we can increase the caloric level up to 200%. Then the total fat that we give can be even higher than in normal formula.

Dr. Heine: Could fluid overload become a problem when aiming for high energy intake?

Dr. Rings: Yes, but it can be restricted in fluid. It is designed in a way that the fluid content is relatively low compared to the ingredients.

Dr. Bayhon: One of the currently advocated nutritional supports is the use of branched chain amino acids for adult patients with hepatic encephalopathy. There are some very encouraging results. They were able to reverse hepatic encephalopathy in as little as 3–5 days and to maximize nutritional support using these branched chain-enriched amino acids. Have you encountered any such results in the use of branched chain amino acids in children?

Dr. Rings: No, I am not an expert in this field, but we have discussed it often. There is no hard evidence in children that these specific amino acids will add to the results that you describe. I went over the literature myself and did not manage to establish it either.

Dr. Fuchs: I have a question about the body composition of either the animal model or children in whom you supply additional energy, protein, and nutrients. Is their body composition equivalent to normal children or do they have a larger fat-free or fat mass? With regard to the pediatric end-stage liver disease (PELD) scoring in which weight is used, a lot of these children have ascites which increases their body weight and which might lead to an underestimation of their undernutrition if using only weight as the indicator. Has anyone looked at using other measures such as mid-upper arm circumference or body composition indexes to further refine the PELD scoring?

Dr. Rings: I want to come back first to the PELD score. It is the height that defines the growth. Weight, which is a very important parameter in clinical management, is not taken into account, otherwise it would be very hard to judge where a child stands at that moment. It is the height to age that is taken into this calculation. With regard to body composition, it is well known that lean body mass is lower in these children, so obviously they have more body fat mass.

Dr. S. Koletzko: It is very important as you pointed out that there is no protein restriction until encephalopathy occurs. We heard this morning that very premature infants receive 4 g protein/kg body weight/day. How much protein/kg do you use in these patients?

Dr. Rings: The protein content can be up to 3.5–4 g in children up to 2 years of age, and we only restrict it to 1–2 g in case of severe encephalopathy. This is usually the case in children with acute liver failure. It is not actually the category of children we are discussing.

Dr. S. Koletzko: Would you comment on the role of ursodeoxycholic acid? Does it do anything to nutrition and fat absorption in these children?

Dr. Rings: Ursofalk is a brand name. When children are cholestatic and their bilirubin levels go up to 50 μmol/l or higher, we give this hydrophilic compound to change their bile composition. We give them a supplement of 15 mg/kg of ursodeoxycholic acid in order to improve the bile flow and thereby also fat absorption. However, this mechanism has not been tested in children to establish if it really helps.

Dr. S. Koletzko: You did not use ursodeoxycholic acid in your model to see whether the absorption of your fatty acids improved or not?

Dr. Rings: We haven't done that yet, but models are now, so it is a nice suggestion.

Dr. B. Koletzko: Could you comment on the composition of the long-chain lipids that you use in your formula? In studies we performed jointly with Dr. Socha in Warsaw, we found a decrease in long-chain polyunsaturated fatty acid metabolites in children with chronic liver disease along with increasing bilirubin levels. This is difficult to explain by malassimilation alone but seems to point to an impairment of essential fatty acid conversion with an increasing degree of cholestasis. This observation raises the question whether cholestatic infants may benefit from an enhanced supply of preformed long-chain polyunsaturated fatty acids.

Dr. Rings: I have no details to answer this question. The formula we use makes use of the normal composition of the long-chain triglycerides. We have not designed another formula. We profile essential fatty acids in the fatty acid spectrum once in a while to see if the children need more of them, in which case we give them additional supplements. It is not a prefixed formula.

Dr. Davidson: Do you modify the formula that you do use from a commercial formula or is it a preparation that you have made up specifically?

Dr. Rings: No, it is a commercial product available in Europe.

Dr. S. Koletzko: How do you provide vitamin E in these patients and how do you monitor whether they get a sufficient amount to avoid hemolysis due to vitamin E deficiency?

Dr. Rings: Monitoring is done by measuring their levels, which we supplement if necessary with water-soluble vitamin E.

Dr. S. Koletzko: The problem is that they often have high cholesterol levels so they might be misleading. I find it very difficult to decide which is the right level in these children. I don't know whether anybody else has an answer.

Dr. Cooke: Although low, the fractional fat absorption rates are still 80–90%. Unless there is a selective malabsorption of a specific mineral or vitamin, deficiency appears unlikely unless requirements are increased significantly.

Dr. Rings: It is not the experience so much, but we tend to test this on a regular basis.

Dr. Milla: Many years ago we showed that in cholestasis, quite profound vitamin E deficiency develops even though the fat absorption rate is reasonably high. It is very difficult to know what is the best way to ascertain vitamin E status. Whilst serum vitamin E can be measured, the effects of deficiency are only apparent at extremely low levels of vitamin E. With regard to visual function, in peripheral nerve conduction studies there are levels well below 5 mmol/l before trouble starts. If the serum level is near the normal range, it seems in practice very unlikely that deficiency symptoms occur. Indeed the original studies that Muller et al. [1] did showed that if their levels increased towards the normal range the nerve conduction defects and visual defects could actually be corrected.

Dr. B. Koletzko: We see the same low levels in cholestatic infants. When we looked at indicators of lipid peroxidation they seemed to be inversely related to vitamin E levels both in untreated patients and in patients treated with water-soluble vitamin E. The level of TBARS is related best to vitamin E corrected for serum lipid concentrations, which makes sense because α-tocopherol is transported by LDL particles. Therefore it seems to me that this may be the best measure to look at the ratios of vitamin E to serum lipids to assess the patient's vitamin E status.

Dr. Milla: Are there good reference ranges for that?

Dr. B. Koletzko: There are reference ranges; I don't know them off hand but they can be found in our publications. But I am not sure whether they are good in terms of defining optimal health outcomes; they are just reference ranges.

Dr. Heine: Vitamin D and vitamin K are important in bone health. In chronic cholestasis the risk of metabolic bone disease is increased. Have you looked whether this nutritional regimen prevents or ameliorates metabolic bone disease?

Dr. Rings: We have not done a very extended study on that. We have a routine of checking bone mineralization yearly and do a DEXA scan about every year or 2. We try to adapt to this problem mostly because the children after transplantation are on prednisone in our schedule and therefore they have an additional risk of bone disease.

Reference

1   Muller DR, Harries JT, Lloyd JK: Vitamin E therapy in abetalipoproteinaemia. Arch Dis Child 1970;45:715.

Cooke RJ, Vandenplas Y, Wahn U (eds): Nutrition Support for Infants and Children at Risk.
Nestlé Nutr Workshop Ser Pediatr Program, vol 59, pp 161–176,
Nestec Ltd., Vevey/S. Karger AG, Basel, © 2007.

Nutrient Requirements of Premature Infants

Ekhard E. Ziegler

Department of Pediatrics, University of Iowa, Iowa City, IA, USA

Abstract

Exact knowledge of the nutrient requirements of premature infants is critically important for the prevention of postnatal growth failure and for improved neurodevelopmental outcome. Methods whereby nutrient requirements can be estimated fall into two categories, factorial methods and empirical methods. Each have their advantages and disadvantages. The factorial methods provide estimates of requirements for protein, energy and a number of other nutrients. The exact methods used can vary but still yield fairly similar results. Factorial methods also permit estimation of the extra nutrients needed for a given degree of catch-up growth, but cannot indicate the extent to which catch-up growth is actually possible. Empirical methods yield estimates of the requirements for protein and energy but not for other nutrients. They often give an indication of what degree of catch-up growth is possible, in addition to providing estimates of the requirements for protein and energy. The advantages of catch-up growth outweigh any possible disadvantages associated with it. The nutrients needed for catch-up growth should therefore always be provided.

Introduction

In recent years it has become apparent that many premature infants, in particular those born with very low birth weight, experience postnatal growth failure [1, 2]. The inadequate nutrient intakes that lead to this growth failure are suspected to be responsible for the impaired neurocognitive development that many premature infants show later in life. This has led to increased efforts to improve nutrient intakes in the hope that improved nutrient intakes will result in improved neurocognitive outcome.

Although it has been known for some time that the nutrient requirements of premature infants are considerably higher than those of infants born at term [3], there has not been much consensus about exactly what the nutrient requirements of premature infants are. The main source of discrepancy has been the different approaches utilized for defining requirements. Another source is the extent to which requirements take into account catch-up growth, of which most preterm infants are capable if given the requisite nutrients. Catch-up growth can occur after intrauterine as well as postnatal growth failure. Because requirements are strongly dependent on body size, they must be defined for specific body weight categories. Estimates of requirements by the factorial approach are weight-specific, but they do not include nutrients needed for catch-up growth. Estimates by the empirical approach typically include nutrients needed for catch-up, but estimates do not apply to infants that are smaller (or larger) than the infants studied.

There is principal agreement that postnatal growth of the premature infant should ideally emulate the growth of the fetus in utero. Such 'normal' growth would be proof of the absence of substantive nutrient deficiency and would provide assurance of unimpaired neurocognitive development. The American Academy of Pediatrics [4] recommends that 'postnatal growth that approximates the in utero growth of a normal fetus of the same postconception age' should be the basis for estimating nutrient requirements.

The fetal model is the basis for estimation of nutrient requirements by the factorial method [5]. Reservations about the fetal model, and about estimates of nutrient requirements based on it, have centered on demonstrated differences in extracellular fluid spaces between the fetus and the premature infant. However, there is no evidence that any other body constituents are affected by birth. There is thus no reason why acquisition of nonaqueous body constituents by the preterm infants could not proceed at the intrauterine rate. Because factorial estimates are based on the fetal model, they pertain to infants who grow at the fetal rate. Nutrient needs for catch-up growth can be estimated by the factorial method only if assumptions are made regarding the extent and speed of catch-up growth. Unlike the empirical approach, the factorial approach provides estimates of requirements for any nutrient for which the content in the fetus is known.

Empirical methods for estimating nutrient requirements depend on establishment of the relationship between intakes of key nutrients, such as protein and energy, and growth. They yield estimates of requirements for protein and energy needed to achieve a specified rate of growth. Empirical methods thus can provide estimates of nutrient needs for growth at the fetal rate as well as accelerated growth, i.e., catch-up growth. Unlike the factorial method, empirical methods do not provide estimated nutrient needs other than protein and energy needs.

Requirements Determined by the Factorial Method

The factorial approach derives nutrient requirements as the sum of two (in the case of parenteral requirements) or three components (in the case of enteral requirements). The largest component, and the component that changes most with body size, is the growth component, i.e., nutrient accretion. The other components are inevitable losses and, in the case of enteral nutrient requirements, efficiency of nutrient absorption.

Determination of the growth component requires knowledge of nutrient accretion with 'normal' growth. Because it is generally agreed that postnatal growth should 'approximate the in utero growth of a normal fetus' [4], the fetus serves as the model from which nutrient accretion is derived. Beginning in the 19th century, the body composition of stillborn infants and infants deceased soon after birth, including premature infants, has been analyzed by a number of investigators. Sparks [6] and Forbes [7, 8] have provided comprehensive summaries of the chemical analysis of some 160 fetuses. Gestational age was not always available, but because most body constituents change as a function of body size (the notable exception being body fat [7]), the data can be used to derive accretion rates even when gestational age is not explicitly known [6, 7]. Ziegler et al. [9] used only data from fetuses with known gestational age for the construction of a 'reference fetus' and derivation of fetal accretion rates. In spite of the differences in approaches (i.e., size vs. age) to the establishment of fetal body composition, nutrient accretion rates derived by the different approaches [6, 7, 9] are actually quite similar [10]. The fetal accretion data presented in table 1 represent a synthesis of the different approaches [6, 7, 9] in combination with contemporary fetal growth data [11]. The data represent our current best estimates of nutrient accretion. In the case of protein, accretion rates shown in table 1 are corrected for presumed inefficiency (90%) of the conversion of dietary protein to body protein. In the case of energy, the accretion value includes the energy cost of growth, estimated by Micheli et al. [12] at 10 kcal/kg/day.

Inevitable losses of protein (nitrogen) occur through desquamation of skin and as urinary nitrogen excretion mostly in the form of urea (desquamation of intestinal cells is accounted for in the correction for efficiency of intestinal absorption). Based on dermal nitrogen losses determined by Snyderman et al. [13], we have assumed average dermal losses of 27 mg/kg/day. Based on published data [14, 15] we have assumed urinary nitrogen losses to be 133 mg/kg/ day. Energy losses comprise resting energy expenditure plus an allowance for miscellaneous expenditures, e.g., occasional cold exposure and physical activity. Based on recent studies [16–18] we have assumed resting expenditure to be 45 kcal/kg/day in infants weighing <900 g and 50 kcal/kg/day in larger infants. Miscellaneous energy expenditures have been assumed to be 15 kcal/kg/day in infants under 1,200 g and 20 kcal/kg/day in larger infants.

Table 1. Estimated nutrient intakes needed to achieve fetal weight gain

	Body weight, g					
	500–700	700–900	900–1,200	1,200–1,500	1,500–1,800	1,800–2,200
Fetal weight gain[a]						
g/day	13	16	20	24	26	29
g/kg/day	21	20	19	18	16	14
Protein (Nx6.25), g						
Inevitable loss[b]	1.0	1.0	1.0	1.0	1.0	1.0
Growth (accretion)[c]	2.5	2.5	2.5	2.4	2.2	2.0
Required intake						
Parenteral[d]	3.5	3.5	3.5	3.4	3.2	3.0
Enteral[e]	4.0	4.0	4.0	3.9	3.6	3.4
Energy, kcal						
Loss	60	60	65	70	70	70
Resting expenditure	45	45	50	50	50	50
Miscellaneous expenditure	15	15	15	20	20	20
Growth (accretion)[f]	29	32	36	38	39	41
Required intake						
Parenteral[d]	89	92	101	108	109	111
Enteral[g]	105	108	119	127	128	131
Protein/energy g/100 kcal						
Parenteral	3.9	4.1	3.5	3.1	2.9	2.7
Enteral	3.8	3.7	3.4	3.1	2.8	2.6

Because nutrient needs are closely related to body weight and weight gain, the nutrient needs apply to all postnatal ages. All values are per kg per day except where noted [modified from 18].

[a]Based on data of Kramer et al. [11].
[b]Urinary nitrogen loss of 133 mg/kg/day [14, 15] and dermal loss of 27 mg/kg/day [13].
[c]Includes correction for 90% efficiency of conversion from dietary to body protein.
[d]Sum of loss and accretion.
[e]Same as parenteral but assuming 88% absorption of dietary protein.
[f]Energy accretion plus 10 kcal/kg/day cost of growth.
[g]Assuming 85% absorption of dietary energy.

Parenteral requirements for protein and energy (table 1) are calculated as the sum of accretion plus inevitable losses. Enteral requirements are calculated as accretion plus inevitable losses corrected for efficiency of absorption, assumed to be 88% for protein and 85% for energy. Requirements (per kg of

Table 2. Requirements for major minerals and electrolytes determined by the factorial method, listed by body weight

	500–1,000 g		1,000–1,500 g		1,500–2,000 g	
	accretion	requirement	accretion	requirement	accretion	requirement
Ca, mg	102	184	99	178	96	173
P, mg	66	126	65	124	63	120
Mg, mg	2.8	6.9	2.7	6.7	2.5	6.4
Na, mEq	1.54	3.3	1.37	3.0	1.06	2.6
K, mEq	0.78	2.4	0.72	2.3	0.63	2.2
Cl, mEq	1.26	2.8	0.99	2.7	0.74	2.5

body weight per day) are presented in table 1 in relation to body weight rather than gestational age because requirements are more closely related to body weight than to gestational age.

Although absolute fetal weight gain (g/day) increases with increasing body size, the fractional fetal weight gain (g/kg/day), as shown in table 1, decreases markedly as a function of weight. In spite of this decrease in the fractional growth rate, the rate of protein accretion remains constant up to a weight of 1,200 g. This is so because the protein content of fat-free body mass increases with increasing body size/age, and this increase offsets the effect of the decrease in fractional growth rate on protein accretion. Energy accretion, on the other hand, increases with increasing body weight. This is due to a marked increase in body fat content, which more than counteracts the decrease in fractional weight gain.

Whereas estimates of requirements for protein are quite firm, estimates of energy requirements are more uncertain. This is in part so because there is a paucity of data regarding resting energy expenditure of small premature infants and, especially, nonresting energy expenditure. Uncertainty also derives from the fact that body fat accumulation of the preterm infant may deviate from that of the fetus without apparent ill consequences for the premature infant. Available energy seems to be prioritized to meeting ongoing needs and is deposited as fat only after all other needs have been met.

Requirements for major minerals and electrolytes derived by the factorial method are summarized in table 2. Although the dermal and urinary losses (not shown in table 2) used in deriving these requirements are based on data from the literature [5], there is considerable uncertainty regarding the minimal urinary losses of electrolytes and of P by premature infants. Also, there is uncertainty concerning the efficiency of intestinal absorption of calcium, which is influenced by multiple dietary and other factors, and there is uncertainty with regard to the amount of bone mineral (Ca, P) that must be deposited in order to maintain bone health. It has become evident that accretion of bone mineral at somewhat less than the fetal rate can be compatible with good bone health, but it is impossible to translate such observations into quantitative estimates of the amounts of dietary calcium and phosphorus needed to maintain bone health.

Requirements Determined by Empirical Approaches

Empirical approaches generally utilize feedings (formulas or human milk) that provide precisely known intakes of energy and protein. Growth and sometimes metabolic balance are used as outcomes. Because requirements are strongly dependent on body size, estimates obtained by the empirical approach apply only to infants that are similar in body size to the infants studied.

Based on analysis of published data, Ziegler [10] demonstrated that in infants weighing more than 1,200 g at birth, weight gain (g/day) increased with increasing protein intake until the latter reached about 3.6 g/kg/day. (There were insufficient data to determine the effect of higher protein intakes.) Intake of energy did not seem to be related to weight gain. A protein intake of 3.6 g/kg/day produced a weight gain of about 30 g/day. Such a weight gain exceeds that of the fetus of comparable weight and thus represents catch-up growth. A protein intake of 3.6 g/kg/day therefore supports a certain amount of catch-up growth.

Kashyap et al. [19–21] performed a series of growth and metabolic balance studies with feedings (human milk, formulas) that varied in protein and energy content. They used the data to derive equations predicting protein and energy intakes necessary to duplicate fetal weight gain. The data were obtained in infants weighing between 1,200 and 2,000 g and thus pertain to infants in this weight range. The authors estimated that protein intake necessary for duplication of fetal weight gain is about 3.0 g/kg/day.

The Life Sciences Research Office (LSRO) [22], based on a comprehensive review of reported nutrition studies of premature infants, concluded that the minimum protein intake of premature infants (weight not specified) is 3.4 g/kg/day with a protein/energy ratio of 2.5 g/100 kcal at the maximum energy intake of 135 kcal/kg/day. The LSRO panel also concluded that a protein intake of 4.3 g/kg/day (with protein/energy ratio of 3.6 g/100 kcal) is without adverse consequences, whereas intakes of 5.0 g/kg/day or higher are likely to be associated with undesirable consequences. It is not clear whether the estimates by the LSRO [22] include allowances for catch-up growth.

Using a variety of endpoints, including growth, body composition and nitrogen balance, Rigo [23] estimated the protein requirements ('advisable recommendation') of infants born at 26–30 weeks' gestation (corresponding

Table 3. Protein requirements (enteral) of premature infants without catch-up

	Weight 800 g		Weight 1,600 g	
	g/kg/day	g/100 kcal	g/kg/day	g/100 kcal
Ziegler (table 1)	4.0	3.7	3.6	2.8
Kashyap et al. [19–21]	–	–	3.0	2.5[a]
Klein [22]	3.4–4.3	2.5–3.6	3.4–4.3	2.5–3.6
Rigo [23]	3.8–4.2	3.3	3.4–3.6	2.8

[a]At energy intake of 120 kcal/kg/day.

to weight of about 800–1,500 g) at 3.8–4.2 g/kg/day (3.3 g/100 kcal) and those of infants born at 30–36 weeks' gestation (corresponding to weight of 1,500–2,700 g) at 3.4–3.6 g/kg/day (2.8 g/100 kcal).

The various estimates of protein requirements are summarized in table 3 for infants with nominal weights of 800 and 1,600 g. It is apparent that there is rather close agreement in spite of the different methods used in arriving at estimates of protein requirements.

Catch-Up Growth

Catch-up growth occurs when an individual, after a period of growth restriction, is returning towards his/her original growth channel. If the growth restriction occurs during a vulnerable period and is severe and/or prolonged, catch-up growth may not be possible or may be incomplete. With lesser degrees of growth restriction, catch-up is likely to occur, provided the requisite amounts of nutrients are provided. To the caregiver, the actual potential for catch-up growth is not known. The caregiver therefore must assume that the potential exists and must provide nutritional support of such a nature as to enable catch-up growth should the potential exist.

Catch-Up Growth after Postnatal Growth Failure

Although all infants experience some weight loss after birth due to adjustment of extracellular fluid spaces, in small premature infants there commonly is actual loss of body substance or at least growth arrest. This severe growth failure is temporary and is typically followed by a period during which growth proceeds, albeit at a slower pace than it would have occurred in utero. There is ample documentation that premature infants usually are capable of at least partial catch-up growth. However, it is not possible to predict with any certainty the degree and the speed with which infants will be catching up. It is quite likely that the extent and speed of catch-up depends on the duration and severity of the preceding growth failure. Catch-up growth requires extra nutrients and will not occur unless the required extra nutrients are provided.

Because of the uncertainties surrounding catch-up growth and the presumed high degree of individual variation, the extra nutrients required for catch-up can be estimated only in general terms. An example will serve to illustrate this. A hypothetical infant weighing 900 g with a modest degree of postnatal growth failure might be able to catch-up and show accelerated weight gain of 23 g/day, which is about 15% higher than the intrauterine rate of 20 g/day. With this, the infant would reach a weight of 1,200 g in 13 days rather than in 15 days, as would occur in utero. This accelerated growth would increase the daily accretion of protein from the intrauterine rate of 2.5 g/kg/day (table 1) to 2.88 g/kg/day and, with inevitable losses unaffected, would increase the parenteral protein requirement from 3.5 to 3.88 g/kg/day. Energy required for growth would increase from 36 to 41.4 kcal/kg/day and the total parenteral energy requirement would increase from 101 to 106.4 kcal/kg/day. The protein/energy ratio would have to increase from 3.5 to 3.65 g/100 kcal. This example illustrates the principle that catch-up growth requires disproportionately more protein than energy and thus increases the required protein/energy ratio of the feeding.

Kashyap et al. [24] used their prediction equations to determine protein and energy requirements for catch-up growth. They estimated that for an infant with a birth weight of 1,400 g to reach a discharge weight of 2,200 g 1 week earlier than would occur at the intrauterine growth rate, protein intake would have to be 3.36 g/kg/day and energy intake 99.6 kcal/kg/day (protein/energy ratio 3.37 g/100 kcal). For the same infant to reach the discharge weight of 2,200 g 2 weeks earlier would require a protein intake of 4.5 g/kg/day and energy intake of 116.8 kcal/kg/day (protein/energy ratio 3.85 g/100 kcal). When subjected to testing in a feeding trial, these predictions were generally found to hold.

Rigo [23] has provided specific advisable protein recommendations for infants with catch-up growth. They are 4.4 g/kg/day (3.4 g/100 kcal) for infants of 26–30 weeks gestational age and are higher than recommendations for infants of the same age without catch-up growth (3.8–4.2 g/kg/day and protein/energy ratio 3.3 g/100 kcal). Similarly, for infants of 30–36 weeks' gestation, the recommended protein intake for those with catch-up (3.8–4.2 g/kg/day, protein/energy ratio 3.3 g/100 kcal) is higher than for those without catch-up growth.

To Catch-Up or Not to Catch-Up?

It has been shown that preterm infants with slow growth due to receiving a nutrient-poor formula have less insulin resistance during adolescence than preterm infants with more rapid growth due to receiving a nutrient-enriched formula [25]. On the basis of this finding it has been suggested that in premature infants rapid growth should be avoided in order to reduce the risk of diabetes later in life. This conclusion may not be warranted because insulin resistance of the more rapidly growing preterm infants was similar to that of term infants [25]. Moreover, the same group [26] had shown previously that the slow-growing premature infants (those receiving the nutrient-poor formula) had substantially lower cognitive achievements in childhood than the faster-growing infants who received the nutrient-enriched formula. These data [25, 26] provide strong evidence for late effects of early nutritional experiences (programming). But they also clearly demonstrate that more rapid growth of premature infants caused by improved nutrient intakes is associated with improved neurocognitive outcome. Morley [27] showed that the rate of weight gain of male premature infants was positively associated with verbal IQ at 7.5–8 years of age and that weight at 9 months of age was positively associated with overall verbal and performance IQ. Thus, there can be no questions that the advantages associated with catch-up growth outweigh any possible disadvantages. Premature infants should always be assumed to be capable of catch-up growth and the extra nutrients required for catch-up growth should be provided.

Catch-Up after Intrauterine Growth Failure

The majority of infants born small for gestational age (SGA) are infants who have experienced intrauterine growth restriction and have the potential for catch-up growth. But the extent, speed and time of onset of catch-up growth are highly variable and unpredictable. In this regard, as in most other regards, catch-up after intrauterine growth restriction is not different from catch-up after postnatal growth failure. Catch-up growth requires nutrient intakes above and beyond those required for normal growth and can occur only if the additional nutrients are provided.

For the purpose of illustrating how the factorial approach can be used to estimate the extra nutrients needed for catch-up growth, requirements for several hypothetical scenarios are shown in table 4. The hypothetical infant is born SGA at 30 weeks gestation weighing 900 g. Shown for comparison are a normally grown (appropriate for gestational age, AGA) infant born at 26 weeks weighing 900 g, and a normally grown infant born at 30 weeks weighing 1,500 g. The assumption is made that the 30-week SGA infant has the body fat (1.5%) of a 26-week infant but has the fat-free body mass composition of a 30-week infant. If the SGA infant grows at the intrauterine rate for a 900-gram AGA infant (20 g/day), the protein and energy requirements are shown in table 4. The main difference between a 26-week AGA and a 30-week SGA infant is a somewhat higher energy expenditure (and hence lower protein/energy ratio) of the SGA infant. This is explained by the more mature composition (i.e., lower water content) of the fat-free body mass of the SGA infant.

We then asked what the protein and energy requirements would be if the SGA infant had partial or complete catch-up by the time of hospital discharge with a weight of 2,200 g. Complete catch-up is not very likely to occur and may not even be possible, but it is used here mainly to illustrate the effect of

Table 4. Nutrient requirements of hypothetical preterm SGA infant with or without catch-up growth; requirements of 26-week and 30-week hypothetical AGA infants are included for comparison

	Gestational age at birth				
	30 weeks[a]	26 weeks	30 weeks	30 weeks	30 weeks
Birth weight, g	900	900	1,500	900	900
Weight status	SGA	AGA	AGA	SGA	SGA
Catch-up[b]	None	–	–	Partial	Complete
Weight gain, g/day	20	20	26	34	46
Parenteral					
Protein, g/kg/day	3.5	3.5	3.2	4.28	5.42
Energy, kcal/kg/day	107	101	109	120	131
Enteral					
Protein, g/kg/day	4.0	4.0	3.6	4.9	6.2
Energy, kcal/kg/day	126	119	128	141	154
Protein/energy, g/100 kcal	3.2	3.4	2.8	3.5	4.0

Requirements estimated for the first 2 weeks of growth, which is assumed to begin with regained birth weight.

[a] Assuming body fat content to be that of a 26-week fetus (1.5%) and composition of fat-free mass to be that of a 30-week fetus (86.8% water, 10.6% protein).

[b] Partial catch-up assumed to reach 1,850 g in 4 weeks, complete catch-up assumed to reach 2,200 g in 4 weeks.

catch-up growth on nutrient requirements. Partial catch-up, on the other hand, whereby the infant makes up about one half of the growth deficit before discharge from the hospital, may occur. Estimates of energy requirements for catch-up growth are based on the assumption that it involves restoration of body fat content to a level commensurate with that of the fetus of similar weight. The data in table 4 show that catch-up growth, whether complete or partial, increases requirements for protein more than requirements for energy. Hence required protein/energy ratios are increased for partial and especially for complete catch-up compared to the 900 g SGA as well as the 900-gram AGA infant. Since otherwise satisfactory catch-up growth could theoretically occur with less than full restoration of body fat, it is possible that energy needs could be less than those shown in table 4 and that protein/energy ratios could be higher.

Conclusions

Exact knowledge of the nutrient requirements of premature infants is critically important for the prevention of postnatal growth failure and ensuring optimal neurodevelopmental outcome. Methods whereby nutrient requirements can be estimated fall into two categories, factorial methods and empirical methods. Either methods have advantages and disadvantages. The factorial methods provide estimates of requirements for protein, energy and a number of other nutrients. Factorial methods permit estimation of the extra nutrients needed for a given degree of catch-up growth, but cannot indicate the extent to which catch-up growth is actually possible. Empirical methods yield estimates of the requirements for protein and energy but not for other nutrients. They often provide estimates of the protein and energy needs for catch-up growth. The advantages of catch-up growth outweigh any possible disadvantages associated with it. The nutrients needed for catch-up growth should therefore always be provided.

References

1 Carlson SJ, Ziegler EE: Nutrient intakes and growth of very low birth weight infants. J Perinatol 1998;18:252–258.
2 Ehrenkranz RA, Younes N, Lemons J, et al: Longitudinal growth of hospitalized very low birth weight infants. Pediatrics 1999;104:280–289.
3 Fomon SJ, Ziegler EE, Vazquez HD: Human milk and the small premature infant. Am J Dis Child 1977;131:463–467.
4 American Academy of Pediatrics Committee on Nutrition: Nutritional needs of low-birth-weight infants. Pediatrics 1985;75:976–986.
5 Ziegler EE, Biga RL, Fomon SJ: Nutritional requirements of the premature infant; in Suskind RM (ed): Textbook of Pediatric Nutrition. New York, Raven Press, 1981, pp 29–39.
6 Sparks JW: Human intrauterine growth and nutrient accretion. Semin Perinatol 1984;8:74–93.
7 Forbes GB: Human Body Composition. New York, Springer, 1987, pp 101–124.
8 Forbes G: Nutritional adequacy of human breast milk for prematurely born infants; in Lebenthal E (ed): Gastroenterology and Nutrition in Infancy. New York, Raven Press, 1989, pp 27–34.
9 Ziegler EE, O'Donnell AM, Nelson SE, et al: Body composition of the reference fetus. Growth 1976;40:329–341.
10 Ziegler EE: Protein requirements of preterm infants; in Fomon SJ, Heird WC, (eds): Energy and Protein Needs during Infancy. New York, Academic Press, 1986, pp 69–85.
11 Kramer MS, Platt RW, Wen SW, et al: A new and improved population-based Canadian reference for birth weight for gestational age. Pediatrics 2001;108:1–7.
12 Micheli JL, Schutz Y, Jéquier E: Protein metabolism of the newborn; in Polin RA, Fox WW (eds): Fetal and Neonatal Physiology. Philadelphia, Saunders, 1992, pp 462–472.
13 Snyderman SE, Boyer A, Kogut MD, et al: The protein requirement of the premature infant. I. The effect of protein intake on the retention of nitrogen. J Pediatr 1969;74:872–880.
14 Saini J, Macmahon P, Morgan JB, et al: Early parenteral feeding of amino acids. Arch Dis Child 1989;64:1362–1366.
15 Rivera JA, Bell EF, Bier DM: Effect of intravenous amino acids on protein metabolism of preterm infants during the first three days of life. Pediatr Res 1993;33:106–111.
16 DeMarie MP, Hoffenberg A, Biggerstaff SLB, et al: Determinants of energy expenditure in ventilated preterm infants. J Perinat Med 1999;27:465–472.
17 Olhager E, Forsum E: Total energy expenditure, body composition and weight gain in moderately preterm and full-term infants at term postconceptional age. Acta Paediatr 2003;92:1327–1334.
18 Ziegler EE, Thureen PJ, Carlson SJ: Aggressive nutrition of the very low birthweight infant. Clin Perinatol 2002;29:225–244.
19 Kashyap S, Forsyth M, Zucker C, et al: Effects of varying protein and energy intakes on growth and metabolic response in low birth weight infants. J Pediatr 1986;108:955–963.

20 Kashyap S, Schulze KF, Forsyth M, et al: Growth, nutrient retention, and metabolic response of low birth weight infants fed varying intakes of protein and energy. J Pediatr 1988;113: 713–721.
21 Kashyap S, Schulze KF, Forsyth M, et al: Growth, nutrient retention, and metabolic response of low-birth-weight infants fed supplemented and unsupplemented preterm human milk. Am J Clin Nutr 1990;52:254–262.
22 Klein CJ: Nutrient requirements for preterm infant formulas. J Nutr 2002;132(suppl): 1395S–1577S.
23 Rigo J: Protein, amino acid and other nitrogen compounds; in Tsang RC, Uauy R, Koletzko B, Zlotkin S (eds): Nutrition of the Preterm Infant, ed 2. Cincinnati, Digital Educational Publishing, 2005.
24 Kashyap S, Schulze KF, Ramakrishnan R, et al: Evaluation of a mathematical model for predicting the relationship between protein and energy intakes of low-birth-weight infants and the rate and composition of weight gain. Pediatr Res 1994;35:704–712.
25 Singhal A, Fewtrell M, Cole TJ, Lucas A: Low nutrient intake and early growth for later insulin resistance in adolescents born preterm. Lancet 2003;361:1089–1097.
26 Lucas A, Morley R, Cole TJ: Randomised trial of early diet in preterm babies and later intelligence quotient. BMJ 1998;317:1481–1487.
27 Morley R: Early growth and later development; in Ziegler EE, Lucas A, Moro G (eds): Nutrition of the Very Low Birthweight Infant. Lippincott, Philadelphia, 1999, p 19.

Discussion

Dr. B. Koletzko: Your data are extremely valuable and give a great basis for orientation of feeding practice. Obviously one would love to have studies with a longer follow-up to test whether your hypothesis regarding the relationship between different levels of intake and outcome can be substantiated. You observe a growth deficit relative to intrauterine growth up to 37 weeks of gestational age. Do you still find the same relative deficit in these infants at 2 or 3 months after expected term birth. Obviously, all infants born at term lose weight after birth and need time to regain weight. Thus I assume that the growth deficit you describe at 37 weeks would be much smaller at 2 weeks after term birth. We do not know whether or not it is important to catch up this growth deficit by 37 weeks, 42 weeks or later. My second question relates to catch-up growth in SGA infants: do we really have any basis to conclude in the length of time a SGA needs to catch up, or even if it should catch up at all? My third question relates to the fascinating studies of Dr. Singhal and Dr. Lucas who reported that long-term outcomes in preterm infants were related to weight change during the first 2 weeks after birth. Do these data allow us to draw conclusions on the feeding of preterm infants? In the first 2 weeks of life the weight change really was mostly weight loss, and I wonder how much of this is related to feeding and how much is related to other factors?

Dr. Ziegler: Catch-up growth certainly continues after discharge. There are follow-up studies that show that even at age 8 years catch-up continues. But as a group, former premature infants are short and have small heads. This reflects practices 15 and 20 years ago; of course I cannot tell you how the babies that we observed in 2005 are going to be. Hopefully they will be better. As a group, premature infants do catch up given appropriate nutrition.

The next question was about SGA infants. I did not address the question whether we should try and make SGA babies catch up. I personally think we should because these infants have undergone a period of undernutrition and the sooner we correct this situation the higher the likelihood that they make up for what they have missed in terms of growth and development. But I know this is controversial and there are arguments against my position.

Your last question was about Dr. Lucas's findings. When he says that split proinsulin levels during adolescence are related to the speed of growth during infancy, he refers to weight change in the first 2 weeks. Both groups at 2 weeks are below birth weight, but those who received the good formula lost less weight since birth than those receiving the bad formula. But what is really important is that the ones with more weight loss also have a low IQ on follow-up. For a while it was thought that accelerated growth should be avoided because of the increased risk of diabetes. I don't think this is justified because slow growth carries the risk of decreased IQ.

Dr. B. Koletzko: But the IQ outcome was really related to weight gain during a different time period of about 30 days after preterm birth, whereas the data on flow-mediated dilatation and split proinsulin were related to weight change during only 14 days.

Dr. Ziegler: I should remind you that Dr. Lucas also had a control group of term breastfed infants who had split proinsulin levels like the fast-growing premature babies.

Dr. Rivera: The data are in some way idealistic. In practice it is sometimes very difficult to achieve this amount of protein intake because premature babies tend to have a lot of complications. You have shown a correlation with protein intake and IQ in those infants.

Dr. Ziegler: Dr. Lucas's data show a correlation between IQ and the degree of undergrowth. The babies who were the most undergrown at discharge had the lowest IQ on follow-up. Now, with regard to your earlier comment, it is really not that difficult to improve protein intake. For instance if you don't have a commercial breast milk fortifier available you can make your own; you can use skim milk powder. We used to do that before commercial fortifiers became available. So, it can be done, perhaps not perfectly but something can be done.

Dr. Fakhraee: Did you check the ammonia level or pH in the babies who got this amount of protein? There are different forms of SGA infants; some are asymmetric and some are symmetric. The symmetric SGA might be due to chromosomal anomalies or other factors like intrauterine infections, and the asymmetric is usually due to malnutrition or placental insufficiency. Did you make any sort of differentiation between these two kinds of SGA infants?

Dr. Ziegler: High ammonia and acidosis are things that were observed in very early studies with extremely high intake of poor quality protein. But in recent studies with higher protein intake there has been no hyperammonemia and no acidosis. There sometimes is a slightly higher BUN which is a normal correlate of protein intake. We see no adverse effects today because the proteins we use are of a much better quality.

With regard to the heterogeneity of the SGA population, I haven't differentiated them. I don't know of anyone who has tried to differentiate the nutrient needs or the growth of these different categories of SGA babies. So I agree with you that it is a heterogeneous group but I don't know what to do about it.

Dr. Cooke: We prospectively compared a protein intake of 3 g/100 kcal with 3.6 g/100 kcal in a group of preterm infants [1]. Infants retained more nitrogen and gained more weight when fed a protein intake of 3.6 g/100 kcal. At the same time, none of the infants developed uremia or metabolic acidosis. These data suggest an intake of 3.6 g/100 kcal better meets protein requirements, as recommended by Dr. Ziegler. However, this study only lasted 2 weeks and longer-term studies are needed to more adequately examine this issue.

Dr. Dhanireddy: It is very hard to argue that babies should grow according to their intrauterine rates when they are not in the uterus; homeostasis is totally different. What data do we have to show that achieving these growth rates would lead to a better outcome? Is the efficiency of energy requirement dynamic in the first several weeks because they are ill, have sepsis, and lung disease, and so even your best estimates may be different from what is needed?

Dr. Ziegler: How do we know that achieving fetal growth gives us better outcomes? We don't know until we have tried to do it. If we achieve fetal growth and still have bad outcomes we can say maybe there are other things causing poor growth. But nobody has achieved fetal growth and until we do, we don't know. My hypothesis is that poor growth and poor neurocognitive outcome are mostly due to inadequate nutrition. I don't know how complications affect caloric requirements, but they certainly do affect growth. Each bout of sepsis slows growth and also affects late outcomes, and each course of steroids causes a brief growth cessation. But there can be no doubt that the main cause of growth retardation is poor nutrition. Premature babies do not have the same amount of body water as fetuses have; they are a little dryer. Should we therefore expect them to grow a little slower than fetuses? I don't think that differences in body water can explain the massive growth failure that we regularly see in premature infants.

Dr. Milla: You have largely been considering short-term morbidity and you alluded to long-term morbidity in quoting Dr. Lucas's data about proinsulin. One of the things you have to think about is whether all preterm infants are the same, whether they all behave in the same way. If you look at the experimental data about perinatal nutrition it is clear that metabolic entrainment occurs and our latest data show that if you continue to be malnourished for a long time after birth, then this together with prenatal malnutrition results in the type of situation Dr. Lucas was describing. Some of his data are diluting your message. Do premature infants need to be handled differently in terms of their nutritional rehabilitation? For example, if they are small for dates born prematurely are they going to have different problems from those that are appropriate for weight?

Dr. Ziegler: What I have shown are data where all babies are lumped together, SGA and AGA. But if I showed you SGA and AGA separately, you would see that the growth curves are the same.

Dr. Milla: I think that is because one is just looking at growth in the short term and in the long term it probably matters whether you become hypertensive or you become diabetic.

Dr. Ziegler: I could not agree more with you but I have no long-term data. The only long-term data we have are from Dr. Lucas.

Dr. Fusch: We are sometimes comparing apples with peaches when we look at preterm babies because they have such different perinatal and postnatal pathology. If an infant is born due to placental disruption or due to chorioamnionitis they behave completely differently, and also their outcome is different. When comparing the SGA children with regard to the difference between symmetric and asymmetric retardation, we have more than two types of children, AGA and SGA; we have at least six subgroups.

Dr. Jochum: How do you estimate the influence of the carbohydrate intake on the protein needs?

Dr. Ziegler: I have no way of estimating the effect of carbohydrate intake on protein needs. The group of Kashyap et al. [2] have shown that carbohydrate and fat differentially affect protein metabolism. But I don't know how to translate this into actual protein requirements.

Dr. Fusch: In the studies by Kashyap et al. there were constant protein intakes and constant calorie intakes at two different levels. They switched the amount of nonprotein calories between more fat and more carbohydrate. With biochemical methods, with stable isotopes and with nitrogen retention, they showed clear differences: nitrogen use was different if more calories were given by carbohydrates than by fat. I don't remember if they showed, as in your experimental set, whether at the end they had different weight gains.

Dr. Fuchs: The outcome you are looking at is growth and I wonder to what extent you have looked at functional outcomes? Even at this young age, have you been able to look at markers of immunity, rates of morbidity and mortality?

Dr. Ziegler: No, I have no such data and I don't know of such data. We all hypothesize that better nutrition improves host defenses, but there are no data. None of the studies that I know of have looked at the outcomes that you ask about. At age 18 months behavioral data have been looked at, this is the earliest age at which it makes sense to look at behavior.

Dr. Thureen: I would like to respond to the question of Dr. Fakhraee regarding types of SGA infants. I believe that IUGR infants are a subset of SGA infants. Unfortunately, many studies have investigated these two groups of infants as a single group. As a result, studies in SGA infants have produced contradictory conclusions because very heterogeneous populations of infants were studied. The extremely growth-restricted infant in utero likely has a very different metabolism than most SGA infants, and thus these two groups need to be studied separately. I think the obstetrical work looking at categorizing the fetal 'metabolic status' using Doppler blood flow and other studies is probably a first start at trying to decide how infants at birth are metabolically very different.

Dr. Beaumier: We are looking at nutrition as though they were term infants, and as if carbohydrate calories from lipids and carbohydrate and protein were independent. What do you think about amino acid as energy used by the fetus ex utero at 32 or 35 weeks for growth? You show that increasing protein intake will improve growth. Is it really just lean mass accretion or amino acid used for calories or something else? Should we think of extremely low birth weight infants as being the same as 1- or 2-month-old babies that are born at term? I don't think we should use the same tools and the same approach.

Dr. Ziegler: I could not agree more with you. I think we should treat the recently born premature infant like a fetus. We should give him parenterally a high carbohydrate and a very high amino acid intake. It has been estimated that the fetus is taking up amino acids at a rate of 5 or 6 g/kg whereas only 2 g/kg are deposited, and so the conclusion is that the remaining amino acids are utilized for energy. I do think we should mimic that in our parenteral nutrition regimen that we apply right after birth. But by the time the infant is fed enterally we have switched over to the typical postnatal regimen where a large part of the calories comes from fat and where the protein intake is barely at the requirement. When I talk about growth, I talk about an infant who has made this transition from the fetal to the postnatal diet.

Dr. Beaumier: But can we confirm that when we switch from parenteral to enteral nutrition that they actually have a different metabolism or a newly adapted metabolism.

Dr. Ziegler: We assume that the infants, when they tolerate enteral feedings, have made the transition or are capable of making the transition. High protein and carbohydrate may be beneficial in enteral feeding. As I pointed out, the phobia of protein is so prevalent and so strong that to propose a higher protein intake would fall on deaf ears. Remember that even protein intakes sufficiently high to meet requirements are not generally accepted.

Dr. Putet: You give some recommendation for an infant growing stably. What about the one who is not growing, what about the metabolic load and some organs like the kidney? The kidney is not mature at all; it is still maturing. What is the metabolic load in the 28-week-old babies and their kidney function? What are the consequences later on at 6–8 months?

Ziegler

Dr. Ziegler: The only consequence I know of is that the kidneys of premature babies with a higher protein intake tend to be larger. Even if there are more serious consequences my priority would still be the brain. In other words, I would be glad to sacrifice some kidney function if it meant that I can salvage the brain.

References

1 Cooke R, Embleton N, Rigo J, et al: High protein pre-term infant formula: effect on nutrient balance, metabolic status and growth. Pediatr Res 2006;59:265–270.
2 Kashyap S, Ohira-Kist K, Abildskov K, et al: Effects of quality of energy intake on growth and metabolic response of enterally fed low-birth-weight infants. Pediatr Res 2001;50:390–397.

Cooke RJ, Vandenplas Y, Wahn U (eds): Nutrition Support for Infants and Children at Risk.
Nestlé Nutr Workshop Ser Pediatr Program, vol 59, pp 177–192,
Nestec Ltd., Vevey/S. Karger AG, Basel, © 2007.

Nutritional Assessment in Preterm Infants

Ian J. Griffin

USDA/ARS Children's Nutrition Research Center and Section of Neonatology,
Department of Pediatrics, Baylor College of Medicine, Houston, TX, USA

Abstract

If the aim of nutritional assessment of preterm infants is to identify suboptimal (or excessive) provision of protein, energy and micronutrients, most currently available methods perform poorly. Assessment of body weight is limited by the confounding effect of fluid status especially in the first few days of life, and measurements of linear growth are relatively imprecise and slow to respond to nutritional changes. Growth assessment is hampered by the lack of an adequate reference standard. Comparisons to historical cohorts of preterm babies are inadequate. As most very low birth weight infants leave hospital below the 10th centile, use of these charts as 'standards' almost guarantees that preterm infants will have poor growth. Growth centiles based on data from newborn preterm infants have certain advantages. However, this is hardly normative data as preterm birth is always an abnormal event. Methods of assessing body composition are largely limited to the research setting, and it remains unclear whether the optimum composition of postnatal growth is one that mimics fetal growth or postnatal growth of the term infant. Biochemical nutritional assessments are of limited utility except in the highest-risk preterm infants, when nutritional inadequacy is likely (severe fluid restriction) or where intake is difficult to assess (use of human milk).

Introduction

Nutritional assessment covers two large and divergent areas. The first is the assessment of the adequacy of the nutrition provided to an individual preterm infant, whilst the second compares nutritional outcomes between different groups. The second is often concerned with assessing the effectiveness of an intervention as part of a research protocol, and may utilize complex outcomes. For example, since 2004 a number of studies have examined the effect of different intakes of glutamate or glutamine in preterm infants.

These studies have examined a variety of outcome measures ranging from growth [1] and plasma amino acid concentrations [2], to amino acid or urea kinetics [3, 4], whole body protein turnover [3], stress hormone and CPR levels [3], and compound functional outcomes such as feeding tolerance [5], necrotizing enterocolitis [1], sepsis [1, 5], and mortality [1]. The only of these measures that might be used to assess the glutamate intake in an individual infant are plasma amino acid concentrations, which are not in routine clinical use, or growth that is likely to be a late and nonspecific finding. The other outcomes are either too difficult or expensive to use (amino acid kinetics, protein/urea turnover), or affected by too many other factors (sepsis, mortality, necrotizing enterocolitis) to be useful in individual assessment. In this review, we will consider the first of these areas: the nutritional assessment of an individual preterm infant.

Growth

Growth is the most common, often the only, ongoing assessment of nutritional outcome in many preterm babies. It implies a coordinated, regulated change in body size and composition.

The Importance of Early Growth

Anyone who has cared for such babies is well aware of the usual pattern of weight change, with an initial loss of weight, followed by a return to positive weight gain, and birth weight being regained by 2–3 weeks of age [6]. In a recent review, Cooke [7] highlights the importance of this early weight loss. He imagines the growth of a hypothetical 27-week 1,007-gram infant who regains their birth weight by 2 weeks (or in a second example by 3 weeks) of postnatal age and thereafter grows parallel to their in utero growth curve. By 37 weeks' corrected gestational age the infant would weigh more than 500 g less than their birth centile, and in the second case about 750 g less. These simulations are not unrealistic. Ehrenkranz et al. [6] examined the growth of 1,660 preterm infants cared for in 12 NICHD research centers in the mid 1990s. The average time to regain birth weight ranged from 11.6 days (SD 6.6) in infants weighing 1,401–1,500 g at birth, to 15.2 days (SD 12.2) in those weighing 501–600 g at birth [6]. In 27- to 28-week-gestation infants it took approximately 2 weeks to regain birth weight, by which time infants weighed approximately 450 g less than their birth centile. In 26- to 27-week infants birth weight was regained by 2–3 weeks of age by which time the weight deficit was about 450 g, a difference that increased to 750 g by 32 weeks' corrected gestational age.

Embleton et al. [8] confirmed the importance of nutrition and growth in the first few weeks of life. In preterm infants ≥31 weeks' gestation weight declined by 1 standard deviation score by 2 weeks of age, and thereafter remained relatively constant. In more immature infants (<30 weeks) weight grew by 1.2 standard deviation score by 3 weeks and afterwards remained fairly constant. Maximum energy (335 kcal/kg) and protein (12 g/kg) deficits were reached by 1 week of age in more mature infants (≥31 weeks). In the less mature (≤30 weeks' gestation) infants similar energy and protein deficits were seen by 1 week of age (406 kcal/kg and 14 g/kg, respectively), but these continued to increase throughout hospitalization reaching 813 kcal/kg and 23 g/kg, respectively, by 5 weeks [8].

It also seems possible that early energy intakes have significant long-term effects. Brandt et al. [9] studied 46 small for gestational age very low birth weight (VLBW) infants. Sixty percent of the infants showed catch-up head circumference (HC) growth, and this was associated with better developmental outcome and higher energy intakes between day of life 2 and 10. Indeed, energy intake on days 2 though 4 were significantly associated with development quotient at 18, 24, 36, 48, 60 and 72 months of age.

Few prospective interventional studies have focused on early manipulations in nutrition. One exception is the study of Wilson et al. [10] who examined the effect of a variety of changes in nutritional practices, and compared the effect of 'aggressive' nutritional support versus the prior 'control' practice. This aggressive support included a variety of measures such as use of higher glucose concentrations, starting parenteral amino acids and lipid earlier, advancing to higher amino acid infusion rates, use of early low-volume trophic feeds, and more aggressive management of hyperglycemia.

The aggressive support led to higher energy, glucose, lipid and amino acid intakes but total fluid intakes were comparable between the two groups. Aggressive nutritional support also reduced the maximum weight loss (5.1 vs. 8.4%), reduced the time to regain birth weight (9 vs. 12 days), improved growth, and reduced the percentage of babies with a weight (38 vs. 56%) or length (33 vs. 57%) less than 3rd centile at discharge or death. Although the 'aggressive' support had an excess of sick babies at birth (judged by the CRIB score) there was no difference in most clinical outcomes between the groups, but for those infants that survived the first week, the odds ratio of bacterial or fungal sepsis was lower in the aggressive nutritional support group [10].

Growth Assessment

Weight
Weight can be easily measured and is the most usual (sometimes the only) growth parameter measured in preterm infants. Its accuracy can be improved by being carried out in as standardized a fashion as possible – naked, disconnected from the ventilator and immediately prior to a feed. However, even small errors can overwhelm 'real' changes in small preterm infants. The presence of an endotracheal tube or a full bladder may lead to larger weight changes than the real underlying growth of small infants.

179

Weight is affected by changes in hydration, a factor that is very important in the first few days of life where total body water usually decreases, or in sick septic babies where edema may be a problem. Term infants typically lose 10% of their body weight in the first few days, and preterm infants may lose 15–20% [11]. Although much of this reflects short-term changes in hydration, up to half the weight lost may be due to mobilization of lean tissue, glycogen and fat stores to compensate for inadequate nutrient intakes in the first few days after birth [11].

Although weight is typically measured daily it is important to consider the weight trend over several days. One way to do this is to calculate the rate of weight gain or weight velocity (in g/kg/day) over several days. This has the advantage that changes in weight velocity are much more sensitive in identifying changes in growth than examining weight plotted on growth curves [7]. Regular assessments of growth velocity averaged over the previous 5 or 10 days can help in the early identification of failure, and in monitoring the response to nutritional interventions.

Linear Growth

Measures of linear growth, such as crown–heel length (CHL), are generally considered the most sensitive measures of the adequacy of nutritional intake [7] and are relatively unaffected by changes in fluid status [11]. CHL is typically measured using a recumbent length board. The infant is placed supine on the board and their shoulders and knees gently pressed into the board. The head is held against a fixed headboard, and a moveable footplate that can slide up the board gently rests against the soles of the feet that are held at 90° to the length board [6, 11].

In a research setting the reproducibility of CHL measurement is good, with a co-efficient of variation of 0.41% and a 95% confidence interval of ±4.5 mm [12]. In other words, if a measurement of CHL is more than 4.5 mm greater than a previous measurement this would be due to chance in only 5% of instances. A difference in CHL measurement of this amount is, therefore, likely to represent real growth. As 4.5 mm represents between 3 and 4 days' CHL growth [6, 12], there seems little to be gained by carrying out CHL measurements more frequently than twice weekly. The reproducibility of CHL measurement in a clinical setting is likely to be worse, as few units have the luxury of having all CHL measurements made by the same team. Given this, the typical clinical practice of weekly CHL measurements seems reasonable.

Ehrenkranz et al. [6] reports serial CHL measurements in preterm infants, showing a steady increase from birth. The average rate of length gain was approximately 1 cm/week [6], significantly greater than the 0.69–0.75 cm/week increase seen in term infants in the first 3 months of life [11].

Due to the difficulties of measuring CHL in preterm infants, other measures of linear growth have been examined including foot length [13], elbow–wrist length [14], crown–rump length [15] and knee–heel length (KHL) [12]. The reproducibility of KHL measurements in a research setting is poorer than CHL reproducibility, with a 95% confidence interval equal to 12–13 days' growth in KHL. Reproducibility is worse in large more vigorous babies, but does improve with practice [12]. KHL growth appears to be nonlinear and to exhibit growth spurts of variable duration that are not related to changes in nutrition [16]. The same, however, may be true of other measures of 'linear' growth.

Head Circumference

HC is measured using a tape measure and is the largest occipital-frontal circumference measured above the brow ridges. Three measures are made, and the largest recorded [6, 11]. HC is a good measure of brain growth and is largely unaffected by changes in fluid status [11].

HC appears to increase at a rate of 0.89–1.00 cm/week in VLBW infants [6], rather more than the 0.5 cm/week seen in term infants during the first year of life. The rate of HC growth tends to increase with increasing postnatal age, with this effect being most apparent in the infants of lowest birth weight [6].

Mid-Arm Circumference

Mid-arm circumference (MAC) is a relatively infrequent measurement in preterm infants. However the data of Ehrenkranz et al. [6] provides useful reference data. MAC growth averaged 0.39–0.45 cm/week in infants weighing between 501 and 1,500 g at birth, although the rate was somewhat less for the 1,401- to 1,500-gram cohort (a pattern also seen for length and HC growth in this population) [6]. MAC decreases during the first 1–2 weeks of postnatal length, presumably reflecting either the changes in hydration or the suboptimal early energy intake seen in such populations. After this, MAC growth accelerates until it reaches a phase of linear rise. This stage is reached earlier in larger infants, beginning at approximately 3–4 weeks in 1,301- to 1,400-gram birth weight infants, but not until 10 weeks in 501- to 600-gram birth weight infants.

Growth Standards for Preterm Infants

In order to measure growth in preterm infants one needs a standard to which to make comparisons. There are three main choices of such a standard: (1) normal fetal growth, (2) growth of a peer group of (preterm) infants and (3) growth of term infants.

(1) Fetal Growth Standards

A variety of fetal growth standards exist, but there are many problems with them [7, 17]. Growth of the fetus can be assessed indirectly using ultrasound measurements, but these are prone to both ultrasound/operator errors as well as errors in the algorithms used to convert ultrasound parameters to weight measurements. Alternatively curves can be estimated using cross-sectional

Table 1. Growth rates from three large studies of birth weight of preterm infants, compared to the data of Lubchenco et al. [19]

Authors	Sample size	Growth rate (27–34 weeks) g/kg/day
Lubchenco et al. [19]	5,635	14.9
Hoffman et al. [20]	1,164,871	11.2 (African American females)
		13.7 (African American males)
		15.4 (Caucasian females)
		15.7 (Caucasian males)
Arbuckle et al. [21]	1,087,629	16.3 (males)
		16.9 (females)
Alexander et al. [22]	3,134,879	20.0

data on the birth weight of 'normal' preterm infants. However, preterm delivery is a highly abnormal event and is often the result of fetal compromise (poor interval growth, signs of fetal distress, ascending infection, multiple gestations) or maternal illness (pregnancy-induced hypertension, HELLP syndrome). Many of these factors may impair placental function and fetal growth and distort the data used to construct growth charts.

Although the American Academy of Pediatrics [18] recommends nutrients to 'approximate the rate of growth and composition of weight gain for a normal fetus of the same post-menstrual age, and to maintain normal concentrations of blood and tissue nutrients' the definition of normal fetal growth is unclear [11, 17]. One of the earliest growth charts is that of Lubchenco et al. [19], based on 5,635 premature babies born at high altitude in Denver, Colo. Based on this dataset, fetal growth was estimated to be about 15 g/kg/day between 27 and 34 weeks' postmenstrual age. Since then a number of other studies have questioned this value [see also 17], the three largest (each studying over 1 million births) are summarized above (table 1).

The more recent studies suggest that the growth rates from the Lubchenco data set are too conservative. It has been suggested that a more appropriate value is 16–17 g/kg/day [17]. Although there may appear to be little difference between growth rates of 15 and 17 g/kg/day these can have a substantial cumulative effect of growth. For a hypothetical 1,007-gram 26-week infant who regains their birth weight by 2 weeks, a growth rate of 17 g/kg/day will equate to a total weight more than 240 g greater by 37 weeks' corrected age compared to if the growth rate had been 15 g/kg/day [7].

Term-born infants also lose weight after birth and take time to regain it; this is not taken in to account in the above calculations. We can calculate the growth rate for a 1,000-gram 27-week infant to catch up with a term-born infant by 44 weeks' postconceptional age, by which time the average weight of term-born males is 4.4 kg [25]. By choosing this time as a target we can account for the initial weight loss that occurs in term infants. The growth rate required for the

Table 2. Growth rate required for a 27-week 1,000-gram infant to catch up with a term infant by 44 weeks' corrected age, depending of the time taken to regain birth weight

Time taken to regain birth weight, days	Required growth rate g/kg/day
7	13.32
14	14.21
21	15.24
28	16.42

preterm infant to catch up with the term-born infant will depend on the time it takes the preterm infant to regain its birth weight (table 2).

If there is a period of poor growth, subsequent rates of weight gain will need to be higher to achieve catch-up, and the effects of this are larger the later the slow growth occurs. For example, if we consider our 27-week 1,000-gram infant who regains birth weight by 2 weeks, a growth rate of 14.21 g/kg/day will ensure catch-up with a term-born infant by 44 weeks. However, if this infant has 5 days without growth (say due to feeds being held for a septic episode) during days of life 40 through 45, the subsequent rate of weight gain to ensure catch-up by 44 weeks' corrected age will be 15.18 g/kg/day. If the same insult occurs between 60 and 65 days of life subsequent growth will need to be 15.54 g/kg/day, 16.32 g/kg/day if it occurs between 80 and 85 days of life, and 19.35 g/kg/day if it occurs between 100 and 105 days of life.

We therefore have targets for postnatal growth ranging from 13–14 g/kg/day to as high as 20 g/kg/day. What is clear is that these lower targets will only be successful if they are achieved every day without fail. They do not allow for a few 'bad days' let alone bad weeks; e.g., when feeds are held for sepsis workup, growth is slow because the infant requires 200 ml/kg/day of fortified human milk rather than the 160–180 ml/kg/day that we expected to be sufficient, and because of the numerous other causes of suboptimal intake [8]. It is also clear that our current goal of growth of 15 g/kg/day is failing to prevent most preterm babies from having suboptimal growth in hospital [8] and being discharged home profoundly growth retarded. Increasing our targets for acceptable postnatal growth to 16–17 g/kg/day [17] seems the least we can do in response to this failure.

(2) Peer Growth Charts

These charts represent the observed growth of historical cohorts of preterm babies. One of the earliest was the growth grid of Dancis et al. [23] published in 1948. This was limited in the gestational age of infants studied (all >29 weeks) and the duration of the study (50 days). As with all such charts it reflects the varied nutritional practices carried out at the time, and is difficult to extrapolate to other populations and nutritional practices. A number of similar charts have been constructed [see 11], including the recent large dataset of Ehrenkranz et al. [6] which included 1,660 VLBW (birth weight ≤1,500 g) infants cared for at 12 NICHD research centers in 1994–1995. Although it provides considerable useful data it reflects nutritional and neonatal practices from that period, and in those centers, that may not be applicable now. In a similar NICHD cohort, growth failure (weight <10th centile at 36 weeks' corrected age) affected between 83 and 100% of VLBW infants depending on birth weight and study center [24]; these postnatal growth standards can therefore at best be considered 'typical' growth rather than optimum growth [11], as an infant growing along their centile line on this chart is almost certain to leave hospital with growth failure.

One advantage of postnatal growth standards is that they allow the weight to be plotted daily [11] and encourage caregivers to focus on growth as an integral part of daily management. However, a baby that is consistently growing along a postnatal chart centile line is no cause for celebration; in the absence of evidence of catch-up growth towards their birth centile, the baby is extremely likely to leave hospital weighing less than the 10th centile.

(3) Term Infant Growth Charts
The US Centers for Disease Control and Prevention and the National Center for Health Statistics have recently produced revised growth centiles for males and females from birth to 20 years of age [25] (see http://www.cdc.gov/growthcharts). Some preterm babies may remain in hospital beyond their expected date of delivery, particularly those with severe chronic lung disease or multiple anomalies. These infants can be plotted on the CDC charts to allow comparison with term-born infants. Growth charts for weight for age, length for age, HC for age, weight for length, and body mass index for age are available for boys and girls between birth and 36 months. These charts probably remain the best way to compare growth of VLBW infants to their term counterparts [26].

Assessment of Body Composition

Much of the preceding discussion has concentrated on issues of weight gain, which will prompt concerns that weight changes may reflect 'only' changes in fat mass or fluid status. The AAP reflects this concern by stating that the goals for nutritional management of preterm infants are 'to approximate the rate of growth *and* composition of weight gain for a normal fetus of the same postmenstrual age' (emphasis added) [27]. It is unclear whether this goal is either achievable or desirable, and if so, how one can assess body composition in the clinical setting.

It is known that the composition of fetal growth changes, with more fat and lean tissue being deposited as gestational age increases [28]. In general, lower protein intakes and higher energy intakes lead to a relative increase in growth of fat mass – a pattern more consistent with the term infant than with the fetus [28]. It remains unclear however what composition of growth is more appropriate for the preterm infants. Unlike the fetus, the preterm infant is transitioning to a situation where considerable amounts of energy are expended on maintaining body temperature, and nutrient supply is changing from a continuous supply of calories to an intermittent supply of more fat-based calories [28]. Given that, it is possible that growth approximating the growth of the term infant (40% fat) is more physiologically sound than that approximating fetal growth (15% as fat). Definite data is, however, lacking. What is clear is that the composition of body weight change can vary widely in response to nutrient intake, even if changes in absolute body weight are very similar [28, 29]. When preterm infants are compared to the reference infant of the same age they have much lower lean mass, lower bone mineral mass but similar fat mass. If comparison is made to the reference infant of the same weight, they have normal lean mass, but increased fat mass and reduced bone mineral mass [30]. It seems likely, therefore, that current nutritional management leads to lower levels of bone mineral and lean tissue growth compared to the reference infant.

The different methods of measuring body composition in preterm infants are reviewed elsewhere [31], although most such techniques remain limited to use in research studies. There are few clinically applicable methods of assessing body composition in individual preterm infants, and those that have been used such as urine creatinine excretion (as a measure of lean mass) [32] and skinfold thickness (as a measure of fat mass) [31] remain unvalidated in preterm infants.

In clinical practice, 'normal' body composition is often assumed if weight, length and HC growth occur in parallel. Precise simple reproducible measures of lean mass and bone mineral mass might help identify interventions that might optimize both quantitative and qualitative aspects of growth, as well as help identify individual preterm infants who might benefit most from these interventions. Similarly, the ability to use methods such as dual X-ray absorptiometry might improve our nutritional management. However, the literature is unclear on what body composition is optimal for the growing preterm infant, and how effective interventions aimed at 'correcting' abnormal body composition might be.

Biochemical Assessments

A wide variety of biochemical measures have been used to assess nutritional adequacy in adults and older children. Some appear to work well in preterm infants, for example serum copper slowly increases with age, and a low serum copper is a useful measure of copper deficiency. Other measures perform much less well, either because the appropriate 'normal' range is unclear, or because they are intrinsically poor measures of status in this age range.

Assessment of Bone Mineral Status

Serum calcium, phosphorus, and alkaline phosphatase are often measured to assess bone mineral status. Serum phosphorus is relatively responsive to dietary changes [33], more so than serum calcium which is under tight homeostatic control. Serum alkaline phosphatase is produced by bone, muscle and intestine. The bone isoform constitutes about 50% of total alkaline phosphatase, and is taken to be a marker of bone formation. Neither total, nor bone, alkaline phosphatase activity are particularly useful measures of bone mineral accretion, and they explain very little of the variability in bone mineral content [33]. Very high alkaline phosphatase levels are usually accompanied by radiological evidence of osteopenia.

One reason that alkaline phosphatase activity continues to be measured is that high levels (>1,200 IU) have been associated with long-term growth failure [18]. It is understandable, therefore, that clinicians would wish to respond to such a finding, for example with calcium and phosphorus supplementation. It is not known, however, whether doing so has any long-term effect on growth.

Routine measurements of calcium, phosphorus, and alkaline phosphatase are probably of limited value. Anecdotally, abnormal findings are rare in most preterm infants (>28 weeks' gestation) who are receiving appropriate levels of preterm formula without fluid restriction. These measurements may be more useful when mineral intakes are less certain (e.g. human milk feeding, fluid restriction).

Assessment of Protein Status

Blood urea nitrogen (BUN) and serum albumin have traditionally been used as a measure of protein status. However, serum albumin has a half-life of 2–3 weeks and a turnover too slow to be a useful way of monitoring the response to nutritional interventions. Theoretically, prealbumin (with a half-life of a few days) and retinol binding protein (with a half-life of about 12 h) would be more responsive. Indeed in a research setting, BUN [34] and retinol binding protein [30] reflect changes in protein intake, whilst serum albumin and total serum protein do not [34].

Routine monitoring of BUN and of serum proteins rarely produces abnormal values in larger (>28 weeks' gestation) formula-fed preterm infants. It is possible that measurement of BUN, serum retinol binding protein or prealbumin may help to identify suboptimal protein intake in subjects whose intake is questionable (e.g. severe fluid restriction) or unclear (human milk-fed infants).

Acknowledgements

This work is a publication of the US Department of Agriculture (USDA)/ Agricultural Research Service (ARS) Children's Nutrition Research Center, Department of Pediatrics, Baylor College of Medicine and Texas Children's Hospital, Houston, Tex. This project has been funded in part with federal funds from the USDA/ARS under Cooperative Agreement No. 58-6250-6-001. Contents of this publication do not necessarily reflect the views or policies of the USDA, nor does mention of trade names, commercial products, or organizations imply endorsement by the US government.

References

1 Poindexter BB, Ehrenkranz RA, Stoll BJ, et al: Parenteral glutamine supplementation does not reduce the risk of mortality or late-onset sepsis in extremely low birth weight infants. Pediatrics 2004;113:1209–1215.
2 van den Berg A, van Elburg RM, Teerlink T, et al: A randomized controlled trial of enteral glutamine supplementation in very low birth weight infants: plasma amino acid concentrations. J Pediatr Gastroenterol Nutr 2005;41:66–71.
3 Kalhan SC, Parimi PS, Gruca LL, Hanson RW: Glutamine supplement with parenteral nutrition decreases whole body proteolysis in low birth weight infants. J Pediatr 2005;146: 642–647.
4 Parimi PS, Devapatla S, Gruca LL, et al: Effect of enteral glutamine or glycine on whole-body nitrogen kinetics in very-low-birth-weight infants. Am J Clin Nutr 2004;79:402–409.
5 van den Berg A, van Elburg RM, Westerbeek EA, et al: Glutamine-enriched enteral nutrition in very-low-birth-weight infants and effects on feeding tolerance and infectious morbidity: a randomized controlled trial. Am J Clin Nutr 2005;81:1397–1404.
6 Ehrenkranz RA, Younes N, Lemons JA, et al: Longitudinal growth of hospitalized very low birth weight infants. Pediatrics 1999;104:280–289.
7 Cooke R: Postnatal growth in preterm infants; in Thureen PJ, Hay WW (eds): Neonatal Nutrition and Metabolism. Cambridge, Cambridge University Press, 2006, pp 47–57.
8 Embleton NE, Pang N, Cooke RJ: Postnatal malnutrition and growth retardation: an inevitable consequence of current recommendations in preterm infants? Pediatrics 2001;107: 270–273.
9 Brandt I, Sticker EJ, Lentze MJ: Catch-up growth of head circumference of very low birth weight, small for gestational age preterm infants and mental development to adulthood. J Pediatr 2003;142:463–468.
10 Wilson DC, Cairns P, Halliday HL, et al: Randomised controlled trial of an aggressive nutritional regimen in sick very low birthweight infants. Arch Dis Child Fetal Neonatal Ed 1997;77: F4–F11.
11 Katrine K: Anthropometric assessment; in Groh-Wargo S (ed): Nutritional Care for High-Risk Newborns, ed 3. Chicago, Precept Press, 2000, pp 11–22.
12 Griffin IJ, Pang NM, Perring J, Cooke RJ: Knee-heel length measurement in healthy preterm infants. Arch Dis Child Fetal Neonatal Ed 1999;81:F50–F55.
13 James DK, Dryburgh EH, Chiswick ML: Foot length – a new and potentially useful measurement in the neonate. Arch Dis Child 1979;54:226–230.
14 Brooke OG, Onubogu O, Heath R, Carter ND: Human milk and preterm formula compared for effects on growth and metabolism. Arch Dis Child 1987;62:917–923.
15 Skinner AM, Battin M, Solimano A, et al: Growth and growth factors in premature infants receiving dexamethasone for bronchopulmonary dysplasia. Am J Perinatol 1997;14:539–546.
16 Kaempf DE, Pfluger MS, Thiele AM, et al: Influence of nutrition on growth in premature infants: assessment by knemometry. Ann Hum Biol 1998;25:127–136.
17 Klein CJ: Nutrient requirements for preterm infant formulas. J Nutr 2002;132:1395S–1577S.
18 Lucas A, Brooke OG, Baker BA, et al: High alkaline phosphatase activity and growth in preterm neonates. Arch Dis Child 1989;64:902–909.

187

19 Lubchenco LO, Hansman C, Dressler M, Boyd E: Intrauterine growth as estimated from live-born birth-weight data at 24 to 42 weeks of gestation. Pediatrics 1963;32:793–800.
20 Hoffman HJ, Stark CR, Lundin FE Jr, Ashbrook JD: Analysis of birth weight, gestational age, and fetal viability, US births, 1968. Obstet Gynecol Surv 1974;29:651–681.
21 Arbuckle TE, Wilkins R, Sherman GJ: Birth weight percentiles by gestational age in Canada. Obstet Gynecol 1993;81:39–48.
22 Alexander GR, Himes JH, Kaufman RB, et al: A United States national reference for fetal growth. Obstet Gynecol 1996;87:163–168.
23 Dancis J, O'Connell J, Holy L: A grid for recording the weight of premature infants. J Pediatr 1948;33:570.
24 Lemons JA, Bauer CR, Oh W, et al: Very low birth weight outcomes of the National Institute of Child Health and Human Development Neonatal Research Network, January 1995 through December 1996. NICHD Neonatal Research Network. Pediatrics 2001;107:E1.
25 Kuczmarski RJ, Ogden CL, Guo SS, et al: 2000 CDC Growth Charts for the United States: methods and development. Vital Health Stat 2002;11:1–190.
26 Sherry B, Mei Z, Grummer-Strawn L, Dietz WH: Evaluation of and recommendations for growth references for very low birth weight (< or =1500 grams) infants in the United States. Pediatrics 2003;111:750–758.
27 American Academy of Pediatrics Committee on Nutrition: Pediatric Nutrition Handbook. Elk Grove Village, American Academy of Pediatrics, 2004.
28 Putet G: Energy; in Tsang RC, Lucas A, Uauy R, Zlotkin S (eds): Nutritional Needs of the Preterm Infant: Scientific Basis and Practical Guidelines. Baltimore, Williams & Wilkins, 1993, pp 15–28.
29 Leitch C, Denne S: Energy; in Tsang RC, Uauy R, Koletzko B, Zlotkin SH (eds): Nutrition of the Preterm Infant: Scientific Basis and Practical Guidelines, ed 2. Cincinnati, Digital Educational Publishing, 2005, pp 23–44.
30 Cooke R, Embleton N, Rigo J, et al: High protein pre-term infant formula: effect on nutrient balance, metabolic status and growth. Pediatr Res 2006;59:265–270.
31 Rigo J, de Curtis M, Pieltain C: Nutritional assessment in preterm infants with special reference to body composition. Semin Neonatol 2001;6:383–391.
32 Rassin DK, Gaull GE, Raiha NC, et al: Protein quantity and quality in term and preterm infants: effects on urine creatinine and expression of amino acid excretion data. J Pediatr Gastroenterol Nutr 1986;5:103–110.
33 Atkinson SA, Tsang RC: Calcium, magnesium, phosphors and vitamin D; in Tsang RC, Uauy R, Koletzko B, Zlotkin SH (eds): Nutrition of the Preterm Infant: Scientific Basis and Practical Guidelines, ed 2. Cincinnati, Digital Educational Publishing, 2005, pp 245–277.
34 Embleton ND, Cooke RJ: Protein requirements in preterm infants: effect of different levels of protein intake on growth and body composition. Pediatr Res 2005;58:855–860.

Discussion

Dr. Rivera: When talking about in utero weight gain we are also idealistically talking about weight gain in relation to growth, because the fetus and the newborn don't come from a necessarily healthy environment. Many of these infants, especially preterm babies, come from an environment in which several factors affect in utero growth. From your point of view what would be ideal?

Dr. Griffin: We know that our babies ex utero are growing at a very different rate than they are in utero, which may mean that the appropriate composition of their body growth has to be different than it would be in utero. Clearly in babies born preterm their growth may not be representative of the growth of a healthy normal fetus, but also their body composition may be different. Because they start at a different developmental stage than the healthy normal fetus, the ideal composition of their subsequent growth might also need to be different.

Dr. Cooke: Should we be talking about growth in absolute terms, grams per day, or as a function of body weight, grams per kilo per day? Current recommendations are that infants gain at a rate which parallels that in utero, i.e. ~17 g/kg/day [1]. Yet, when body weight is suboptimal, e.g. the small for gestational age or postnatally growth-retarded infant, the infant falls progressively away from the intrauterine curve despite a gain of ~17 g/kg/day. Growth rates should be expressed in absolute terms at a rate which at least parallels that in utero, perhaps even greater if an infant is to achieve their original birth weight percentile.

Dr. Griffin: Historically the reason for expressing growth in grams per kilogram per day was the Lubchenco data that say that the number was pretty consistent from 27–34 weeks. You are right, grams per day may be more appropriate but the targets are constantly moving. As it is much easier to remember 15 g/kg/day than 8 or 10 different targets depending on what week of life the baby is. Practically I think we need to make a compromise and stick with grams per kilogram per day.

Dr. Cooke: Maybe this is one of the reasons we don't do so well. Growth is not consistent throughout gestation, in either rate or composition [2]. Averaging it over a period, then relating needs to suboptimal body weight, may ensure that the infant receives too little or too much at the wrong time, hence poor growth that is commonly observed in these infants.

Dr. Griffin: That is right but even if we take relatively conservative goals for protein and energy intake and goals that are much lower than Dr. Ziegler presented early on, we are consistently failing to meet those intake goals, as your data from Newcastle show [3]. I think our first goal should be to meet those intake goals and then see if we still have the problem.

Dr. Cooke: Preterm infants fed a nutrient-enriched formula after hospital discharge achieve a rate and a composition of growth similar to the term infant at the same corrected age [4, 5]. Whether it is possible to achieve this earlier in life is not clear. Until the protein and energy requirements are better defined we are unlikely to do so.

Dr. Putet: You showed us the weight gain composition of the fetus between 25 and 30 weeks gestational age and in this composition there is a lot of water, 75–80%. Does postnatal growth need this amount of water? As far as there are protein deposition and lean mass, the same as in utero, can we accept the idea that the premature infant may grow on his own curve, minus 2 deviation standards up to 36 weeks for instance? At this time the water content of the weight gain composition of the fetus is much less and the baby will catch up by that time. Your aim was to wait for up to 44 weeks. What do you feel about this?

Dr. Griffin: You are right, if our goal is to match the body composition of the fetus then all our babies need a lot more total body water and I don't think that practically or clinically it is anything that any of us want to do. Comparing ex utero with in utero is more helpful.

Dr. Saavedra: What should our targets be? Whatever the target we aim for, should it be a minimum or an ideal target? To what extent is the conservative approach to increasing feedings related to falling short of reaching our targets, , particularly given the fear of necrotizing enterocolitis? Many people are convinced that either going too fast or giving a high caloric density is associated with the risk of necrotizing enterocolitis. Does this actually contribute to this very slow increment of feedings in the first couple of weeks?

Dr. Griffin: Necrotizing enterocolitis is the disease that neonatologists have an understandable fear about: in the morning the baby is completely well, and 2 h later the entire bowel is dead; this fear modifies everybody's behavior to feeding. Neonatologists are also very attached to specific numbers and one of these numbers is 20 ml/kg/day, which is how much you increase feeds. Of course there are now randomized control data that advancements of 30 ml/kg/day are probably just as safe and lead to full feeds sooner and more rapid reattainment of birth weight [6] as 20 ml/kg/day. But this number is just so engrained in neonatologists that I don't know of anybody who is doing 30 g/kg/day. I also think that because of the fear of necrotizing enterocolitis this cautiousness could well be counterproductive. Fear of feeding the baby for the first 4 or 5 days of life (or even longer) will result in a sick gut as well as an ailing baby, and it would not be a big surprise that feeding is then sometimes not successful.

Dr. Dhanireddy: You have shown various ways of plotting growth. Can you recommend a growth chart or should we ask the obstetrician to send his intrauterine growth chart and continue to follow that? Maybe our goal should be to match intrauterine growth rather than use the Lubchenco growth charts or various others.

Dr. Griffin: I think a lot of those fetal grids are based on preterm baby cohorts. I don't really think that they are very informative as it gives a false sense of security. Calculations of growth velocity and particularly trying to project those forward in time to say growth continuation at this rate is what is wanted at the time of discharge, or at the time of term, will perhaps give us a clearer idea.

Dr. Dhanireddy: There is no growth velocity chart?

Dr. Griffin: No there isn't, but it is easy enough to calculate.

Dr. Hentschel: You mentioned several biochemical markers of how to follow infants that are poorly growing. Does amino acid analysis play a role in a poorly growing infant if you consider keeping that infant on parenteral amino acid solutions?

Dr. Griffin: I don't think amino acid concentrations are useful except in very rare circumstances – very high protein intake (to avoid toxicity) or as a research tool.

Dr. Cooke: In children and adults, when protein intake is low so is blood urea nitrogen (BUN), unless renal or fluid status is compromised [7]. Although the situation is less clear-cut in preterm infants [8], a more recent study by our group suggests that there is a clear relationship between protein intake and BUN in the otherwise normal preterm infant [9]. In effect, BUN can be used as a measure of the adequacy of protein intake, an area that has recently been addressed by Ziegler et al. [10]. I wonder if Dr. Ziegler would like to comment?

Dr. Ziegler: The relationship between protein intake and BUN in premature infants unfortunately is not very tight. We used it anyway because monitoring BUN has its advantages. If the BUN is very low, one can be sure that protein intake is inadequate, and if the BUN is very high, it would be prudent to reduce protein intake.

Dr. Haschke: Now I am confused. What is a good reference for BUN? Is it the breastfed infants during the first 2 months of life, the healthy term breastfed infant? What should it be?

Dr. Cooke: I really was thinking of an adequacy of protein intake in relationship to BUN. What do we use in the preterm infants? We know that BUN in the first 48–72 h of life probably is a better reflection of renal function and it changes with time. Later on, when we vary protein intake in preterm infants there is a linear relationship. A cutoff is chosen, and as you well know working with Dr. Ziegler for a long time, nobody could decide whether we should be aiming for 2–4 mmol. We saw a large group of preterm infants receiving fortified human milk, and their BUN ran at 1–2 mmol which to me is low. Translating that into milligrams per deciliter, I am thinking of 6 mg/dl less. By using this arbitrary cutoff, I increase intake in these babies and the BUN increases and the growth velocity improves.

Dr. Ziegler: We don't have standards for urea concentration in the first 2 or 3 weeks of life for the premature infant. There are many factors that influence BUN. The glomerular filtration rate starts very low and increases gradually so by 3 weeks on average infants reach a normal glomerular filtration rate. Hydration status and protein intake are just some factors that influence BUN. So we don't have standards, but we know that if BUN is very low, the interpretation is inadequate protein intake, and if it is very high then we would reduce protein intake, regardless of the actual reason for the high BUN. But the real question that I want to ask is how do you increase protein intake in practice?

Dr. Griffin: In practice we would give more energy and protein – more formula in formula-fed babies or more fortified breast milk (or more multi-component supplementation) in human milk-fed babies. We would rarely increase protein independently of energy so usually they would both go together and it's a moot point whether energy or protein is the issue because our response to that is going to be the same. For babies who are profoundly fluid restricted we would occasionally use modular protein supplements but overwhelmingly the response would be to increase the volume or density of formula or fortified expressed breast milk.

Dr. Fusch: Skin-fold thickness is not so bad for preterm and term infants and can be easily made and the measurements are quite reliable. It seems that nutrition is more or less adequate or approaching adequacy. In the data from Ulm a large variation exists between different neonatal units in Germany regarding when and at what body weight children are discharged. There are considerable differences even if the discharge age is standardized. What is the current practice in the different units for adjusting the amount of feed? Often the amount of feed the baby should get enterally is not calculated everyday but if the amount has been the same for 3 consecutive days then the staff is alerted and feeding is increased. I would like to know how often this happens and if this can explain some of these effects, especially in infants growing stably who have a reduced risk of necrotizing enterocolitis?

Dr. Griffin: When we write feeding orders, we do it everyday but that is not optimal because we make rounds in the morning and the baby was measured the night before. So we are always half a day behind their actual weight but it is a consistent half a day. If we think we should give 120 kcal/kg/day that is mostly based on yesterday's weight, not on today's weight.

Dr. Putet: I agree that urea is a very good marker when it is low. When the premature infant is getting 130 kcal/kg/day we do not increase the volume; we just increase the protein intake if urea is below 2 mmol because we believe that it is really the protein which is deficient. We use only human milk fortifier.

Dr. Cooke: I was thinking about your question on weight. Should we use actual or expected weight to estimate nutrient intake? Many preterm infants are growth retarded, either at birth or postnatally. Intakes and target growth rates related to a suboptimal weight will always underestimate the needs and growth potential of these infants [11]. Perhaps what we should be using is expected rather than actual weight as Dr. Griffin points out.

References

1 Klein CJ: Nutrient requirements for preterm infant formulas. J Nutr 2002;132:1395S–1577S.
2 Ziegler EE, Thureen PJ, Carlson SJ: Aggressive nutrition of the very low birthweight infant. Clin Perinatol 2002;29:225–244.
3 Embleton NE, Pang N, Cooke RJ: Postnatal malnutrition and growth retardation: an inevitable consequence of current recommendations in preterm infants? Pediatrics 2001;107: 270–273.
4 Cooke RJ, McCormick K, Griffin IJ, et al: Feeding preterm infants after hospital discharge: effect of diet on body composition. Pediatr Res 1999;46:461–464.
5 Cooke RJ, Griffin IJ, McCormick K, et al: Feeding preterm infants after hospital discharge: effect of dietary manipulation on nutrient intake and growth. Pediatr Res 1998;43:355–360.

6 Caple J, Armentrout D, Huseby V, et al: Randomized, controlled trial of slow versus rapid feeding volume advancement in preterm infants. Pediatrics 2005;114:1597–1600.
7 Heimberger DC: Adulthood; in Shils ME, Shike M, Ross AC, et al (eds): Modern Nutrition in Health and Disease. Philadelphia, Lippincott Williams & Wilkins, 2006, pp 830–842.
8 Boehm G, Muller DM, Beyreiss K, Raiha NC: Evidence for functional immaturity of the ornithine-urea cycle in very-low-birth-weight infants. Biol Neonate 1988;54:121–125.
9 Cooke R, Embleton N, Rigo J, et al: High protein pre-term infant formula: effect on nutrient balance, metabolic status and growth. Pediatr Res 2006;59:265–270.
10 Arslanoglu S, Moro GE, Ziegler EE: Adjustable fortification of human milk fed to preterm infants: does it make a difference? J Perinatol 2006, in press.
11 Cooke RJ: Postnatal growth in preterm infants; in Thureen P, Hay W (eds): Neonatal Nutrition and Metabolism. Cambridge, Cambridge University Press, 2006, pp 47–57.

Cooke RJ, Vandenplas Y, Wahn U (eds): Nutrition Support for Infants and Children at Risk.
Nestlé Nutr Workshop Ser Pediatr Program, vol 59, pp 193–208,
Nestec Ltd., Vevey/S. Karger AG, Basel, © 2007.

Early Aggressive Nutrition in Very Preterm Infants

Patti J. Thureen

University of Colorado Health Sciences Center, Denver, CO, USA

Abstract

Despite numerous advances in the nutrition of preterm infants, the increasing survival at lower birth weights is resulting in a new frontier of extrauterine nutritional support of these vulnerable infants. The extremely low birth weight infant has endogenous energy to maintain energy balance for only 3–4 days without an exogenous energy supply. Nevertheless, many clinicians are still hesitant to introduce substrates at high rates early in life secondary to concerns of intolerance and toxicity. Current feeding practices appear to be resulting in significant postnatal growth failure in very preterm neonates. Optimizing nutritional support in these infants is critical to avoiding adverse growth and neurological outcomes. There is a need for scientifically based feeding strategies to achieve normal in utero growth rates postnatally. Important areas for research include determination of safe and efficacious upper limits of energy and amino acid intake, identification of markers for protein toxicity, better characterization of the effect of various neonatal illnesses and the neonatal stress response on nutritional metabolism, development of enteral feeding strategies that will allow for more rapid enteral feeding advance while reducing the risk of necrotizing enterocolitis, and understanding the benefits and risks of both over- and undernutrition in the extremely low birth weight infant.

Rationale for and against Early Aggressive Nutrition

Despite numerous advances in nutrition of preterm infants over the past decade, the increasing survival at lower birth weights is resulting in a new frontier of extrauterine nutritional support of these vulnerable infants. Extremely low birth weight infants (ELBW, i.e. <1,000 g in weight) have unique metabolic substrate requirements, predicted by high protein turnover rates, high metabolic rates, and high glucose utilization rates. The ELBW infant has endogenous energy reserves of only about 200 kcal, enough to

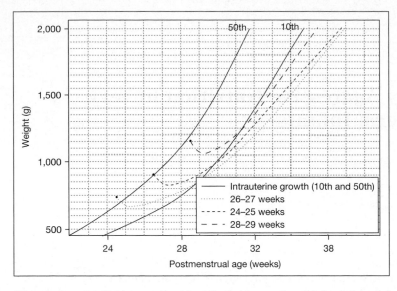

Fig. 1. Longitudinal growth of hospitalized very low birth weight infants [2, with permission].

maintain energy balance for only 3–4 days without an exogenous energy supply. Nevertheless, many clinicians are still hesitant to introduce substrates at high rates early in life secondary to concerns of intolerance and toxicity. In addition, there have been few studies demonstrating significant advantages to an aggressive approach. Several arguments for an aggressive approach include: (1) preventing a decrease in nutrient supply to the nutritionally vulnerable ELBW infant, (2) there are data suggesting improved developmental outcomes with early protein intake [1], (3) nationally and internationally, nutritional strategies for very preterm infants are resulting in postnatal growth failure from which the neonate does not recover by hospital discharge [2–4] (fig. 1), and (4) this postnatal growth failure is associated with increased risk of poor developmental outcome in very preterm infants [5, 6].

A commonly recommended standard for providing comprehensive postnatal nutrition to very preterm infants is one that duplicates normal in utero human fetal growth at the same gestational age [7]. This long-standing recommendation by the American Academy of Pediatrics has not included guidelines about how this should be achieved, however, and there is no data in the literature to support or refute this recommendation. Based on the significant variation in clinical practice, attaining a targeted rate of weight gain in very preterm infants is likely to be accomplished by very different nutritional strategies and without consideration of 'quality' of weight gain [8, 9].

Replicating body composition of the fetus of the same gestational age as the preterm infant may be a more desirable nutritional goal. However, this necessitates an appreciation of the differences between normal fetal nutrition and commonly used postnatal nutritional practices in very preterm neonates. Amino acid uptake by the fetus is far in excess of that needed to meet accretion requirements; the excess amino acids are oxidized, contributing significantly to fetal energy production. However, amino acids are delivered to the preterm neonate in the first several weeks of life at low rates that are significantly less than required to provide for normal rates of fetal protein accretion. Glucose delivery to the fetus is determined by the maternal glucose concentration and occurs at a rate that reflects fetal glucose utilization for energy production. Fetal glucose utilization also occurs at relatively low plasma insulin concentrations. In the preterm newborn glucose usually is administered at higher rates than the fetus receives in utero, frequently producing hyperglycemia and plasma insulin concentrations that are significantly higher than those seen in the fetus. In addition, high glucose delivery rates to the preterm infant are likely to contribute to fat deposition. At 50–60% of gestation there is little fetal lipid uptake and this only gradually increases towards term. In contrast, in the very preterm newborn infant lipid is commonly provided as an energy source in amounts that exceed in utero delivery rates, contributing to adipose tissue production much earlier in development and in excess of rates that occur gradually over the third trimester of fetal development.

Clearly, current nutritional practices in preterm infants (high energy intakes of lipid and glucose accompanied by low protein intakes) contrast with the nutrient supplies that the normally growing fetus receives (high amino acid uptake with just sufficient uptake of glucose and lipid). The risks and benefits of these different nutritional patterns for the very preterm infant are not known.

Strategies for Delivering Parenteral Substrates to ELBW Neonates

Protein

Maximal weight-specific protein gain throughout life occurs prior to 32 weeks' gestation. Thus, amino acid requirements are high in the fetus and very preterm infant in order to provide for the exceptionally high fractional protein synthetic and growth rates at this early developmental age. Infants who receive only supplemental glucose lose 1% of protein stores each day, and this may be even greater in very preterm newborns. If the target nutritional intake in the very preterm newborn is to achieve fetal protein accretion rates, then early amino acid administration is critical to avoid protein malnutrition. The quantity of postnatal amino acid administration that is required to produce fetal rates of protein accretion has not been determined, but appears to be at least 3–4 g/kg/day [10].

Protein accretion is also affected by energy intake. Energy is required for both protein metabolism and deposition. Not only are relative protein accretion rates higher in the ELBW infant, but also are relative protein synthetic and breakdown rates, both of which are energy-dependent processes. Synthesis-to-gain ratios in ELBW infants may be as high as 5:1. It has clearly been shown in preterm infants that at the same protein intake, increasing energy intake increases protein accretion rate up to a maximal energy intake of 100–120 kcal/kg/day. This relationship, however, is curvilinear, with most of the effect of energy on protein gain taking place at less than 50–60 kcal/kg/day [11]. In contrast, increasing protein intake leads to increased protein accretion at nearly all energy intakes above 30–50 kcal/kg/day. Such observations support the need for much higher protein intakes than these infants normally receive and indicate that protein gain will be greatest with protein, not energy, intake.

Energy

In order to prevent breakdown of endogenous energy stores, enough energy must be given to at least provide for energy expenditure. From data collected in ventilated ELBW infants in the first days of life, resting metabolic rate is approximately 40 kcal/kg/day. Approximately 20% of basal metabolic rate is accounted for by protein metabolism, or about 4–5 kcal/g protein. The energy cost of protein accretion is the sum of the energy stored (4 kcal/g) plus the metabolic cost of protein gain, which is estimated to be approximately 10 kcal/g protein. Therefore, energy intake to meet energy requirements for protein accretion should be at least 10 kcal/g protein gained. Studies indicate that protein growth in most ELBW infants probably occurs when amino acid intake rates are at or above 1.0–1.5 g/kg/day. Therefore, minimal total energy intake should equal resting metabolic rate plus 10 kcal/kg of infant weight for each gram per kilogram of protein intake above 1 g/kg. For a relatively stable, ventilated ELBW infant in the first days of life, this would give a minimal energy requirement of approximately 50 kcal/kg/day of energy intake at an amino acid intake of 2 g/kg/day, and 60 kcal/kg/day at an amino acid intake of 3 g/kg/day. This theoretical calculation supports the clinical observation that most infants will be in a positive protein balance at 2 g/kg/day of protein intake when given at least 50–60 kcal/kg/day of energy.

In the absence of protein intake, glucose is likely a more effective energy substrate in preventing protein breakdown than is fat, though the impact of the composition and amount of the energy source on protein metabolism remains controversial in ELBW infants. Optimal glucose/lipid intake ratios that maximize protein accretion have not been determined in the neonatal population. However, it is worth considering that the fetus at comparable gestational age to the ELBW infant uses primarily glucose and not lipid as a nonprotein energy source. Furthermore, as discussed above, the fetus also takes up at least twice the amino acid load that it requires for net protein accretion and the balance is oxidized, providing energy. However, it is not clear if amino acids can be used as an energy source in ELBW infants in early postnatal life.

Glucose

In terms of maximal glucose intake, the general consensus has been to avoid hyperglycemia. The upper limit of the normal glucose concentration has not been defined in preterm infants, although many references use the value of 7 mmol/l (126 mg/dl). Common clinical practice is to tolerate glucose concentrations of up to 8.3–11.1 mmol/l (150–200 mg/dl), but the safety and consequences of this practice are unknown. The most common reason given for avoiding significant hyperglycemia is the risk for osmotic diuresis with secondary dehydration and metabolic instability. However, a recent review suggests that this is relatively uncommon [12]. In infants who are normoglycemic, we consider the upper limit of glucose administration to be that which meets the maximal glucose oxidative capacity. This is the glucose intake above which glucose exceeds the energy needs of the body and the excess glucose is converted to fat. Glucose conversion to fat is an energy-inefficient process that results in increased energy expenditure, increased oxygen consumption, and increased carbon dioxide production. This is an undesirable effect in all parenterally fed very preterm infants, but a particular concern in infants with existing lung disease. Chessex et al. [13] have shown that ventilated preterm infants with early and mild bronchopulmonary dysplasia receiving increased glucose intake do increase their carbon dioxide production, but this is compensated for by increasing their respiratory drive. However, this may not occur in infants with significant lung disease. The rate of glucose administration that exceeds the maximal glucose oxidative capacity is not completely known in neonates, but probably is above 11–13 mg/kg/min (~18 g/kg/day) [14, 15].

Lipid

Minimal intravenous lipid intakes should be targeted to prevent essential fatty acid (EFA) deficiency particularly in view of their critical role in postnatal brain development. Preterm infants have very limited endogenous lipid stores [16]. EFA deficiency develops by 4–5 days after birth if exogenous fat is not given and can be prevented with as little as 0.5 g/kg/day lipid (estimates range from 0.25 to 1.0 g/kg/day). Other benefits of intravenous lipid include its role as a high-density energy source (which can be provided by the peripheral venous route due to its isotonicity with plasma) and as a vehicle for facilitating delivery of fat-soluble vitamins. Optimal intravenous lipid intake above that which prevents EFA is controversial and has resulted in different lipid administration strategies among neonatal intensive care centers. Early use and/or rapid advancement of lipid emulsions in the preterm infant has been cautious, however, because of concerns for potential development of several possible complications, including lipid intolerance, potential interference with immune function, impaired bilirubin metabolism and adverse effects on pulmonary function. There has been no recent evidence, though, that these concerns have been seen with the modest infusion rates of 0.5–1.0 g/kg/day that are commonly used today. A recent review comparing 'early' (≤5 days of age) versus 'late' (>5 days of age) initiation of parenteral lipids, which included 5 studies in 397 neonates, demonstrated no significant statistical differences between groups in the primary outcomes of growth rates, death, and chronic lung disease or the secondary outcomes, including several pulmonary disorders [17]. The authors concluded that early parenteral lipid administration could not be recommended for benefits of short-term growth or prevention of morbidity and mortality. However, there appears to be no clear contraindication to starting intravenous lipid infusions within the first day of life in most preterm infants, and there is a benefit in terms of ameliorating or preventing EFA deficiency. Clearly there is a critical need for more definitive information regarding the conditions under which intravenous fat administration should be limited.

Early Parenteral Nutrition Studies in ELBW Neonates

The first comprehensive, prospective, randomized, controlled trial of 'aggressive' versus 'conservative' nutrition in 125 relatively sick neonates weighing <1,500 g at birth was conducted in the 1990s by Wilson et al. [18]. Infants in the aggressive intake group were sicker, were started on earlier enteral nutrition (day 2 vs. day 5 in the control group), parenteral amino acids (day 1 vs. 3), and parenteral lipid (day 2 vs. 5). Nutrients were advanced more quickly and to higher maximal intakes in the aggressive nutrition group, and insulin was used if hyperglycemia developed. In terms of outcomes, there were no differences between groups in survival, hospital stay, days to full enteral feeding, and incidence of necrotizing enterocolitis (NEC), bronchopulmonary dysplasia, sepsis, cholestasis, and osteopenia. There was a significant improvement in weight gain at discharge from hospital in the aggressive intake group, though both groups demonstrated significant postnatal growth failure with discharge weight less than the 10th percentile of their standard growth curves.

A number of studies have focused on early protein administration in preterm infants. These studies have demonstrated that infusion of amino acids with glucose as early as the first day of life decreases protein catabolism. In general, 1.5–2.0 g/kg/day of protein intake is sufficient to avoid catabolism in neonates. In terms of the upper limits of protein intake, if the goal is to achieve intrauterine rates of protein deposition, then requirements of up to 3.8–4.0 g/kg/day of protein intake just to provide sufficient amino acids for protein accretion

Table 1. Estimated nutrient intakes needed to achieve fetal weight gain

	Body weight, g				
	500–700	700–900	900–1,200	1,200–1,500	1,500–1,800
Fetal weight gain[a]					
g/day	13	16	20	24	26
g/kg/day	21	20	19	18	16
Protein (Nx6.25), g					
Inevitable loss[b]	1.0	1.0	1.0	1.0	1.0
Growth (accretion)[c]	2.5	2.5	2.5	2.4	2.2
Required intake					
Parenteral[d]	3.5	3.5	3.5	3.4	3.2
Enteral[e]	4.0	4.0	4.0	3.9	3.6
Energy, kcal					
Loss	60	60	65	70	70
Resting expenditure	45	45	50	50	50
Miscellaneous expenditure	15	15	15	20	20
Growth (accretion)[f]	29	32	36	38	39
Required intake					
Parenteral[d]	89	92	101	108	109
Enteral[g]	105	108	119	127	128
Protein/energy, g/100 kcal					
Parenteral	3.9	4.1	3.5	3.1	2.9
Enteral	3.8	3.7	3.4	3.1	2.8

Because nutrient needs are closely related to body weight and weight gain, the nutrient needs apply to all postnatal ages. All values are per kg per day [19, with permission].
[a]Based on data of Kramer et al. [31].
[b]Urinary nitrogen loss of 133 mg/kg/day [32, 33] and dermal loss of 27 mg/kg/day [34].
[c]Includes correction for 90% efficiency of conversion from dietary to body protein.
[d]Sum of loss and accretion.
[e]Same as parenteral but assuming 88% absorption of dietary protein.
[f]Energy accretion plus 10 kcal/kg/day cost of growth.
[g]Assuming 85% absorption of dietary energy.

have been estimated for ELBW infants [19] (table 1). In a randomized trial of early 'low' versus 'high' parenteral amino acid intake, it was shown that increased parenteral amino acid intakes for approximately 24 h produced short-term increases in protein growth in preterm infants [20]. This prospective, randomized study included 28 infants (mean weight 946 ± 40 g; SEM) who received either 1 g/kg/day (low amino acid intake) versus 3 g/kg/day (high amino acid intake) in the first days of life. Efficacy was determined by protein balance, and was significantly lower in the 1 versus 3 g/kg/ day amino acid intake groups by both nitrogen balance and leucine-stable isotope methods.

In terms of potential toxicity with the higher amino acid intake, there were no significant differences between groups in the amount of sodium bicarbonate administered, the degree of metabolic acidosis, or the blood urea nitrogen (BUN) concentration. When compared with plasma amino acid concentrations of normally growing 2nd and 3rd trimester human fetuses who were sampled by cordocentesis the normal fetal amino acid concentrations for both essential and nonessential amino acids were equal to those in the 3 g/kg/day group (except for threonine and lysine, which were significantly lower than seen in the fetus), but were at least twice the concentrations in the 1 g/kg/day group. More recently, in a large cohort of infants <1,500 g (n = 135 infants) te Braake et al. [21] compared 2.4 g/kg/day amino acids starting on the first day of life versus a stepwise increase over the first 3 days of life, and confirmed the safety (BUN and amino acid concentrations) and efficacy (nitrogen balance) of both strategies. Thus, in the short term it appears such amino acid delivery rates to the neonate are safe and beneficial, though the long-term effects have not been evaluated.

In the past several years initiation of 3 g/kg/day of parenteral amino acid intake in the first 1–2 days of life has become routine in many neonatal intensive care units. Nevertheless, a number of clinicians are hesitant to prescribe this rate of amino acid infusion because of concerns about potential amino acid toxicity. Currently there are no definitive clinical markers of toxicity from protein intake. In general, many clinicians follow BUN levels. However, a recent study in preterm infants showed no correlation between amino acid intake and BUN concentration [22]. Although gradually increasing amino acid intake over the first several days of parenteral nutrition is often advocated, there is no evidence that this specifically promotes tolerance of amino acids [21]. Clearly, further studies are needed to determine if even higher amino acid intakes are safe and efficacious when administered to very preterm neonates.

Role of Insulin in Enhancing Growth with Parenteral Nutrition

Exogenous insulin is most commonly used to control early hyperglycemia in very preterm infants. However, informal surveys suggest that there are a number of centers that use insulin in preterm neonates receiving parenteral nutrition for the purpose of enhancing growth. Insulin has been shown to successfully lower glucose levels and to increase weight gain without undue risk of hypoglycemia [23–25]. It is presumed that improved weight gain is secondary to both increased glucose utilization and improved protein balance in infants receiving parenteral nutrition. However, little is known about the effects of intravenous insulin infusions and relative hyperinsulinemia on the quality of weight gain and on counterregulatory hormone concentrations and the possible effects of these concentrations.

Administration of intravenous amino acids has been shown to decrease glucose concentrations in ELBW infants, presumably by enhancing endogenous insulin secretion. In the above study by Thureen et al. [20], an approximate doubling of insulin concentration occurred in the high versus low amino acid intake study group. The much lower incidence of neonatal hyperglycemia following the earlier postnatal introduction of parenteral amino acids was reported by Micheli et al. [26], and may be due to increased insulin secretion. It is known that enteral feeding also stimulates insulin release in infants. Since instituting a policy of early 'high-dose' parenteral amino acids, glucose intake rates at a maximum of 12 mg/kg/min and early minimal enteral feeding (MEF), we have virtually no significant hyperglycemia in preterm neonates, and insulin use is rare in our nurseries.

Contribution of Enteral Feeding to a Strategy of Early Aggressive Nutrition

An 'early aggressive' approach to nutrition benefits from early introduction of small-volume enteral nutrition (also referred to as MEF) in order to (1) provide trophic benefits of nutrient stimulation to the gut, (2) allow for a more comprehensive package of nutrient administration, and (3) avoid prolonged parenteral nutrition. The most common reason for delayed initiation and limited advancement of enteral feedings in preterm infants is the concern for increasing the risk of NEC. Clearly, there often is reason to cautiously initiate enteral feeding in very preterm infants soon after birth because of the known immaturity of a number of physiological and hormonal systems at early gestational ages. However, early enteral feeding prevents gut atrophy, stimulates maturation of the gastrointestinal system, may actually enhance eventual feeding tolerance, and may reduce the incidence of NEC, especially when colostrum and human milk are used. Most importantly, there is no evidence that MEF increased the risk for development of NEC [27]. Thus early MEF appears to have a role in early aggressive nutrition. Unfortunately, because of the concern for NEC, there is a paucity of definitive studies to guide early enteral feeding beyond the early use of MEF in very preterm neonates. Several small physiological studies give clues to best feeding practices, but do not provide comprehensive strategies for enteral feedings. Meta-analyses of enteral feeding practices are often not conclusive because there are an enormous number of variables in existing studies that make comparisons among studies difficult, and generalizations about safety and efficacy problematic. There are a number of enteral feeding trials with a decreased incidence of NEC as the primary outcome, but most of these are underpowered and not definitive. Clearly more research is needed in this area.

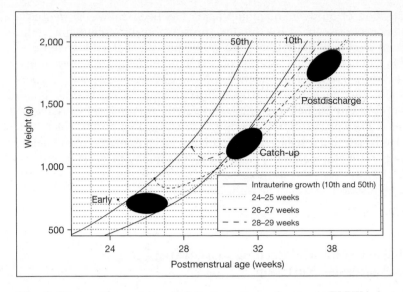

Fig. 2. Three phases of growth faltering commonly seen in ELBW infants.

Aggressive Nutrition beyond the Early Neonatal Period: Is Postnatal Growth Failure Inevitable?

As noted above, a number of studies over the past 10 years would suggest that postnatal growth failure is unavoidable in ELBW infants. Many of the nutritional intervention studies to date have focused on delivering increased quantities of nutrients in the first 2–4 weeks of life. Clearly, this has decreased the catabolism seen prior to this type of intervention, and in some cases has resulted in improved weight gain. Growth faltering can occur at numerous time points during hospitalization, and solving the postnatal growth failure problem in this population will require different nutritional strategies at different time points. Figure 2 suggests there are at least three phases of growth faltering commonly seen in ELBW infants: (1) the several weeks immediately after birth when neonates are the most fragile, (2) the intermediate time period when infants are commonly slowly advanced to full enteral nutrition, but which could potentially represent an opportunity for significant catch-up growth, and (3) the postdischarge phase. There is currently little data regarding strategies to either prevent or reduce the incidence of growth faltering during these latter growth phases [28], and even less data regarding the risks and benefits of catch-up growth. Both human and animal investigations indicate that undernutrition, particularly insufficient protein intake, during critical development periods may adversely affect long-term linear growth, neurodevelopmental outcomes, and general health. In contrast, overfeeding and/or positive crossing of growth percentiles may be associated with adverse later-life health outcomes such as obesity and type-2 diabetes [29, 30]. These contrasting responses to the amount (over- vs. undernutrition) and the timing of specific approaches to neonatal nutrition raise a number of as yet unanswered questions regarding postnatal nutrition of the very preterm infant.

References

1   Lucas A, Morley R, Cole TJ: Randomised trial of early diet in preterm babies and later intelligence quotient. BMJ 1998;317:1481–1487.
2   Ehrenkranz R, Younes N, Lemons J, et al: Longitudinal growth of hospitalized very low birth-weight infants. Pediatrics 1999;104:280–289.
3   Carlson SJ, Ziegler EE: Nutrient intakes and growth of very low birth weight infants. J Perinatol 1998;18:252–258.
4   Embleton NE, Pang N, Cooke PJ: Postnatal malnutrition and growth retardation: an inevitable consequence of current recommendations in preterm infants? Pediatrics 2001;107:270–273.
5   Latal-Hajnal B, von Siebenthal K, Kovari H, et al: Postnatal growth in VLBW infants: significant association with neurodevelopmental outcome. J Pediatr 2003;143:163–170.
6   Saigal S, Stoskopf BL, Streiner DL, et al: Physical growth and current health status of infants who were of extremely low birth weight and controls at adolescence. Pediatrics 2001;108:407–415.
7   American Academy of Pediatrics Committee on Nutrition: Nutritional needs of low-birth-weight infants. Pediatrics 1985;76:976–986.
8   Olsen IE, Richardson DK, Schmid CH, et al: Intersite differences in weight growth velocity of extremely premature infants. Pediatrics 2002;110:1125–1132.
9   Bloom TB, Mulligan J, Arnold C, et al: Improving growth of very low birth weight infants in the first 28 days. Pediatrics 2003;112:8–14.
10 Kashyap S, Heird WC: Protein requirements of low birthweight, very low birthweight, and small for gestational age infants; in Raiha NCR (ed): Protein Metabolism during Infancy. Nestle Nutrition Workshop Series. Vevey, Nestec, New York, Raven Press, 1994, vol 33, pp 133–146.
11 Micheli JL, Schutz Y: Protein; in Tsang RC, Lucas A, Uauy R, Zlotkin S (eds): Nutritional Needs of the Preterm Infant, Scientific Basis and Practical Guidelines. Pawling, Caduceus Medical Publishers, 1993, pp 29–46.
12 Hey E: Hyperglycaemia and the very preterm baby. Semin Fetal Neonatal Med 2005;10: 377–387.
13 Chessex P, Belanger S, Bruno P, et al: Influence of energy substrates on respiratory gas exchange during conventional mechanical ventilation of preterm infants. J Pediatr 1995;126: 619–624.
14 Van Aerde JEE, Sauer PJJ, Pencharz PB, et al: Effect of replacing glucose with lipid on the energy metabolism of newborn infants. Clin Sci 1989;76:581–588.
15 Piedboeuf B, Chessex P, Hazan J, et al: Total parenteral nutrition in the newborn infant: energy substrates and respiratory gas exchange. J Pediatr 1991;118:97–102.
16 Koletzko B: Parenteral lipid infusion in infancy: physiological basis and clinical relevance. Clin Nutr 2002;21(suppl 2):53–65.
17 Simmer K, Rao SC: Early introduction of lipids to parenterally-fed preterm infants. Cochrane Database Syst Rev 2005;2:CD005256.
18 Wilson D, Cairns P, Halliday H, et al: Randomized controlled trial of an aggressive nutritional regimen in sick very low birthweight infants. Arch Dis Child 1997;77:F4–F11.
19 Ziegler EE, Thureen PJ, Carlson SJ: Aggressive nutrition of the very low birthweight infant. Clin Perinatol 2002;29:225–244.
20 Thureen PJ, Melara D, Fennessey PV, et al: Effect of low versus high intravenous amino acid intake on very low birth weight infants in the early neonatal period. Pediatr Res 2003;53: 24–32.

21 te Braake FWJ, Van Den Akker CHP, Wattimena DJL, et al: Amino acid administration to premature infants directly after birth. J Pediatr 2005;147:457–461.
22 Ridout E, Diane Melara D, Rottinghaus S, et al: Blood urea nitrogen concentration as a marker of amino acid intolerance in neonates with birthweight less than 1250 grams. J Perinatol 2005;25:130–133.
23 Kanarek KS, Santeiro ML, Malone JI: Continuous infusion of insulin in hyperglycemic low-birth-weight infants receiving parenteral nutrition with and without lipid emulsion. JPEN J Parenter Enteral Nutr 1991;15:417–420.
24 Collins JW Jr, Hoppe M, Brown K, et al: A controlled trial of insulin infusion and parenteral nutrition in extremely low birth weight infants with glucose intolerance. J Pediatr 1991;118:921–927.
25 Thabet F, Bourgeois B, Putet G: Continuous insulin infusion in hyperglycaemic very-low-birth-weight infants receiving parenteral nutrition. Clin Nutr 2003;22:545–547.
26 Micheli J-L, Schutz Y, Junod S, et al: Early postnatal intravenous amino acid administration to extremely-low-birth-weight infants; in Hay WW Jr (ed): Seminars in Neonatal Nutrition and Metabolism. Columbus, Ross Products Division, Abbott Laboratories, 1994, vol 2, pp 1–3.
27 Tyson JE, Kennedy KA: Trophic feedings for parenterally fed infants. Cochrane Database Syst Rev 2005;3:CD000504.
28 Ernst KD, Radmacher PG, Rafail ST, et al: Postnatal malnutrition of extremely low birth-weight infants with catch-up growth post-discharge. J Perinatol 2003;2:477–482.
29 Singhal A, Fewtrell M, Cole TJ, Lucas A: Low nutrient intake and early growth for later insulin resistance in adolescents born preterm. Lancet 2003;361:1089–1097.
30 Sabita U, Thomas EL, Hamilton G, et al: Altered adiposity after extremely preterm birth. Pediatr Res 2005;57:211–215.
31 Kramer MS, Platt RW, Wen SW, et al: A new and improved population-based Canadian reference for birth weight for gestational age. Pediatrics 2001;108:1–7.
32 Saini J, Macmahon P, Morgan JB, et al: Early parenteral feeding of amino acids. Arch Dis Child 1989;64:1362–1366.
33 Rivera JA, Bell EF, Bier DM: Effect of intravenous amino acids on protein metabolism of preterm infants during the first three days of life. Pediatr Res 1993;33:106–111.
34 Snyderman SE, Boyer A, Kogut MD, et al: The protein requirement of the premature infant. I. The effect of protein intake on the retention of nitrogen. J Pediatr 1969;74:872–880.

Discussion

Dr. Rivera: What was the mean rate of growth and weight gain in those infants with early feeding? Were you able to measure the IQ of those babies with this type of approach?

Dr. Thureen: These studies were very short-term investigations that did not address long-term growth rates or developmental outcome. A more recent study we are doing indicates that early protein administration correlates with increased growth at 2 months of age. Poindexter et al. [1] recently showed that early amino acid administration to very preterm infants was associated with better growth and fewer infants with small head circumference at 36 weeks postmenstrual age. Clearly more studies are needed to assess growth and neurodevelopmental outcomes after early high protein administration to this population.

Dr. Fakhraee: We see some small babies <1,000 g who cannot tolerate D10W and usually we must use insulin. What is your opinion on that? With regard to minimal enteral feeding, what is the incidence of jaundice?

Dr. Thureen: We have seen a dramatic decrease in the incidence of hyperglycemia in our very preterm infants since starting early parenteral amino acids and early minimal enteral feeding, both of which likely stimulate endogenous insulin secretion. Clearly there are still a few infants who need exogenous insulin to treat significant hyperglycemia even with early amino acids and enteral feedings. We do not, however, use insulin as a 'nutritional adjuvant' to enhance growth in infants without hyperglycemia since the possible adverse effects of such a strategy have not been sufficiently studied. Since the mid 1980s a number of studies have shown that minimal enteral feeding decreases the incidence and/or severity of jaundice.

Dr. Fakhraee: Actually I meant they cannot tolerate more than 4 mg/kg/min. We see it very often in the babies <1,000 g.

Dr. Thureen: The incidence of hyperglycemia varies dramatically and in different units it goes from 1 to 2% up to almost 100% of the infants, and in general those are infants who have high glucose infusion rates. Clearly you are talking about infants who don't have high glucose infusion rates and I am not sure whether there are other stress factors that might contribute to hyperglycemia. We look at these infants on a case by case basis to really to try to decide what other factors are affecting this because you should not be having that degree of hyperglycemia in infants closed to 1,000 g. Clearly there is a lot of data on 24- to 25-week-old infants showing that no matter what you give them they still remain hyperglycemic. These infants are fed in most units and go on insulin to try to control the degree of hyperglycemia.

Dr. Fakhraee: You mentioned lipid infusion in severe infection. What is your definition of severe infection? What are the contraindications that you consider for minimal enteral feeding? Is there any contraindication to starting minimal enteral feeding?

Dr. Thureen: We didn't go through each of those relative contraindications of lipid, but for infection there is a lot of evidence, at least in vitro, that lipid decreases neutrophil function and so there is some concern that giving high lipid intakes in a child who is septic could make things worse.

Dr. Fakhraee: Is there any contraindication to start early minimal feeding?

Dr. Thureen: We do not start minimal enteral feedings if an infant has significant hypoxic events, pressor support >5–10 μg/kg/min, clinical instability such as with significant sepsis, situations associated with decreased blood flow such as hypotension or clinically significant patent ductus arteriosus, or in infants with large aspirates or recurrent abdominal distention. In infants who are IUGR or those who have had hypoxia we are starting to assess superior mesenteric artery blood flow patterns in response to test feeds of 1–3 ml/kg, and we hope this will help us define which infants are at risk with even a minimal enteral feeding.

Dr. B. Koletzko: In your study comparing amino acid intakes of 1–3 g that provide very valuable results, you chose to start providing amino acids only at about 24 h of age.

Dr. Thureen: We did not choose to start amino acids at 24 h of age but rather at birth. However, when we did that study, it took 24 h to order and receive that solution. Now we always have available a 'stock' amino acid solution that is stable and stored in the unit and we currently use this as the initial intravenous fluid after birth in all preterm neonates.

Dr. B. Koletzko: That may already answer my question because in the ESPGAN guidelines on pediatric parenteral nutrition published at the end of 2005 [2] we encourage people to start intravenous glucose with amino acids right from birth. Why do you use the wording 'aggressive nutrition' for safe and efficacious early enteral nutrition? As a pediatrician I have a problem with that. I wouldn't call it 'aggressive' but just patient oriented and in fact probably less aggressive than starving a patient. Maybe if one would change terminology the practice could be even more widespread.

Dr. Thureen: When we started our study of 1 versus 3 g/kg/day of amino acid intake in very preterm infants early in life, most neonatologists around the world were starting infants on 1 g/kg/day of amino acids followed by a very slow advance of amino acid intake. Many clinicians considered 3 g/kg/day to be a dangerously high intake at which to start so we used the term 'aggressive' to acknowledge this concern. Now this intake is widely felt to be safe and demonstrates a number of clinical benefits. But you are right, it is semantic, and I agree with your suggestion to call it 'effective or intensive nutrition support'.

Dr. Vento: Could you comment on the conditionally essential amino acids, the L-cysteine, taurine or L-arginine which in certain circumstances, especially in very low birth weight infants or in low gestational age, could have some influence on their development?

Dr. Thureen: As you mentioned, there is a group of amino acids that may not be considered essential until there is a critical situation and they become 'essential'. I believe we need a better understanding of the conditions under which these amino acids need to be supplied. The whole area of nutrition in specific diseases or during critical illness in preterm infants needs further investigation.

Dr. Saavedra: One of the difficulties that we have even after starting minimal enteral feeding is the rate of advancement that follows. There are two factors that we always see, mostly directed to this concern of potential NEC: using low concentration energy formulas and the apparent signs of intolerance. What is your position regarding concentration advancement versus volume advancement, bolus versus continuous gastric feedings?

Dr. Thureen: Unfortunately, all enteral feeding decisions are based on the fear of developing NEC. With the exception of hyperosmolar feeds, there is little evidence that certain feeding practices produce NEC. It is likely that many factors other than feeding contribute to NEC such as adverse alteration of gut flora secondary to excessive use of antibiotics, altered gut integrity, cytokine release, inflammatory responses and infections. I believe that the one thing that is becoming more evident is that the best enteral feeding to prevent NEC is breast milk. There is no evidence that dilute formulas prevent NEC, and in my opinion, they are contraindicated because they result in decreased caloric intake. Most 'intolerance' in very preterm infants is secondary to the poor GI motility seen in preterm infants, not to early NEC. Studies by Berseth and Nordyke [3, 4] suggest that giving feeds over longer periods (we use a 'slow bolus' over 30–60 min), breast milk and nondilute formulas, enhances gastric emptying and distal motor activity. In addition, bolus feedings stimulate a physiological pattern of hormone release that may not be seen with continuous feeds. We usually reserve continuous feeds for infants with reflux symptoms where smaller volume feedings are but one part of our strategy to decrease reflux. Data suggest that the rate of volume advance has little to do with the development of NEC [5, 6]. Unfortunately, most studies regarding feeding strategies and the development of NEC are statistically underpowered to provide sufficient data on which to guide feeding practices.

Dr. Dhanireddy: The question of 'good BUN' and 'bad BUN' intrigues me. Frequently these extremely low birth weight babies have azotemia and we are struggling to decide whether is it too much protein. At what point would you cut back on the protein or slow down on progression?

Dr. Thureen: As I discussed in my presentation, our studies have not shown a significant correlation between amino acid intake and BUN levels [7]. Because of my concern with protein toxicity I have consulted with a number of metabolic and renal specialists. Their concern for toxicity focuses on encephalopathy, which occurs with BUN levels nearing 80–100 mg/dl. However, in neonatology our concern is that an elevated BUN level may reflect an inability to metabolize protein. My practice is to decrease amino acid administration when the BUN level approaches 35 or 40 mg/dl or when there is an unexplained significant metabolic acidosis since, although many things contribute to both a high BUN level and to metabolic acidosis, decreasing amino acid intake is one thing I can modify that could be having an adverse effect. Some of my colleagues tolerate BUN levels of up to 50–60 mg/dl. In my experience, BUN levels above 40 mg/dl are unusual at 3 g/kg/day protein intake, but I know a number of neonatologists who are now starting to administer much higher parenteral amino acid intakes.

Dr. Haschke: As long as one has a continuous supply for the fetus or during continuous parenteral and enteral nutrition, it is clear that we do not have toxic concentrations of amino acids. As soon as we move to bolus feeding, it is quite different because here, the time between feeding and blood sampling for amino acid determination plays a big role. So sometimes one may miss a high amino acid concentration if blood is not taken at the right moment. We had this problem in one study when we were looking at high protein formulas for premature infants where the amino acid concentrations were taken exactly at a certain time point after feeding and it is clear that they vary considerably. There are differences, for example depending on whether blood sampling for amino acid determination occurs 1 or 3 h after feeding.

Dr. Thureen: I do very few enteral feeding studies and actually Dr. Cooke can address this much better than I can. It is a concern, especially as people start to advocate higher protein intakes in enteral feedings. It is an excellent point that we have to be careful with enteral feeding, especially when people are doing supplementation of enteral feeding. It is a very wide practice which could be dangerous without looking at amino acid levels for instance.

Dr. Cooke: In the absence of an inborn error of metabolism, we are unsure what plasma amino acids mean. Reference values are not fully established for the preterm infant. In effect, what is high, therefore what is acceptable or unacceptable remains to be determined.

Dr. Thureen: I have seen some studies where amino acid concentrations have been high enough that our metabolic specialist said it could be potentially neurotoxic. Dangerous levels of various amino acids have not been well established.

Dr. Cooke: Can I comment on BUN. In the absence of associated anomalies, e.g. renal dysfunction, and/or metabolic anomalies, such as acidosis or hyperammonemia, we really don't know how to interpret 'high' BUN. BUN is to total parenteral nutrition as gastric residuals are to enteral feeds, we get concerned but it alone is not a reason to discontinue parenteral nutrition.

Dr. Fusch: There is some effect of BUN on plasma osmolality. It is one of the most important contributors. As long as you have stable conditions it might be of less importance, but if BUN is changing quickly I don't know what will happen.

Dr. Cooke: It doesn't change that much. It is fairly consistent and we are talking about levels of 20, 30, 36 mg/dl. None of these children develop a BUN above 40 mg/dl or ~6 mmol and I think that is the crucial issue.

Dr. Benavides-Hernandez: The perinatal period is an important moment of metabolic programming. It is clear that aggressive nutritional support is beneficial in the short term and in neurologic outcome. I would like to know if you followed the patients or if you have any estimation of the long-term effect regarding overweight, renal function, and serum lipids?

Dr. Thureen: No, and I personally don't do follow-up studies because the population at the hospital cannot easily be followed. But I think those are very important questions that need to be addressed, as well as those that Dr. Alan Lucas and others have put forth regarding nutrition and postnatal metabolic programming.

Dr. Beaumier: I would like to echo your reference about early protein and the benefit of having no more hyperglycemia because we have been doing that with 2.5 g and we have no more hyperglycemia. A question about lipids: what are your guidelines for advancement?

Dr. Thureen: We monitor triglyceride concentrations and try to keep them less than 150 mg/dl. There is evidence that the more gestationally immature infants, small for gestational age infants, and infants with systemic infection have lower lipoprotein lipase activity and thus less lipid tolerance. Since triglyceride levels can be unpredictable in very preterm infants, we monitor blood levels with each advance in lipid volume to be certain the levels are at a safe range. We administer intravenous lipids over 24 h when possible because of evidence that lipids are better tolerated if given over a longer period of time.

Dr. Heine: We usually aim for a balance between carbohydrate and fat calories of about 50:50, in the older infants at least. In your experience, which proportion of glucose calories versus lipid calories do you apply?

Dr. Thureen: I think most neonatologists are still using 45–50% caloric intake as lipid. I am sure it is different in different institutions, but that is also our practice.

Dr. Heine: Does this also apply in very premature infants?

Dr. Thureen: We gradually advance lipid as tolerated in this population up to 45–50% calories as lipid.

References

1 Pointdexter BB, Langer JC, Dusick AM, et al: Early provision of parenteral amino acids in extremely low birth weight infants: relation to growth and neurodevelopmental outcome. J Pediatr 2006;148:300–305.
2 Koletzko B, et al: Guidelines on Paediatric Parenteral Nutrition of the European Society of Paediatric Gastroenterology, Hepatology and Nutrition (ESPGHAN) and the European Society for Clinical Nutrition and Metabolism (ESPEN). J Pediatr Gastroenterol Nutr 2005;41(suppl 2):S1–S87.
3 Berseth CL: Effect of early feeding on maturation of the preterm infant's small intestine. J Pediatr 1992;120:947–953.
4 Berseth CL, Nordyke C: Enteral nutrients promote postnatal maturation of intestinal motor activity in preterm infants. Am J Physiol 1993;264:G1046–G1051.
5 Rayyis SF, Ambalavanan N, Wright L, Carlo WA: Randomized trial of 'slow' versus 'fast' feed advancements on the incidence of necrotizing enterocolitis in very low birth weight infants. J Pediatr 1999;134:293–297.
6 Kennedy KA, Tyson JE, Chamnanvanakij S: Rapid versus slow rate of advancement of feedings for promoting growth and preventing necrotizing enterocolitis in parenterally fed low-birth-weight infants. Cochrane Database Syst Rev 2000;2:CD001241.
7 Ridout E, Melara D, Rottinghaus S, Thureen PJ: Blood urea nitrogen concentration as a marker of amino acid intolerance in neonates with birthweight less than 1250 grams. J Perinatol 2005;25:130–133.

Cooke RJ, Vandenplas Y, Wahn U (eds): Nutrition Support for Infants and Children at Risk.
Nestlé Nutr Workshop Ser Pediatr Program, vol 59, pp 209–211,
Nestec Ltd., Vevey/S. Karger AG, Basel, © 2007.

Discussion

Following the presentation on 'Human Milk Fortification' by G. Putet

Dr. Haschke: Could you elaborate a little bit on protein quality? Nowadays we should consider not only the protein quantity in human milk, but also protein quality, because we know that the quality changes rapidly. The whey fraction decreases after a couple of weeks and the nutritive quality of the milk might not be the same immediately after birth and later on because the composition of the protein differs. Are there any studies on this, or could you speculate on how this could affect the real intake values of nutritive and nonnutritive protein?

Dr. Putet: The only thing I really know is that the whey to casein ratio of the human milk is changing. The more mature the milk is the more this ratio will change to around 50 to 50 and will not stay at 60 to 40.

Dr. Puplampu: I would like to know what type of protein was used to fortify human milk. You mentioned dextrose maltose being one of the ingredients, but what about the others, particularly protein, and what type of protein?

Dr. Putet: In the various studies I showed there were different human milk fortifiers. So from one study to another the human milk fortifier was not at all the same. Most of the time they were either Enfamil or Eoprotein.

Dr. Netrebenko: You showed the higher osmolarity of human milk fortifiers. Have you seen any adverse effect of this kind of feeding?

Dr. Putet: There have been several studies showing that when the osmolarity of the fluid given per os is above 550 mosm it may be dangerous for the baby and provoke necrotizing enterocolitis. This is why we have to be careful that the osmolarity is not too high.

Dr. Netrebenko: So it means that these fortifiers are not very safe for preterm babies?

Dr. Putet: They are safe. What I showed is that human milk fortifiers may increase the osmolarity of human milk to a certain level. This level has not been shown to increase necrotizing enterocolitis. When this kind of human milk is used and some drugs are added at the same time, the osmolarity may increase a bit more. So caution must be taken to dilute the drugs with enough human milk.

Dr. Beaumier: You talked mainly about protein but in earlier talks we heard that protein is missing. Perhaps we should think about having a higher protein concentration. What would the effect of the combinations human milk and human milk fortifier be on protein? What is the source of calories added. Currently, and I am talking only for North America, we are using carbohydrate- and lipid-predominant fortifiers. Is there any preference? We just heard from Dr. Thureen that increased carbohydrate above 18 g/day might have a detrimental effect due to lipogenesis. Looking at the carbohydrate content of human milk and the carbohydrate-predominant fortification, a couple of calculations will give a value in the 20–22 range.

Dr. Putet: Most of the human milk fortifiers contain energy with dextrin maltose or lactose, lipids and minerals, vitamins and some oligoelements. It is important to know that they contain minerals to be able to know what the result on calciuria is when this fortifier is added. With human milk fortifier the carbohydrate load is not that much; at the most it may be 8 cal/dl. I don't think there is any consequence of that because if they are given at 180 ml/kg/day the total amount of carbohydrate will not be that high. If they are given at a much higher volume intake, the protein intake and total energy intake will perhaps be a little too high. I don't know of any study comparing the effect of 50/50 energy supplementation with lipids or dextrin maltose with human milk fortifier or of any comparison of lipids and carbohydrate in very low birth weight infants.

Dr. Dhanireddy: When we add the fortifiers to human milk, what is the impact on the bioavailability of the various nutrients? Frequently these babies are on continuous feeds through plastic tubing. Does that alter the absorption of nutrients?

Dr. Putet: Human milk fortifier may change the capacity for retention but not the bioavailability. For instance if a human milk fortifier which has the correct amount of phosphorus is added, then the calcium retention of human milk will increase because at the same time there will be a little more phosphorus. Therefore the impact of the fortifier on calcium phosphorus balance must be measured or known. It is more the retention which has to be looked at rather than the bioavailability, because most of the time the bioavailability, which means metabolizable nutrients, will not change; it may increase but it will not change in infants.

Adding human milk fortifier by syringe will not change the amount of nutrients. We know that there may be protein losses or energy losses within a syringe, but by adding human milk fortifier the percentage of nutrients remaining within the syringe will not change.

Dr. Kamenwa: We have been talking about food allergy in babies and I was just wondering whether the protein macromolecules used to fortify human milk may be a potential risk for sensitizing these preterm babies?

Dr. Putet: When human milk is fortified and used within a few hours, the osmolarity will not increase. Attention must be paid to the osmolarity of the drugs added to the fortifier. If the fortified human milk is left for 24 h, the osmolarity will increase a little.

Dr. Fusch: Does the introduction of cow's milk products in the fortifier increase the risk of sensitization?

Dr. Putet: With the introduction of cow's milk protein the risk may increase. There are now some partially hydrolyzed human milk fortifiers and very soon there will be human milk fortifiers with totally hydrolyzed protein.

Dr. Haschke: There is one fortifier presently on the market which is based on extensively hydrolyzed protein, so there is no risk of sensitizing an infant to cow's milk protein. For other formulas which include intact proteins, the question might be valid but nobody has really studied this.

Dr. Putet: You are right, there is a human milk fortifier with cow's milk, total protein, and partial protein like the one we use, but it is not yet available in every country.

Dr. Costalos: When a premature baby is breastfed by its mother it is getting enough milk when breastfeeding is continuous. If breastfeeding continues after 1 month the protein or sodium content decreases even if the baby is getting his mother's milk. This must be taken into consideration. For 1 month it is all right but after that something must be done.

Dr. Fusch: We know what we are putting into the milk when we use the fortifier. But we do not know what the basis of the individual mother's milk is. Sometimes we see babies who do not grow with a 5% fortifier and even when the fortifier is increased up to 7.5%, which has not been studied or recommended, the baby does not grow either. Then we switch to normal preterm infant formula and the baby grows. How often do you think the mother's milk does not have a high enough energy or protein content?

Dr. Putet: It will always be difficult to measure the protein content of human milk. We can only rely on what is generally accepted. Even in the first or second week of life some mother's milk has a very low protein content, 1.2 or 1.3 g/dl, some others will stay at 1.8 g/dl. So most of the time it is very difficult to add human milk fortifier from one meal to another. This is why it is better to give the fortifier for the whole day; the error will be much less.

Dr. von der Weid: Microbiological growth after reconstitution of human milk fortifier appears after 48–72 h. Like any powdered infant formula, the product must be consumed as soon as possible after reconstitution, especially in the case of sensitive premature infants. I am surprised to see that bacterial growth in human milk was maintained in the fridge at 4°C, a temperature at which bacteria normally do not grow. What kind of bacteria was detected in these samples?

Dr. Putet: You are not totally right because in France I am know that mothers who live a certain distance from the hospital keep their expressed breast milk in the fridge and bring it to the hospital. So I would say the time of 48 h is right if we are sure that the fridge temperature is not too high, and this may explain why it was not growing. When expressed breast milk is put in the fridge at 4°C, even though there are some colonies at the beginning, most of the time a decrease in the number of colonies will be seen over the first 24 h. Even if it is kept for a longer time it will be stable. Studies have shown that if it is kept up to 48 h there will be no growth. If the fridge is at 8°C or more there may be growth.

Cooke RJ, Vandenplas Y, Wahn U (eds): Nutrition Support for Infants and Children at Risk.
Nestlé Nutr Workshop Ser Pediatr Program, vol 59, pp 213–228,
Nestec Ltd., Vevey/S. Karger AG, Basel, © 2007.

Postdischarge Nutrition of Preterm Infants: More Questions than Answers

Richard J. Cooke

University of Tennessee Center for Health Sciences, Memphis, TN, USA

Abstract

Postnatal growth retardation is inevitable in preterm infants, the more immature the infant the greater the degree of postnatal growth retardation at hospital discharge. After hospital discharge, several studies have shown that growth is poorer in preterm infants fed a standard term formula than those fed a nutrient-enriched infant formula. This is not surprising because term formulas are designed to meet the requirements of the term infant, not the more rapidly growing preterm infant. After hospital discharge, breastfed infants do not grow as well as their formula-fed counterparts. Yet, there are no randomized controlled trials comparing growth in breastfed infants who did and did not receive nutrient supplementation. If mature human milk is designed to meet the needs of the term infant then breastfed preterm infants may also benefit from nutrient supplementation. Questions persist about nutritional support of preterm infants after discharge. What is the ideal composition of a postdischarge formula? Given the wide heterogeneity in nutritional status of preterm infants at hospital discharge and the difference in growth rates and composition between girls and boys, it is not clear that one formula can or will meet the nutritional needs of all infants. Studies in which infants were fed a nutrient-enriched formula to ≥ 6 months' corrected age show the most consistent advantage while those in which the nutrient-enriched formula was fed to ≤ 2 months' corrected age had no effect on growth. Whether this is a reflection of the duration of feeding or not is unclear. Further studies are needed to examine this issue. To date, little attention has focused on the role and/or effects of complimentary feeds these infants. Complimentary feeds will confound the effects of any study examining postdischarge growth in preterm infants. However, they may also be an important adjunct in meeting nutritional needs of these high-risk infants. Further studies are also needed to examine this issue.

Copyright © 2007 Nestec Ltd., Vevey/S. Karger AG, Basel

Introduction

Several studies have examined postnatal growth in preterm infants during the initial hospital stay and noted that most preterm if not all very low birth weight infants are growth retarded at hospital discharge [1–7]. In studies where nutritional intake was measured, recommended dietary intakes took time to establish and infants accrued a significant nutrient deficit that was directly related to the growth deficit [1–5].

In studies where intake was not measured poor growth was related to poorer clinical outcomes [6, 7]. This is not surprising because it takes time to establish recommended dietary intakes in the infant with a complicated neonatal course. Once established, intake may be interrupted during episodes of clinical instability further increasing the nutrient deficit. However, other factors may underpin the development of growth retardation in these infants.

Current recommendations are that the rate of weight gain parallel that of the fetus of the same gestational age once birth weight has been regained [8, 9]. Yet, an infant of 27 weeks' gestational age weighing ~1,000 g at birth who regains birth weight by 2 weeks of age and grows at the intrauterine rate will weigh ~540 g less than the fetus and be growth retarded. If current recommendations are met most, if not all, very low- birth weight infants will be growth retarded at hospital discharge.

Current recommendations assume requirements are similar for all preterm low birth weight infants [8, 9]. However, Ziegler [10] has noted that protein and energy requirements change with advancing gestation and a formula with a protein:energy ratio of 3.0 g/100 kcal, that is currently recommended for preterm infants, will not meet the needs of the very low birth weight infant.

Recommended dietary intakes are based on needs for maintenance and normal growth [8, 9]; no allowance is made for recovery or 'catch-up' growth [11]. In the study of Embleton et al. [3], the accrued protein deficit, i.e., need for recovery, varied from 15 to 25 g/kg/day. To recoup this deficit before hospital discharge, an additional 0.5–1.0 g/kg/day would be required, further confusing the issue.

Although many factors contribute to the development of postnatal growth retardation and the degree of postnatal growth retardation will vary, depending upon the level of immaturity of the infant, one point is clear: close attention must be paid to nutritional support and growth of these infants in the first 12–18 months of life.

Postdischarge Nutritional Support of the Preterm Infant

Several studies have examined postdischarge growth in preterm infants [12–18]. Although some 'catch-up' growth has been observed, preterm infants do not grow as well as their term counterparts. There are several possible reasons for this.

Current in-hospital feeding practices ensure that preterm infants are malnourished and growth retarded at initial hospital discharge. A 'critical epoch' of growth may, therefore, have been missed. Preterm infants also have greater morbidity than term infants during the first year of life [19–23] and intercurrent illness will affect growth, irrespective of whether they are admitted to hospital or not.

Until relatively recently, little attention had been paid to nutritional factors in the pathogenesis of this problem. In most early studies, infants were fed either human milk or a term infant formula after hospital discharge [12–18]. Both feeding regimens are designed to meet nutritional needs of the term rather than the rapidly growing preterm infant. Infants, therefore, were partly underfed during the first 6–12 months of life.

Lucas et al. [24] randomized preterm infants (birth weight ≤1,800 g, gestational age ≤34 weeks; n = 16/group) to be fed either a term formula or a nutrient-enriched infant formula after hospital discharge. Those fed the nutrient-enriched formula grew better and had better bone mineralization at 3 and 9 months' corrected age [25]. However, Chan et al. [26] were unable to show any differences in growth between preterm infants fed a term formula and those fed either a nutrient-enriched or preterm infant formula after hospital discharge.

Cooke et al. [27–29] randomized otherwise 'normal' preterm (≤1,750 g birth weight, ≤34 weeks' gestation) infants to one of three feeding groups: one group (n = 49) was fed a nutrient-enriched infant formula between discharge and 6 months, the second (n = 54) group a term formula between discharge and 6 months and the third (n = 26) a nutrient-enriched formula between discharge and term and a term formula between term and 6 months' corrected age.

The results are presented in figures 1 and 2. Infants fed the nutrient-enriched formula between discharge and 6 months had lower volumes, similar energy but greater protein intake than the other groups (fig. 1). Increased protein intake was paralleled by greater serum urea nitrogen, weight and length gains, which, in turn, were reflected by greater body weight, length, head circumference, lean mass and absolute (g) but not fractional fat (%) mass (fig. 2). No consistent differences were detected in growth or body composition between the second and third groups.

Initial analyses indicated that effects on growth were predominantly in boys. A subsequent analysis, when data were converted to z-scores, is revealing and is presented in figure 3. Between birth and discharge, z-scores for body weight fell in boys in both treatment groups. Between discharge and 6 months, z-scores were consistently greater in boys fed the preterm formula. The pattern is exactly the same in girls, indicating that girls also benefited when fed the nutrient-enriched formula.

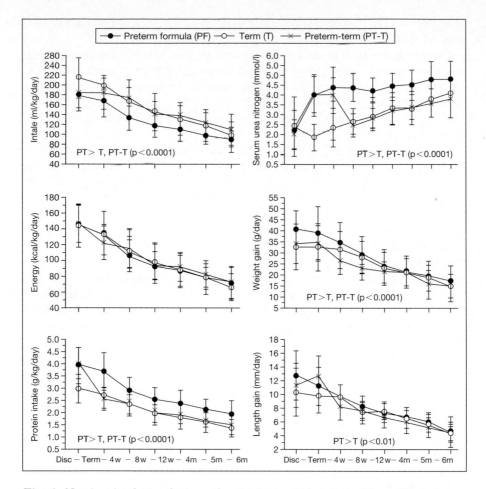

Fig. 1. Nutrient intakes and serum chemistries in study infants. Disc = Discharge.

Carver et al. [30] randomized preterm infants (<37 weeks, ≤1,800 g) to be fed either a nutrient-enriched formula (n = 67) or a term formula (n = 56) between discharge and 12 months' corrected age. Infants were stratified according to birth weight (<1,250, ≥1,250 g). No differences were detected in energy intake but protein intake was greater in infants fed the nutrient-enriched formula. Growth was also better, particularly in infants <1,250 g who were heavier, longer and had a greater head circumference at 6 months' corrected age.

Lucas et al. [31] randomized a group of preterm infants (<37 weeks, <1,750 g) to be fed either a nutrient-enriched (n = 113) or term (n = 116) formula between discharge and 9 months' corrected age. Infants fed the enriched formula grew better, i.e., they were heavier and longer at 9 months

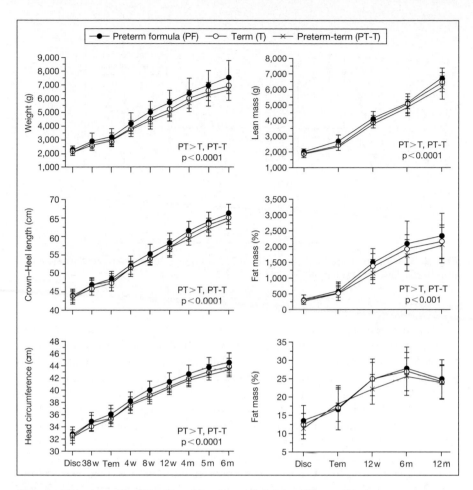

Fig. 2. Growth and body composition in study infants. Disc = Discharge.

and longer at 18 months than infants fed the term formula, an effect that was more marked in boys than girls. No differences were detected in neurodevelopmental outcome between the treatment groups.

De Curtis et al. [31] randomized a group of preterm infants (<35 weeks' gestational age, birth weight of <1,750 g) to be fed either a nutrient-enriched formula (n = 16) or a standard term formula (n = 17) between hospital discharge at ~37 weeks and ~2 months' corrected age. No significant differences were detected in the volume of formula intake but protein and energy intakes were greater in infants fed the nutrient-enriched formula. No differences were detected in growth or body composition between the treatment groups.

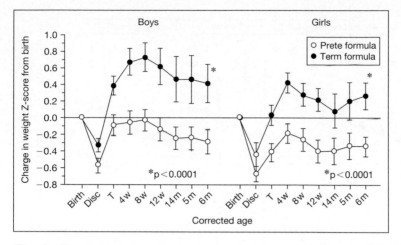

Fig. 3. Grwoth in study infants, expressed as a change in standard deviation scores from birth. Disc = Discharge; T = term.

Litmanovitz et al. [33] randomized a group of very low birth weight infants to be fed a nutrient-enriched (n = 10) or standard term (n = 10) formula between hospital discharge and 6 months' corrected age. No differences were detected in growth, bone strength and/or bone turnover between the treatment groups.

Henderson et al. [34] recently did a systematic review examining the use of a caloric and protein-enriched formula for improving growth and development following hospital discharge. These authors concluded that there is 'little evidence that feeding' with nutrient-enriched formulas 'affected growth and development'. As such, their conclusions merit scrutiny.

Energy and protein contents of the nutrient-enriched formulas varied from 72–80 kca/100 ml and 1.8–2.2 g/100 ml, as did the duration of intervention, term to 12 months, and sample sizes used, 20–229, while some studies stratified for degree of immaturity and/or sex and others did not. Given the differences in study design and sample sizes it is not clear that they are entirely comparable.

The first outcome variable evaluated was 'growth during the trial period'. The results of one study were used, that of de Curtis et al. [32], wherein the sample size was 33 and hardly representative. The endpoint was gain in weight, crown–heel length and head circumference between 36 weeks and 2 months' corrected age. Yet, growth velocity changes rapidly during this time (see fig. 1) and that which is averaged over a 12-week period may not reflect early but significant differences between the groups [27].

The second endpoint was 'longer-term growth', i.e., weight, length and head circumference at 6, 9 and 18 months' corrected age. Data from only one study was used at 6 months [33] and one at 9 months [31], again not entirely

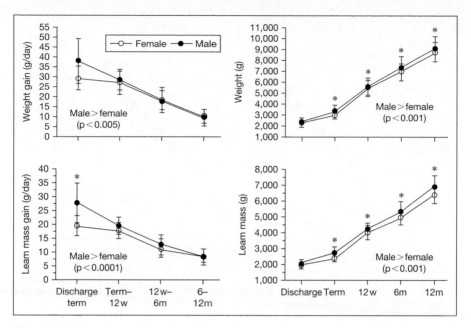

Fig. 4. Body composition in girls and boys fed the preterm infant formula. Disc = Discharge; T = term.

representative. The third endpoint was neurodevelopmental outcome at 18 months. The meta-analysis included the studies of Lucas et al. [31] and Cooke et al. [28], a sample size of 358 infants. No differences were detected between infants fed the standard and nutrient-enriched formula, a valid conclusion under the circumstances.

The conclusions drawn by Henderson et al. [34] on 'growth' but not on development, therefore, must be questioned. A closer look at these studies is revealing. In the study of Cooke et al. [27–29], one group was fed the nutrient-enriched formula to term and no growth advantage was detected. In the study of de Curtis et al. [32], the nutrient-enriched formula was fed to 2 months and no growth advantage was detected. Yet, in the studies with an adequate sample size, where the nutrient-enriched formulas were fed to 6 [27–29], 9 [31] and 12 [30] months, growth was better, suggesting that duration of feeding is an important consideration.

In the studies of Cooke et al. [27–29], Carver et al. [30] and Lucas et al. [31] infants were stratified according sex. In these studies, the effect of diet was greatest in males. This is not surprising because boys are programmed to grow faster and accrete more lean mass [35] and, therefore, benefit from a higher protein-to-energy ratio. This is illustrated in figure 4 where boys fed the nutrient-enriched formula grew faster and accreted more lean mass than girls fed the same formula [29].

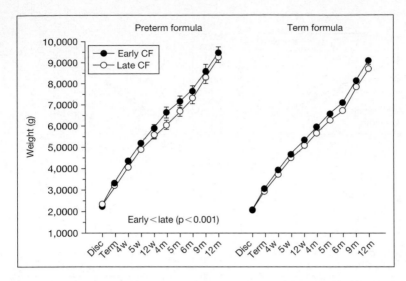

Fig. 5. Growth in infants weaned before (early CF) and after (late CF) 4 months corrected age. Disc = Discharge.

In the study of Carver et al. [30] infants were stratified according to birth weight, <1,250 and 1,250–1,800 g. Infants <1,250 g also seemed to benefit more from the nutrient-enriched formula. This also is not surprising. At hospital discharge, the more immature the infant, the greater the accrued nutrient deficit, the more likely the infant is to benefit from a postdischarge nutrient-enriched formula.

An additional consideration is the introduction of complimentary feeds (CF). All of these studies were performed at a time when CF is introduced. Yet, none of these studies provided any information on the timing of introduction and/or the nature of the CF or the possibility that CF affected the amount of formula consumed.

In the study of Cooke et al. [27–29], it was hypothesized that if intake more adequately met requirements, then infants fed the nutrient-enriched formula would be satisfied longer and CF would be introduced later.

A wide variation was noted in the timing of the introduction of CF and no differences were detected in corrected age between infants fed the nutrient-enriched formula and those fed the term formula (66 ± 34 vs. 61 ± 29 days).

It is recommended that CF not be introduced before 4 months' corrected age [36]. Infants were, therefore, stratified into those who were fed CF before and after 4 months. Infants who were fed CF early were heavier (fig. 5), longer and had a greater head circumference (data not presented) than those who were fed CF later, irrespective of which formula was fed. Thus, infants who were fed CF early may be inherently different from those who were fed CF later.

In summary, results from larger studies suggest that preterm infants, particularly males and very low birth weight infants, grow better when fed a nutrient-enriched formula following discharge until 6 months' corrected age or beyond. Better growth primarily reflects increases in lean body mass.

The Breastfed Infant

Before hospital discharge, preterm infants fed human milk do not grow as well as infants fed nutrient-enriched formulas [37, 38]. It is, therefore, recommended that human milk be fortified with additional nutrients [9]. Growth improves but it is still not as good as in those fed a preterm infant formula [2]. Why is this?

Fortifiers differ in nutrient composition and it is unclear whether any really meet requirements. This, perhaps, is not surprising because the composition of human milk varies widely [39], is rarely measured and there is no way of knowing what the infant is really receiving. If intake less adequately met requirements, then the accrued nutrient deficit is greater and growth is poorer.

After hospital discharge, breastfed infants also grow more poorly than those fed nutrient-enriched formulas [26, 31, 40]. This again is not surprising. Mature human milk is designed to meet the needs of the term infant and not the preterm infant. Breastfed infants are generally fed fortified human milk before discharge, have accrued a greater nutrient deficit. In effect their needs for 'recovery' are also greater.

There are other aspects of concern for these infants. Infants fed unsupplemented human milk not only have poorer growth but also anomalies in bone mineral accretion and metabolism [26, 31, 40] which can be related to outcome in the short term, e.g. osteopenia [41] and fractures [42] and long term, e.g. poorer linear growth [43].

In a study examining growth and body composition after hospital discharge, infants fed a term formula had poorer bone and increased fat accretion when compared to those fed an enriched-nutrient formula [44]. Wauben et al. [40] have also noted poorer bone and increased fat accretion in infants fed human milk compared to a nutrient-enriched formula.

These data support the idea that 'we are what we eat'. When mineral intake is inadequate infants are at risk for deficiencies in mineral accretion. If the protein-to-energy intake is inadequate then, as in term infants [45], infants will accrete less lean but increased fat mass. Whether either anomaly in some way alters 'programming' and, therefore, health in adult life remains to be determined.

Outstanding Issues

Questions remain about the feeding of nutrient-enriched formulas to preterm infants during the first year of life. The first relates to formula composition. What is the ideal composition of these formulas? Will one formulation meet the varying needs of a heterogeneous group of growth-retarded infants? Will one formulation meet the needs of girls and boys?

There are major differences in energy, protein, mineral and micronutrient content between formulas used in previous studies. While most studies showed a growth advantage the magnitude of effect varied, the study with the most consistent growth advantage was closest to that of a regular preterm formula [27–29].

How long should these formulas be fed? In studies where the nutrient-enriched formula was fed to term or 2 months no advantage was noted. However, in studies where a nutrient-enriched formula was fed to 6, 9 and 12 months the most consistent advantage was noted. Whether 6 is better than 9 or 12 months or vice versa remains unclear.

The introduction of CF is an important confounding variable when assessing the effects of nutrient-enriched formulas on growth and developmental outcome. The timing, nature and contribution of CF must be clearly documented and/or controlled when examining outcome in this nutritionally vulnerable group of infants.

Breastfed infants might benefit from additional nutrient supplementation, achieving this, however, is problematic. Fortifiers could be used. Alternatively, a nutrient-enriched formula might also be fed once breastfeeding is fully established. Breastfeeding during the day supported by nutrient-enriched formula at night might not only improve growth but also prolong breastfeeding in these infants.

References

1 Wilson DC, Cairns P, Halliday HL, et al: Randomised controlled trial of an aggressive nutritional regimen in sick very low birthweight infants. Arch Dis Child Fetal Neonatal Ed 1997;77: F4–F11.
2 Carlson SJ, Ziegler EE: Nutrient intakes and growth of very low birth weight infants. Perinatology 1998;18:252–258.
3 Embleton NE, Pang N, Cooke RJ: Postnatal malnutrition and growth retardation: an inevitable consequence of current recommendations in preterm infants? Pediatrics 2001;107:270–273.
4 Clark RH, Thomas P, Peabody J: Extrauterine growth restriction remains a serious problem in prematurely born neonates. Pediatrics 2003;111:986–990.
5 Olsen IE, Richardson DK, Schmid CH, et al: Intersite differences in weight growth velocity of extremely premature infants. Pediatrics 2002;110:1125–1132.
6 Ehrenkranz RA, Younes N, Lemons JA, et al: Longitudinal growth of hospitalized very low birth weight infants. Pediatrics 1999;104:280–289.
7 Cooke RJ, Ainsworth SB, Fenton AC: Postnatal growth retardation: a universal problem in preterm infants. Arch Dis Child Fetal Neonatal Ed 2004;89:F428–F430.

8 AAPCON: Nutritional needs of preterm infants; in Kleinman RE (ed): Pediatric Nutrition Handbook. Elk Groove Village, American Academy of Pediatrics, 1998, pp 55–88.
9 Klein CJ: Nutrient requirements for preterm infant formulas. J Nutr 2002;132:1395S–1577S.
10 Ziegler, EE, Thureen PJ, Carlson SJ: Aggressive nutrition of the very low birthweight infant. Clin Perinatol, 2002;29:225–244.
11 Heird WC: Determination of nutritional requirements in preterm infants, with special reference to 'catch-up' growth. Semin Neonatol 2001;6:365–375.
12 Ernst JA, Bull MJ, Rickard KA, et al: Growth outcome and feeding practices of the very low birth weight infant (less than 1500 grams) within the first year of life. J Pediatr 1990;117:S156–S166.
13 Casey PH, Kraemer HC, Bernbaum J, et al: Growth patterns of low birth weight preterm infants: a longitudinal analysis of a large, varied sample. J Pediatr 1990;117:298–307.
14 Fitzhardinge PM, Inwood S: Long-term growth in small-for-date children. Acta Paediatr Scand Suppl 1989;349:27–34.
15 Fenton TR, McMillan DD, Sauve RS: Nutrition and growth analysis of very low birth weight infants. Pediatrics 1990;86:378–383.
16 Kitchen WH, Doyle LW, Ford GW, Callanan C: Very low birth weight and growth to age 8 years. I. Weight and height. Am J Dis Child 1992;146:40–45.
17 Kitchen WH, Doyle LW, Ford GW, et al: Very low birth weight and growth to age 8 years. II. Head dimensions and intelligence. Am J Dis Child 1992;146:46–50.
18 Ross G, Lipper EG, Auld PA: Growth achievement of very low birth weight premature children at school age. J Pediatr 1990;117:307–309.
19 McCormick MC, Shapiro S, Starfield BH: Rehospitalization in the first year of life for high-risk survivors. Pediatrics 1980;66:991–999.
20 Hack M, Caron B, Rivers A, Fanaroff AA: The very low birth weight infant: the broader spectrum of morbidity during infancy and early childhood. J Dev Behav Pediatr 1983;4: 243–249.
21 Navas L, Wang E, de Carvalho V, Robinson J: Improved outcome of respiratory syncytial virus infection in a high-risk hospitalized population of Canadian children. PICNIC. J Pediatr 1992;121:348–354.
22 Thomas M, Bedford-Russell A, Sharland M: Hospitalisation of RSV infection in ex-preterm infants – implications for RSV immune globulin. Arch Dis Child 2000;83:122–127.
23 Wang E, Law B, Stephens D: Pediatric Investigators Collaborative Network on Infections in Canada (PICNIC) prospective study of risk factors and outcomes in patients hospitalised with respiratory syncytial viral lower respiratory tract infection. J Pediatr 1995;126: 212–219.
24 Lucas A, Bishop NJ, King FJ, Cole TJ: Randomised trial of nutrition for preterm infants after discharge. Arch Dis Child 1992;67:324–327.
25 Bishop NJ, King FJ, Lucas A: Increased bone mineral content of preterm infants fed with a nutrient enriched formula after discharge from hospital. Arch Dis Child 1993;68:573–578.
26 Chan GM, Borschel MW, Jacobs JR: Effects of human milk or formula feeding on the growth, behavior, and protein status of preterm infants discharged from the newborn intensive care unit. Am J Clin Nutr 1994;60:710–716.
27 Cooke RJ, Griffin IJ, McCormick K, et al: Feeding preterm infants after hospital discharge: effect of dietary manipulation on nutrient intake and growth. Pediatr Res 1998;43:355–360.
28 Cooke RJ, Embleton ND, Griffin IJ, et al: Feeding preterm infants after hospital discharge: growth and development at 18 months of age. Pediatr Res 2001;49:719–722.
29 Cooke RJ, McCormick K, Griffin IJ, et al: Feeding preterm infants after hospital discharge: effect of diet on body composition. Pediatr Res 1999;46:461–464.
30 Carver JD, Wu PY, Hall RT, et al: Growth of preterm infants fed nutrient-enriched or term formula after hospital discharge. Pediatrics 2001;107:683–689.
31 Lucas A, Fewtrell MS, Morley R, et al: Randomized trial of nutrient-enriched formula versus standard formula for postdischarge preterm infants. Pediatrics 2001;108:703–711.
32 De Curtis M, Pieltain C, Rigo J: Body composition in preterm infants fed standard term or enriched formula after hospital discharge. Eur J Nutr 2002;41:177–182.
33 Litmanovitz I, Dolfin T, Arnon S, et al: Bone strength and growth of preterm infants fed nutrient-enriched or term formula after hospital discharge. Pediatr Res 2004;55:274A.
34 Henderson G, Fahey T, McGuire W: Calorie and protein-enriched formula versus standard term formula for improving growth and development in preterm or low birth weight infants following hospital discharge. Cochrane Database Syst Rev 2005;2:CD004696.

35 Rawlings DJ, Cooke RJ, McCormick K, et al: Body composition of preterm infants during infancy. Arch Dis Child Fetal Neonatal Ed 1999;80:F188–F191.
36 Kleinman RE: American Academy of Pediatrics recommendations for complementary feeding. Pediatrics 2000;106:1274.
37 Tyson JE, Lasky RE, Mize CE, et al: Growth, metabolic response, and development in very-low-birth-weight infants fed banked human milk or enriched formula. I. Neonatal findings. J Pediatr 1983;103:95–104.
38 Gross SJ: Growth and biochemical response of preterm infants fed human milk or modified infant formula. N Engl J Med 1983;308:237–241.
39 Atkinson SA, Alston-Mills B, Lonnerdal B, Neville MC: Major minerals and ionic constituents of human and bovine milks; in Jensen RG (ed): Handbook of Milk Composition. San Diego, Academic Press, 1995, pp 593–622.
40 Wauben IP, Atkinson SA, Shah JK, Paes B: Growth and body composition of preterm infants: influence of nutrient fortification of mother's milk in hospital and breastfeeding post-hospital discharge. Acta Paediatr 1998;87:780–785.
41 Lucas A, Brooke OG, Baker BA, et al: High alkaline phosphatase activity and growth in preterm neonates. Arch Dis Child 1989;64:902–909.
42 Koo WW, et al: Sequential bone mineral content in small preterm infants with and without fractures and rickets. J Bone Miner Re, 1988;3:193–197.
43 Fewtrell MS, Prentice A, Cole TJ, Lucas A: Effects of growth during infancy and childhood on bone mineralization and turnover in preterm children aged 8–12 years. Acta Paediatr 2000;89:148–153.
44 Brunton JA, Saigal S, Atkinson SA: Growth and body composition in infants with bronchopulmonary dysplasia up to 3 months corrected age: a randomized trial of a high-energy nutrient-enriched formula fed after hospital discharge. J Pediatr 1998;133:340–345.
45 Fomon SJ, Ziegler EE, Nelson SE, Frantz JA: What is the safe protein-energy ratio for infant formulas? Am J Clin Nutr 1995;62:358–363.

Discussion

Dr. Chubarova: When I was a teenager we were told to introduce solid foods for premature babies much earlier than term babies and mostly it was cereals, but I am not sure it improved growth. If you suggest introducing solid foods earlier, what foods are you talking about?

Dr. Cooke: It doesn't change that much. It is fairly consistent and we are talking about levels that are in the range of 20, 30 or 36 mg/dl. None of these children develop a BUN above 40 mg/dl or ~6 mmol and that is the crucial issue.

Dr. Beaumier: About the principle of giving the mothers a rest when the babies are very hungry and actually eating all the time. We came across an idea to actually express breast milk and fortify it at least twice a day. This can be given to the baby by someone other than the mother and she can rest. You talked about supplementation as a growth avenue but what about long-chain polyunsaturated fatty acids (LCPUFAs), what about other nutrients that you haven't mentioned in your talk?

Dr. Cooke: We focused on protein-energy malnutrition because we think that is the rate-limiting step in preterm infants, particularly boys [1]. The nutrient-enriched formulas have LCPUFAs and deficiency appears unlikely. One issue that I have not raised is iron status in these infants. In our original study, we compared two levels of iron intake, 0.5 and 0.9 mg/100 ml of formula [2]. There were no differences in iron nutritional status during the first year of life between the groups. However, we would support the idea that post-discharge formulas contain a minimum level of 0.9 mg/100 ml.

Dr. Fusch: Was zinc the same?

Dr. Cooke: Zinc nutritional status was not evaluated in these infants but it could also be an area of concern. However, no infant failed to thrive but grew at growth rates similar to the term infant at the same corrected age [1].

Dr. Griffin: I just have a comment to make about the complementary feed issue, just to remind people that there is a randomized control trial of complementary feeding post-discharge in preterm babies [3]. A strategy of using weaning foods with higher energy and protein densities (and more iron and zinc) leads to better catch-up growth, which is interesting, as it suggests that if there is a critical period for growth in these infants it is probably a lot broader than we might initially have thought.

Dr. Puplampu: Some children who were initially breastfed and then introduced to formula later reject beast milk. Is it possible that the weight gain noticed in children fed fortified breast milk could be due to water retention caused by the phosphate content?

Dr. Cooke: I do not think so. Term infants fed marginal levels of protein upregulate volume so that both protein and energy intake increase. Weight gain improves, reflecting increased fat rather than lean mass accretion [4]. A similar scenario also appears to occur in preterm infants fed supplemented human milk [5]. Weight gain most likely reflects increased fat and lean mass accretion.

Dr. Costalos: I think it is wrong to put babies of 1,000 and 2,000 g together. I don't think babies of 2,000 g, unless they are IUGR, really need formula. We just completed a 2-year study giving babies post-discharge formula and a lot of them really grew very fast but we didn't select the babies. The ones who are going to need this post-discharge formula are babies under 1,000 g and IUGR babies. If we put them all together perhaps they unnecessarily get too many calories. Coming back to the cereals which were mentioned before, there was a study where cereals were introduced to these babies at the age of 13 weeks and they had a better head growth at the age of 1 year, which is perhaps important.

Dr. Cooke: Nutritional status is quite variable at hospital discharge, the smaller and more immature the infant at discharge the greater the degree of malnutrition [6]. It may be simplistic to assume that one formulation will meet the needs of all preterm infants. To date, studies have focused on infants weighing ≤1,750 g at birth, with boys and those weighing ≤1,250 g seeming to benefit most. Yet we must start somewhere and this is just the beginning for all appropriately grown infants weighing ≤1,750 g at birth. I really can make no recommendations on the small for gestational age infant.

Dr. Van Dael: Knowing that there is still a lot of science to be done on preterm optimal nutrition, how would you react to the fact that some governments lay down particular nutritional requirements for preterm formulas. Take India for example, where they say that the protein composition should be 30% casein and 70% whey, and in China where there is no particular recommendation for preterm formulas but where a preterm formula needs to comply with term infant formula compositions.

Dr. Cooke: I am not really sure how to answer this question. If and when a government rules on this issue then one would hope that nutritional expertise has already been obtained and is the basis for the ruling. I am also not sure how many infants weighing ≤1,000 g are surviving in either India or China and/or whether it is a major health care consideration.

Dr. Putet: I am a little confused about the terms of post-discharge formula and term formula because we should perhaps think more about the protein content and calorie content. Some discharge formulas have the same caloric content or same protein content as some term formulas. You showed data in which the main difference was the protein intake. Can you comment on the fact that the 4-month infant who is drinking milk can modulate the volume intake, making the most important thing not perhaps the caloric intake but the protein intake? We know in term infants that by increasing the protein intake of the formula a little with the same energy intake they will grow better, they will be taller and weigh more at 1 year of age. So the question is what is the most important protein or energy intake knowing that the baby will modulate according to the total energy of the day?

Dr. Cooke: Energy content is really what determines intake. However, when protein intake is marginal the volume of intake is further increased to increase protein intake. In effect, infants will gain more weight, the gain primarily reflecting fat rather than lean mass [4]. Protein content, when it is low, is also important.

Dr. Haschke: We had a Nestlé Nutrition Workshop 1 year ago at Half Moon Bay in California, in which long-term outcome was the major topic. One message which I still remember from Dr. Lucas was 'grow fast pay later'. How long should we feed such formulas? Nobody so far has really evaluated the long-term positive or negative outcome of feeding such formulas with a high protein content for up to 9 or 12 months. I fully agree with the concept of the need of the premature infant for catch-up growth until it has reached a certain weight, let's say the birth weight of the term infant. Assuming that the body composition is not too different from that of a term infant, why are we continuing to feed these infant formulas without looking at the long-term outcome? It might be, with a high protein intake, that we stimulate certain growth factors which later on result in increased fat accumulation of the body. So far nobody knows this and I strongly feel that we have to be very careful, in particular on how long we should recommend feeding these formulas.

Dr. Cooke: Poor nutrition can be directly related to poorer neurodevelopmental outcome in preterm infants [7]. The idea that 'by growing fast you may pay later' is interesting. It is based upon data showing higher proinsulin levels, a measure of insulin resistance, in preterm infants fed a nutrient-enriched diet compared to those fed a lower nutrient diet during early life [8]. However, proinsulin levels in the enriched group were similar to a reference group of term breastfed infants indicating that those fed the nutrient-enriched diet were at no greater risk, while those fed the lower-nutrient diet were at lower risk compared to the reference infants. I agree with you, the key issues are what we should feed, how long we should feed it and what measures of outcome should we be looking at. It should be noted that infants in our original study had a body weight and composition similar to the term infant at the same corrected age [1].

Dr. Fuchs: I am curious as I see that you use weight for age, length for age and head circumference as your growth indexes. But I don't understand why you don't use weight for length. If your sample sizes are large enough, then it is not so important, but the sample sizes in the cited studies are really small enough that it does make a difference.

Dr. Cooke: When we aim to rehabilitate severely malnourished children that are not preterm infants, we aim for an ideal weight for height and then when we overshoot that, that is when we get concerned. If we get an obese child, that may impact the question programming.

Dr. Fuchs: Let me comment. If you could measure body composition would you think that it is a better reflection of the degree of leanness or fatness, than weight for length?

Dr. Cooke: I am not sure but my interpretation of the data is that with DEXA lean mass is measured more accurately than fat mass. Our original concern related to energy intake and the possibility of excess energy storage in infants fed the nutrient-enriched formula, so we used it to assess fat mass.

Dr. Aly: As I understood fortification is important but how can it be done properly? Can we conclude that most premature babies weighting 1,500 g and more can depend upon the preterm formula as an added nutrient to the mother's milk, in case it is available, or even as a single mode of feeding after discharge?

Dr. Cooke: There are no randomized control trials examining post-discharge intervention in breastfed preterm infants. In principle, term human milk was designed for the term infant. As such it does a marvellous job but it was never designed for the preterm infant. We, therefore, must be circumspect when advising a breastfeeding mother whose infant is not 'thriving'.

Dr. Aly: No, I mean could we depend upon the preterm formula as a single mode of feeding for these preterm babies? In some countries after discharge of preterm babies, it is difficult to prescribe fortification for reasons of sterilization, availability, cost, etc. It is much easier to prescribe a preterm formula which has the right composition, is easy to prepare, and gives high energy and protein intake. So why can we not make this conclusion?

Dr. Cooke: We need the data that outcomes are better in infants supplemented with preterm formula than in non-supplemented breastfed preterm infants after hospital discharge before we can make a recommendation. In an infant who is not thriving then one might study the BUN. If it is low then supplementation with a preterm formula might be appropriate.

Dr. Beaumier: Should we still look at actual growth, weight, length and so on, or should we look at functional outcome? What is the difference when as an adult the patient has actually gained 2 cm or not, but is bright and healthy? It goes along with what you were saying about the comments of Dr. Lucas 'grow fast pay later', and how is this related to adult nutrition? We must not forget that the American diet is not good, and we prepare babies for a good diet but as adults they have a bad diet.

Dr. Cooke: To date, we focused on anthropometric and developmental outcomes. But relating poor growth to poor development is less than clear-cut, in that it is confounded by the effects of immaturity on the developing CNS. We need to be able to relate growth to more immediate measures of outcome, e.g. immunologic function, so that intervention can be instituted and evaluated. We really do not know what level of growth retardation is significant.

Dr. Griffin: I just wanted to make a comment about the 'grow fast pay later' theory. There really are almost no data for or against this being a legitimate concern in preterm babies. If you take a step back and look at the Barker hypothesis, the babies that do badly are small at birth, they are small at 1 year of age and they are big after 4 years of age, and that is an entirely different growth pattern than we see in our babies. Our babies are born generally appropriately sized, but then they become profoundly malnourished. When we intervene the best event is, if they are going to catch up, they will catch up by about 1 month corrected age. Obviously you don't want to continue and make them fat later on. This is an entirely different pattern of growth to those high risk Barker hypothesis babies.

References

1 Cooke RJ, McCormick K, Griffin IJ, et al: Feeding preterm infants after hospital discharge: effect of diet on body composition. Pediatr Res 1999;46:461–464.
2 Griffin IJ, Cooke RJ, Reid MM, et al: Iron nutritional status in preterm infants fed formulas fortified with iron. Arch Dis Child Fetal Neonatal Ed 1999;81:F45–F49.
3 Marriott LD, Foote KD, Bishop JA, et al: Weaning preterm infants: a randomised controlled trial. Arch Dis Child 2003;88:F302–F307.
4 Fomon SJ, Ziegler EE, Nelson SE, Frantz JA: What is the safe protein-energy ratio for infant formulas? Am J Clin Nutr 1995;62:358–363.
5 Wauben IP, Atkinson SA, Shah JK, Paes B: Growth and body composition of preterm infants: influence of nutrient fortification of mother's milk in hospital and breastfeeding post-hospital discharge. Acta Paediatr 1998;87:780–785.

6　Embleton NE, Pang N, Cooke RJ: Postnatal malnutrition and growth retardation: an inevitable consequence of current recommendations in preterm infants? Pediatrics 2001;107: 270–273.

7　Lucas A, Morley R, Cole TJ: Randomised trial of early diet in preterm babies and later intelligence quotient. BMJ 1998;317:1481–1487.

8　Singhal A, Fewtrell M, Cole TJ, Lucas A: Low nutrient intake and early growth for later insulin resistance in adolescents born preterm. Lancet 2003;361:1089–1097.

Cooke RJ, Vandenplas Y, Wahn U (eds): Nutrition Support for Infants and Children at Risk.
Nestlé Nutr Workshop Ser Pediatr Program, vol 59, pp 229–231,
Nestec Ltd., Vevey/S. Karger AG, Basel, © 2007.

Concluding Remarks

I will briefly summarize the part on allergy and gastrointestinal disease before we go on with the last three talks on nutrition in the preterm baby. The first part of the meeting focused on allergy and Dr. Wahn gave us an introductory lecture showing the complex interaction between the genetic background and the environmental determinants leading to allergic manifestations and to the allergic phenotype, and several times he certainly stressed the importance of cats.

After that Dr. Nowak-Wegrzyn showed us very nicely how fundamental research opens new perspectives for patients. She focused on the characterization of many allergenic food proteins that are under investigation for allergy therapy, and she also said that differences in allergenic epitope recognition patterns may be associated with resistance and the severity of food allergy.

Dr. Beyer taught us how different methods have now been developed to determine the allergenicity of different HA formulas, and that new approaches are being developed to generate immunotherapy for allergy as we also mutate proteins.

Then we went back to daily clinical practice with Dr. von Berg who showed us the concept of hypoallergenicity for atopy prevention. Again the fact was stressed that only those products should be used which have been clinically tested. She showed that both those testing partial and extensive hydrolysates can be effective. Usually 3 years after the intervention there is a reduction in atopic dermatitis as well as the partial and extensive hydrolysates. She said that perhaps partial hydrolysates reduce atopic dermatitis via the induction of tolerance.

This brings us to the last talk on allergy which was by Dr. Lack who focused on the oral tolerance concept. He showed us that he wanted to induce tolerance for inhalants and food allergens rather with high than low dose antigen. In fact he further developed the window principle to give the right antigen at the right dose at the right moment, and with that strategy he would in fact induce tolerance and prevent allergenization.

If you want to reduce allergenicity, you have to give something with the best tolerance. The problem is that with amino acids you are at the lowest allergenicity and also the lowest tolerance induction, and a balance in-between needs to be found.

Ulrich Wahn

Concluding Remarks

So this moves us to the second part of the symposium which focused on gastrointestinal disorders. Dr. Ruemmele told us about chronic enteropathy and looked at it from a molecular basis. He developed the concept of several congenital enteropathies, microvillous atrophy, and showed the very interesting relation between these enteropathies and cow's milk protein enteropathy; he in fact broadened the topic to the first part of the symposium.

Dr. Fuchs talked about the clinical aspect of chronic enteropathy and he showed that there are many causes of chronic enteropathy, but they differ between the developed and the developing world. Chronic enteropathy in developing countries is still a major cause of death in children, more than 1 million per year, and there is a direct interaction between intestinal mucosal injury, malnutrition and impaired immunity. Recovery is dependent on the proper nutritional management and the rehabilitation of that nutrition.

Dr. Milla then had a talk on the transition from parenteral to enteral nutrition. He stated that in intestinal failure parenteral nutrition is lifesaving but also potentially dangerous. Enteral nutrition needs to be introduced at the earliest opportunity, stressing the old knowledge again that if the gut works it must be used but also not too optimistically because minimal enteral feeding must also be used to increase the volumes fairly gradually and total parenteral nutrition must be minimized to the lowest level possible. By introducing enteral feeding intestinal adaptation is optimized, but of course remaining aware of the underlying gastrointestinal disease and not forgetting to treat that. He also showed us new data on experience gained in his hospital with the newly developed elements of diet which directly influence inflammation and food tolerance, offering additional tools.

What I tried to do was to speak about the relation between feeding and gastrointestinal enteropathy and introduce the concept of functional food, stressing that food is more than calories and simple nutrients, that those nutrients can also have a function, and we discussed this in relation to lipids and nucleotides. There was a lot of discussion about probiotics in different indications, and strain specificity of probiotics was certainly stressed. In Brussels we have also had some experience with the new semi-elemental diet in children with less severe conditions than in London. We have shown the efficacy and also that the formula was well tolerated and accepted.

Then before lunch Dr. Davidson gave his talk on stressed mucosa. He showed that many diseases very frequently affect gastrointestinal function by altering barrier function. Especially with the breath test he showed that non-invasive techniques may provide a better way to assess the effects of stress and also a simple way to assess interventions.

Dr. Rings said that cholestasis is important and causes growth failure, and therefore it is a challenge for survival. Because of the increasing waiting time for liver transplant there is a need to improve the nutrition of these children because it is clear that they have a better outcome when their nutritional condition is improved. He showed us very nice models of how this optimal nutrition in cholestatic infants can be reached.

Finally all the speakers and chairpersons of both parts of the symposium thank the organizers for the beautiful meeting.

Yvan Vandenplas

First of all let me say how very grateful I am to Doctors Ekhard Ziegler, Ian Griffin, Patti Thureen and Guy Putet for coming and giving their presentations here. Collectively, we tried to cover the important aspects of the nutritional support of preterm infants with minimal overlap.

Dr. Ziegler discussed the determination of nutrient requirements in preterm infants and, in so doing, made several key points. The first was that protein requirements are substantially greater than we previously thought. The second was that the ratio of protein:energy requirements are not consistent throughout gestation and are greater in the smaller more immature (closer to 3.6–3.8 g/100 kcal) than the more mature (3.0–3.3 g/100 kcal) infant.

Dr. Griffin discussed the assessment of nutritional outcome in the preterm infant and made the following points. Although growth assessment is crucial, reference cohorts for postnatal growth, in absolute or compositional terms, are not widely accepted for preterm infants. He also noted that outside the research setting there are no reliable measures of body composition. Finally, he noted that biochemical assessments of nutritional adequacy are rarely of use in guiding nutritional interventions in most preterm babies.

Dr. Thureen addressed the issue of aggressive nutrition in preterm infants. Contrary to popular opinion she demonstrated that early parenteral nutrition with a protein intake of 2–3 g/kg/day is well tolerated by preterm infants in the first 24–36 h of life and is associated with better glucose tolerance. She also indicated that increased blood urea nitrogen of itself is not a good measure of protein tolerance but more a measure of adequacy of renal function and/or energy intake during early life.

Dr. Guy Putet discussed human milk fortification. What he highlighted was the uncertainty in this area for preterm infants. Most fundamentally he pointed out that not all fortifiers are the same and that supplementation with different fortifiers may produce different results in terms of growth. He highlighted the need for further studies in this area.

My talk focused on the post-discharge nutritional support of preterm infants. It is clear that preterm infants are growth retarded at initial hospital discharge and benefit when fed a nutrient-enriched formula during the first 6–12 months of life. What remains unclear are the optimum composition and duration of feeding of post-discharge nutrient-enriched formulas. What also remains unclear is whether breastfed infants would also benefit from nutrient supplementation, particularly those who are not thriving during the first year of life.

Richard J. Cooke

Subject Index

233

Subject Index

Subject Index